Diagnosis and Management of Breast Tumors

Michael O. Idowu
Priti A. Shah
Mary Helen Hackney
Margaret M. Grimes
Charles Edward Geyer, Jr.
Douglas W. Arthur
Harry D. Bear
Editors

Diagnosis and Management of Breast Tumors

A Practical Handbook and Multidisciplinary Approach

Springer

Editors
Michael O. Idowu
Department of Pathology
Virginia Commonwealth University
Health (VCU HEALTH)
Richmond, VA
USA

Priti A. Shah
Department of Radiology
Breast Imaging Section
Virginia Commonwealth University
Health (VCU HEALTH)
Richmond, VA
USA

Mary Helen Hackney
Division of Hematology Oncology
and Palliative Care
Department of Internal Medicine
Virginia Commonwealth University
Health (VCU HEALTH)
Richmond, VA
USA

Margaret M. Grimes
Department of Pathology
Virginia Commonwealth University
Health (VCU HEALTH)
Richmond, VA
USA

Charles Edward Geyer, Jr.
Division of Hematology Oncology
Department of Internal Medicine
Virginia Commonwealth University
Health (VCU HEALTH)
Richmond, VA
USA

Douglas W. Arthur
Department of Radiation Oncology
Virginia Commonwealth University
Health (VCU HEALTH)
Richmond, VA
USA

Harry D. Bear
Division of Surgical Oncology
Department of Surgery
Virginia Commonwealth University
Health (VCU HEALTH)
Richmond, VA
USA

ISBN 978-3-319-57725-8 ISBN 978-3-319-57726-5 (eBook)
DOI 10.1007/978-3-319-57726-5

Library of Congress Control Number: 2017953372

Printed on acid-free paper

This Springer imprint is published by Springer Nature
The registered company is Springer International Publishing AG
The registered company address is: Gewerbestrasse 11, 6330 Cham, Switzerland

This book is dedicated to my wife, Funmilola Ayodele (Aduke) and children, Michelle and Ethan - you all make the efforts worth it. I also wish to acknowledge Professor Bola O. Osifo, Dr. Celeste N. Powers, and Dr. David S. Wilkinson, for their invaluable and influential roles in my career.

Michael O. Idowu

I dedicate this book to my family, particularly my parents Anil and Varsha; my dear and ever supportive husband, Snehal; my mentor, colleague, and friend, Dr. Gilda Cardeñosa; my colleague and confidant, Dr. Tiffany Tucker; a team of skilled, compassionate, unwavering technologists and clerical staff; and the countless patients from whom I have learned so much.

Priti A. Shah

I wish to dedicate this to my wife Christine and my 3 sons, who have supported me from the start of my career. I also want to acknowledge the inspiration of my three most influential role models: my Father, S. Elmer Bear, DDS, who set an example of dedication to his profession and to his patients; Dr. Bernard Fisher, who demonstrated the joy of moving the field of breast cancer treatment forward through clinical research; and Dr. Walter Lawrence, Jr., who encouraged me to "get involved."

Harry D. Bear

Foreword

The sheer number of benign and malignant breast lesions and the options available for the management of breast cancer may appear daunting. Even in the setting of a unified, multidisciplinary team, there may be some disconnect among its members (namely, pathology, radiology, medical oncology, surgical oncology, and radiation oncology). For example, radiologists and pathologists may be unaware of specific surgical, chemotherapeutic, or radiotherapy approaches and management techniques (i.e., "what happens next"). Similarly, the oncologists (medical, surgical, and radiation) may be unfamiliar with the diagnostic challenges encountered by radiologists and pathologists. *The lack of clarity to the often asked question of "what next" or "what are they going to do next" may sometimes lead to ambiguous diagnosis and possibly suboptimal management of the patient.* The specialties involved in the initial diagnosis (radiology and pathology) may consider the rest of the management of patients "not their headaches," mostly due to limited awareness of "what happens next."

We believe that it would be ideal for all members of the multidisciplinary team, including the patient's primary care provider, to have a basic understanding of the entire process, from work-up to completion of treatment, including diagnostic and therapeutic options, approaches, and techniques.

With this in mind, this text aims to present a practical and concise handbook on the approach to diagnosis and management of breast diseases written by subspecialty experts for quick reference by trainees and general practitioners. There are comprehensive reference texts on the criteria for diagnosis and algorithm for management of breast diseases. This text aims to bridge the gap of "what next" and foster an understanding of the diagnosis and management of breast tumors.

The Editors

Preface

This book focuses on the approach to the diagnosis and management of common breast lesions or tumors. There are generous illustrations and figures to enhance readers' appreciation of the lesions and processes being discussed. Medical students, trainees, and physicians involved in diagnosis and management of breast diseases will find relevant, practical points for their education and practice.

The book is divided into two parts. Part 1 is divided into five chapters. Each chapter is written by subspecialty experts. Chapters 1 and 2 discuss the radiologic and pathologic approach to diagnosis of breast lesions, respectively. Chapters 3, 4, and 5 address the surgical oncology, medical oncology, and radiation oncology approaches to management, respectively.

Part 2 focuses on the radiologic and pathologic diagnosis of selected breast lesions with emphasis on radiologic-pathologic correlation. Entities such as fibroepithelial lesions, papillary lesions, proliferative lesions, invasive carcinomas and miscellaneous lesions are highlighted. There are ample images to illustrate criteria used to assess and categorize each lesion presented. In addition to radiologic-pathologic correlation, Chap. 9 further highlights management approach and treatment options for invasive carcinomas.

It is our hope that this text will enhance appreciation for the multidisciplinary approach to the diagnosis and management of common breast lesions and provide some clarity for trainees and community/general practitioners on the question of "what next?".

The Editors

Contents

List of Contributors

Todd C. Adams, MD Department of Radiation Oncology, Virginia Commonwealth University Health (VCU HEALTH), Richmond, VA, USA

Douglas W. Arthur, MD Department of Radiation Oncology, Virginia Commonwealth University Health (VCU HEALTH), Richmond, VA, USA

Harry D. Bear, MD, PhD Division of Surgical Oncology, Department of Surgery, Virginia Commonwealth University Health (VCU HEALTH), Richmond, VA, USA

Christopher Chipko, MD Department of Radiation Oncology, Virginia Commonwealth University Health (VCU HEALTH), Richmond, VA, USA

Charles Edward Geyer, Jr., MD Division of Hematology Oncology, Department of Internal Medicine, Virginia Commonwealth University Health (VCU HEALTH), Richmond, VA, USA

Margaret M. Grimes, MD, MEd Department of Pathology, Virginia Commonwealth University Health (VCU HEALTH), Richmond, VA, USA

Mary Helen Hackney, MD, MS, FACP Division of Hematology Oncology and Palliative Care, Department of Internal Medicine, Virginia Commonwealth University Health System (VCU HEALTH), Richmond, VA, USA

Michael O. Idowu, MD, MPH Department of Pathology, Virginia Commonwealth University Health (VCU HEALTH), Richmond, VA, USA

Valentina Robila, MD, PhD Department of Pathology, Virginia Commonwealth University Health (VCU HEALTH), Richmond, VA, USA

Nicholas Serrano, MD Department of Radiation Oncology, Virginia Commonwealth University Health (VCU HEALTH), Richmond, VA, USA

Priti A. Shah, MD Department of Radiology, Breast Imaging Section, Virginia Commonwealth University Health (VCU HEALTH), Richmond, VA, USA

Jaime A. Singh, MD Department of Pathology, Virginia Commonwealth University Health (VCU HEALTH), Richmond, VA, USA

Hetal Vachhani, MD Division of Hematology Oncology, Department of Internal Medicine, Massey Cancer Center, Virginia Commonwealth University Health (VCU HEALTH), Richmond, VA, USA

Part I

Overview of Evaluation and Management of Breast Diseases

1 Overview of Radiologic Quality Assurance and the Imaging Evaluation of Breast Lesions

Priti A. Shah

Quality Assurance in Breast Imaging

Although the field of radiology as a whole is subject to many levels of regulation and accreditation, breast imaging, and specifically mammography, is a subspecialty subject to rigorous standards of care that are legally mandated in the United States. Two major entities collaboratively regulate breast imaging in the interests of quality and safety. Responding to issues and inconsistencies in matters pertaining to patient care and image quality, the American College of Radiology (ACR) developed the Mammography Accreditation Program in the late 1980's as a means of periodic peer review and feedback from experts for improvement [1, 2]. Secondly, the Mammography Quality Standards Act (MQSA) was enacted by Congress in the 1990's to set national quality standards through specific regulatory requirements that were established by the Food and Drug Administration (FDA) for mammography [1, 3]. Under MQSA, all facilities that provide mammography services in the United States must be inspected by the FDA every year, earn accreditation by an FDA approved body (which includes the ACR, and the states of Arkansas, Iowa, and Texas) every 3 years, and be certified by Health and Human Services every 3 years. Mammography facilities under the Department of Veterans Affairs, while not included in MQSA, undergo accreditation by the ACR to maintain the same standards of care [2]. Through the interplay between these agencies' directives, every aspect of a mammography practice is overseen, including but not limited to technologist, radiologist, and physicist training, equipment quality control, radiation safety, image quality, result documentation and communication practices, and patient outcomes.

P.A. Shah, MD
Department of Radiology, Breast Imaging Section,
Virginia Commonwealth University Health (VCU HEALTH), Richmond, VA, USA
e-mail: priti.shah@vcuhealth.org

M.O. Idowu et al. (eds.), *Diagnosis and Management of Breast Tumors*,
DOI 10.1007/978-3-319-57726-5_1

Some practical aspects of patient care by breast radiologists are also regulated. For example, it is required by MQSA that patients are provided a written summary of their mammogram results in non-medical terminology. This is separate from the radiology report that is sent to the referring clinician. Because of MQSA, this direct communication with patients has been the standard of care before the days of web-based patient portals and widespread campaigns in medicine promoting patient-centered care.

The breast radiologist is also responsible for establishing radiological – pathological concordance and directing patient management based on a biopsy result, unlike for other image guided biopsies, or for other practitioners. In this way, breast imagers are uniquely subject to standards not legally required by non-radiologists. For example, a radiologist and a surgeon can both perform a core needle breast biopsy, however, the former must document and track the results, patient follow-up, and outcomes; and this data (among others) is then used to calculate individual and practice statistics that comprise a medical audit subject to review by the FDA. Recall rates, biopsy recommendations, true and false positives and negatives, re-biopsy rates, invasive cancer detection, positive predictive values, and so on are measured against established benchmarks, and routinely assessed. Part of this is because of the self-directed nature of the breast imaging work up that leads to procedures—there must be an internal system of checks and balances—but the main goal is to provide quality and consistency of patient care, with appropriate follow up.

Nearly contemporaneous to the inception of the MQSA was the creation of the Breast Imaging Reporting and Data System (BI-RADS) by the American College of Radiology [4, 5]. In the vein of creating guidelines for clear reporting and monitoring patient outcomes, BI-RADS is a quality assurance system most relevant to our referring clinicians with regard to the communication of findings and recommendations for management by the radiologist through, for example, standardized reports and categorization of follow-up. By using BI-RADS, the radiologist can generate specific, concise, consistent reports via a lexicon of approved terms, with clear, concise recommendations from defined assessment categories to allow for meaningful, clinically relevant consultation (Table 1.1).

Table 1.1 Breast imaging lexicon: examples of finding descriptors (mammography) [5]

Masses	Shape: round, oval, irregular Margins: circumscribed, obscured, microlobulated, spiculated, indistinct Density: high density, equal density, low density, fat containing
Calcifications	Morphology (suspicious): amorphous, coarse heterogeneous, fine pleomorphic, fine linear, branching Distribution: grouped, regional, diffuse, linear, segmental

Breast imaging lexicon - assessment categories, likelihood of malignancy, and management recommendation [5]:

0—Incomplete: need additional imaging evaluation or prior study for comparison
1—Negative: ~0% likelihood of malignancy, recommend routine screening
2—Benign finding (e.g.. cyst): ~0% likelihood of malignancy, recommend routine screening
3—Probably benign finding (e.g., probable fibroadenoma, focal parenchymal asymmetry): <2% likelihood of malignancy, recommend 6-, 12-, and 24-month follow-up; after which, if stable, finding is considered benign (BI-RADS 2)
4—Suspicious: 2–10% likelihood of malignancy (4a, low suspicion); 10–50% likelihood of malignancy (4b, moderate suspicion); 50–95% likelihood of malignancy (4c, high suspicion), biopsy recommended
5—Highly suggestive of malignancy: >95% likelihood of malignancy, biopsy recommended
6—Known biopsy-proven malignancy, treatment plan recommended

When used appropriately, each descriptor or combination thereof connotes a differential diagnosis and a level of suspicion. For example, a description of an oval low density mass with circumscribed margins suggests a specific differential diagnosis (perhaps a cyst, fibroadenoma, or papilloma), one that is vastly different from that implied by a description of an irregular dense mass with spiculated margins (such as an intermediate nuclear grade invasive ductal carcinoma or invasive lobular carcinoma). However, it is important to note that there is considerable inter-reader variability in choice of descriptors and terms even within the lexicon, possibly because of differences in perception and overlap in imaging features [6, 7].

There is some flexibility in these assessment categories to allow for the nuances of actual patient care. For example, a subareolar abscess is a benign finding, but short interval follow-up might be recommended to ensure resolution; a patient with a known malignancy may undergo imaging follow-up if she is not a surgical candidate. When used appropriately, the lexicon enables the radiologist to provide a meaningful report that guides patient care. Terms like "clinical correlation advised" are discouraged in favor of concrete recommendations and actions.

Screening and Its Controversies

By definition, *a screening mammogram is for the routine surveillance of breast cancer in an asymptomatic patient.* It is comprised of two (nearly) perpendicular low-dose x-rays of each breast: a craniocaudal (CC or top-to-bottom) and a medial-lateral oblique (MLO or side-to-side) view. Two images of each breast are the standard of care to be able to include as much tissue in the image as possible; studies have shown a 25–45% increase in cancer detection when two views are obtained compared with one [8]. This is because inherent in how the patient is positioned, each view has a "blind spot" that has the potential of excluding some tissue—even with superb technique, for example, a CC view may exclude some superior tissue, and an MLO view may miss far medial tissue.

The specifics of frequency and age of initiation of screening mammography are controversial. As with any screening program, the goal is early detection: to find early stage cancer that is more susceptible to less aggressive treatments and therefore has the best prognosis and survival. With breast cancer, the 5-year survival rate for localized disease at diagnosis can be up to 98.8%, and 12-year survival up to 95% with tumors smaller than 1cm at diagnosis [9, 10].

The national benchmark for overall sensitivity of mammography is 86.9%, and specificity 88.9% [11, 12]. Mammography is not a perfect test (is there a perfect test in medicine?); however, it is one of the most studied tests in medicine, resulting in a large volume of data, from but not limited to randomized control trials, that consistently shows a significant (at least 30%) decrease in mortality when done annually in average-risk women over 40, through early detection, with decades of follow-up [13–17]. Part of the advantage of mammography is its ability to detect microcalcifications associated with stage 0 disease (intraductal cancer or ductal carcinoma in situ) better than any other imaging modalities, even in women with dense breast tissue. This is because DCIS often manifests as microcalcifications, the detection of which is optimized by the radiographic technique used in mammography (low-dose, high-resolution imaging). Starting at age 40 is recommended because the incidence of breast cancer doubles in women ages 35–39 to ages 40–45 years old, and cancers grow more aggressively in these women than in postmenopausal patients [9, 18, 19]. Although cancers in postmenopausal women may be more indolent, causing some to favor less frequent screening in these patients, increasing age is a risk factor, and so earlier detection may allow for less aggressive treatment options that are better tolerated in the setting of other health problems that may come with age.

Recent changes in screening guidelines are not based on new or refuting data, but rather on a shift of attention away from the benefits of mammography to its potential harms (see below). Simply put, for women of average risk, the US Preventive Services Task Force (USPSTF) recommends biannual screening mammography for women ages 50–74, stating that the net benefit is moderate. For women younger than 50, the position of the USPSTF is that the decision to screen should be an individual one based on values of potential benefits versus potential harms and that the net benefit for women in this group is small. And for women older than 74, the current evidence is deemed "insufficient" to assess the balance of benefits and harms [20].

The American Cancer Society now advises that women should have the opportunity to begin screening at age 40 if they choose, and that mammography be done annually between 45 and 54; women over 54 can be screened every other year or annually, depending on personal preferences [21].

The changes in guidelines, and the controversies, stem from new attention on issues such as patient anxiety, radiation, false positives, and invasive procedures and their complications [22]. These are important topics; however, as discussed below, they do not outweigh the proven benefits of mammography when it comes to early detection and survival.

There is conflicting data regarding short term and long term effects of the anxiety related to mammography, however, there is evidence that women are still willing to return yearly even after a false positive; the apprehension is not incapacitating, nor does it outweigh the desire to "know" one's status regarding breast cancer [23, 24]. Direct, radiologist-led patient education about screening and breast cancer has also been shown to decrease anxiety through increased patient knowledge and feelings of empowerment [25]. Lastly, significant portion of this anxiety is attributed to waiting for results, and the fear of the unknown. But rather than discourage mammograms for this reason, there are ways to shorten the interval between screening, recall, diagnosis, and biopsy that serve to alleviate this component of anxiety [26]. As outlined above, radiologists are legally required to provide the patient with her imaging results, which is routinely done the same day in the case of a diagnostic workup. But practices may opt to do this even with screening studies, even if only at the specific request of the patient. Our practice routinely accepts add-ons and walk-in patients for screening and diagnostic studies and offers same-day ultrasounds and biopsies. We have an agreement with our pathologists to receive biopsy results the next day, and the radiologist provides those results directly to the patient at that time. If cancer is diagnosed, we immediately schedule the patient for a surgical consultation, and the patient is seen within the week. While this can make for unpredictable workflow, efforts by the entire team to streamline the process are seen as being in the best interest of the patients.

All x-rays use radiation. However, there is no data showing that the radiation from yearly mammograms is a cause of breast cancer. In the spectrum of medical tests, mammography is considered low dose [27, 28]. A standard four-view mammogram (two views of each breast) is approximately 1/7 of the radiation received from natural background sources annually, such as the air, water, and soil in our environment [29]. Moreover, as outlined above, all mammography facilities in the United States are required to undergo routine inspection and accreditation by entities such as the FDA and American College of Radiology: practices are regularly and systematically monitored with regard to equipment, safety, quality, radiation dose, and technologist and physician training. So even though mammography uses radiation, the vast, proven benefits of early detection outweigh the theoretical risks from the relatively small dose of radiation, a dose which is kept in check.

With regard to false positives in mammography, in addition to monitoring data such as equipment and dose, mammography facilities are also required to track measures such as patient outcomes and physician performance. Among many national benchmarks, the acceptable "abnormal interpretation rate" for *screening mammography* is 5–12% [12]. While this may seem high, the number of patients receiving a normal or benign result is, by definition, substantially higher: about 90 percent of screening patients get a clean bill of health. Of the 5–12% of patients recalled, the vast majority will also be "cleared" with additional mammographic views and/or ultrasound. Of the remaining, biopsy rates are less than 2 percent; benchmarks for acceptable PPV for biopsies performed are 20–45% for screening-detected abnormalities and 30–55% for palpable findings [12]. Many breast imagers work hard to minimize recalling patients, and even lower recall rates and higher positive predictive values can be acheived through better technologist and physician training [30]. For example, for about a decade, the collective callback rate in our practice was less than 10% and our PPV for biopsies 50–60%. Double reading has also been shown to decrease call backs [31, 32]. In addition to better training and collaboration, advances in technology can contribute to lowering recall rates and false positives. 3-D mammography, or tomosynthesis, is an example of this. Instead of a single, "flat," 2-dimensional image, these 3-D studies provide the radiologist with multiple separate thin (1 mm) "slices" through the entire thickness of the breast that can be evaluated layer by layer. This can decrease the effect of summation or superimposition of normal structures encountered more frequently with the traditional (2-D) mammogram, thereby decreasing false positives, and allow for the increased detection of invasive cancers [33–35].

With regard to the potential harm of invasive procedures, when a biopsy is necessary, there are opportunities to minimize local trauma and, therefore, associated discomfort and possible complications. Imaging-guided core needle biopsies are less invasive than surgical biopsies, can be done in the same exam room as the mammogram or ultrasound, and require no IV or general anesthesia, nor advanced preparation (such as fasting or stopping anticoagulation) by the patient. *The complication rate of imaging-guided needle biopsy is <1%, which includes bleeding, infection, and tissue damage* [36, 37]. Even then, there are opportunities for improvement. For example, smaller gauge, spring-loaded biopsy needles may be used instead of larger, vacuum-assisted ones in certain circumstances. Physician skill and more precise techniques can allow for taking fewer, "high-yield" samples (my mentor once said that theoretically, you only need one core to make the diagnosis—which drives me to make each pass count to this day). Using a patient-centered and specific approach to decide which patients may or may not benefit from placement of a marker clip, which is routinely placed at the biopsy site by almost all radiologists and requires a two-view post-procedure mammogram to confirm its location, may obviate the cost, extra time, and radiation associated with this part of the procedure.

In these ways, the potential harms of screening can be addressed and overcome, rather than being used as excuses to discourage annual mammography. To discourage or possibly limit access to this lifesaving test going forward may undo all of the gains in early detection and survival made previously.

It is important to reiterate here that the controversies in screening guidelines are with regard to the average-risk patient. Most organizations still agree that women who are high risk (see below) should start annual screening at 40 or earlier based on their risk factors such as age of onset of cancer in a first-degree relative.

Diagnostic Imaging

As the name would imply, *diagnostic imaging is typically reserved for the workup or diagnosis of a specific sign or symptom of the breast or axilla or to evaluate an abnormality on a screening mammogram.* Common clinical examples include a "lump" felt on physical exam, skin changes, focal pain, and spontaneous nipple discharge. In most practices, diagnostic imaging involves a combination of additional mammographic views and/or ultrasound, and the evaluation is tailored to the patient based on the findings at each step of the process. This "work-in-progress" approach keeps the radiologist alert, and, as he/she must (by MQSA) provide results directly to the patient in lay language, requires that the radiologist "own" his/her assessment and plan.

Without getting into the technical aspects of diagnostic workups, some of the additional mammographic images include *spot compression views* at the area of radiographic concern and full paddle views done at different angles than standard screening views. Altering the angle at which tissue is seen, and further compressing the breast in the specified area, can reduce the potential masking effect of normal overlapping tissue and allows for confirmation, improved visualization, and localization (for possible ultrasound or biopsy) of the finding in question. In the case of a mass, confirming it in two (perpendicular) planes is integral to the BI-RADS definition of a mass. If the suspected finding "disappears," it may be attributed to tissue overlap at the time of screening, and no further workup may be needed. As an analogy, for example, when we take our laundry out of the washer, it is often "balled up." When spread on the clothesline, we see that there was never really a "ball" in it. The radiologist may perceive a "mass" or "lump" at screening that "spreads out" as normal tissue once viewed from a different angle, and further, focal compression is applied. If a finding persists/is confirmed on spot compression views, ultrasound may be undertaken, particularly in the evaluation of a mass, architectural distortion, or focal asymmetry.

Calcifications are further evaluated with *magnification views* because of their size. These views use different patient positioning and technical factors than standard screening or spot compression views to optimize contrast and resolution and minimize the effect of superimposed tissue—all paramount when assessing structures smaller than a millimeter. Ultrasound is not usually useful in further characterization of microcalcifications. The detection and work up of breast calcifications is further outlined below.

Breast Density

Breast tissue is composed of fatty, fibrous, and glandular tissue. These elements vary in proportion from person to person and sometimes between breasts in the same patient (see discussion on asymmetry below). The amount and combination of types of tissue are under genetic and hormonal influences, and though it can change somewhat during a lifetime, it is simply how an individual woman's breast is made.

Fatty tissue is radiolucent, translating to a higher sensitivity for mammography to detect small cancers, since invasive cancers (most often, masses) are typically equal or higher density than breast tissue. Fibrous and glandular tissue, sometimes termed together as fibroglandular tissue, is more opaque or "dense" radiographically. So it follows that the more fibrous and glandular the tissue, the denser the breast tissue appears, and the more challenging it is to detect a small cancer. It is the old polar bear in a snowstorm analogy, hence the decreased sensitivity of mammography in dense breasts (Figs. 1.1 and 1.2). To add to this limitation in detection, studies also show a mild to moderate increase in cancer risk incurred by having predominantly dense tissue, the mechanism of which is still unclear [38].

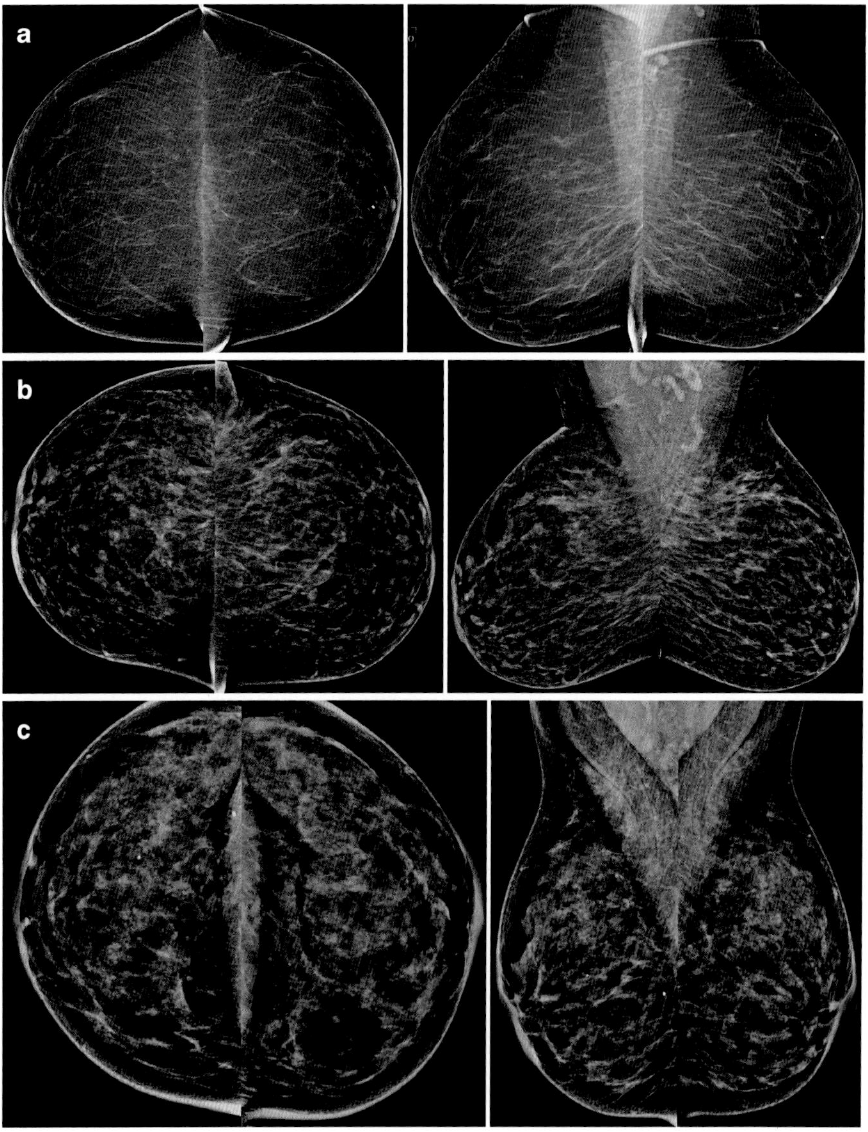

Fig. 1.1 Breast composition as defined by the ACR BI-RADS mammography lexicon [36]. (**a**) Almost entirely fatty. (**b**) Scattered areas of fibroglandular density. (**c**) Heterogeneously dense. (**d**) Extremely dense

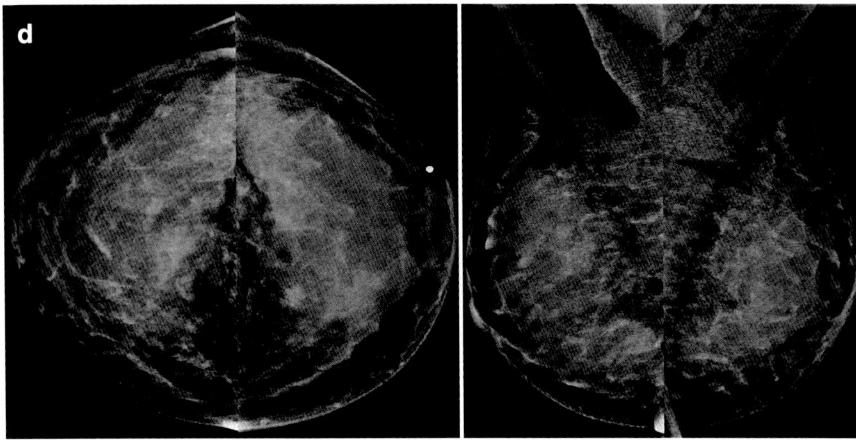

Fig. 1.1 (continued)

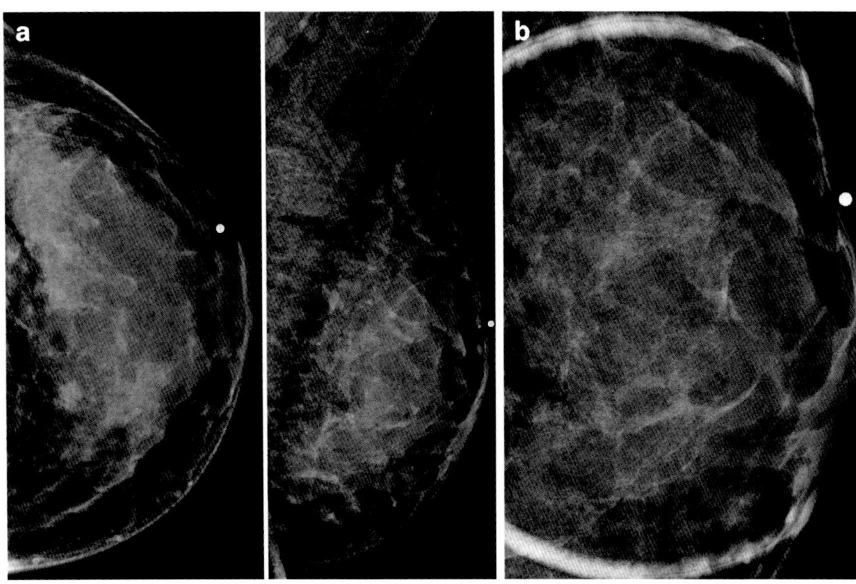

Fig. 1.2 Lowered sensitivity of the detection of masses in extremely dense breast tissue. 40-year-old woman with family history of premenopausal breast cancer. (**a**) Standard and (**b**) spot compression views done for a "lump" in the left breast (marked with a metallic BB on the skin) do not clearly show a mass. (**c**) Targeted ultrasound demonstrates an irregular mass, biopsy of which yielded invasive ductal carcinoma, high nuclear grade

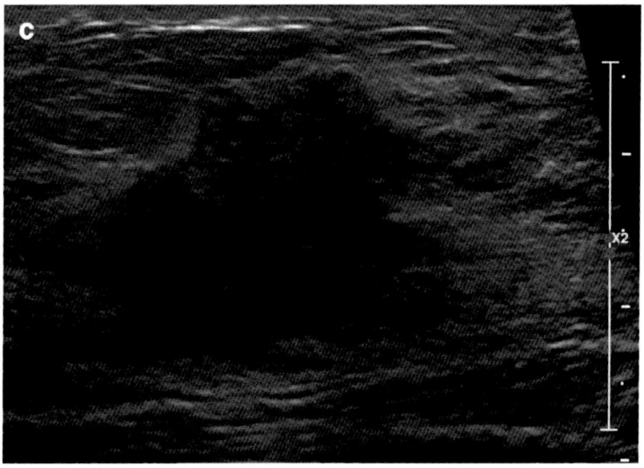

Fig. 1.2 (continued)

The lowered sensitivity of mammography combined with increased cancer risk associated with dense tissue has driven patient advocates and politicians to establish state laws requiring radiologists to directly inform patients about their breast density in more than half of the United States—known as breast density notification legislation. The goal of this is to provide women information to allow them to make more informed decisions regarding screening and breast health. At our institution, the statement added to result letters reads:

> Your mammogram demonstrates you have dense breast tissue. Dense breast tissue is very common and is not abnormal. However, dense breast tissue can make it harder to find cancer on a mammogram and may also be associated with an increased risk of breast cancer. This information about the result of your mammogram is given to you to raise your awareness. Use this information to talk to your doctor about your own risks for breast cancer. At that time, ask your doctor if more screening tests might be useful, based on your risk.

Of note, by MQSA requirements, density information has always been included in the radiology report that is sent to the ordering clinician; it is only in recent years that individual states are mandating this information be included in the patient result letter as well.

However, the benefit of this information is not as clear cut as it seems and has given pause to radiologists and patients alike, especially amidst the controversies about screening guidelines. Some radiologists' threshold for classifying tissue as "dense" is when the mammogram is > 50% dense. This was further divided into categories of "heterogeneously dense" (51–75%) or "extremely dense" (>75%) by older editions of the BI-RADS lexicon; the current edition does not provide percentage guidelines, reflecting that the majority of radiologists make this assessment subjectively [39]. As would be expected, there is much (documented) inter- and intraobserver variability in breast density assessments [40]. Software programs exist to objectively quantify dense tissue; however, these are in large part investigational, and currently not in routine clinical practice. Secondly, density is also affected by radiographic technique. For example, if the image is undercompressed or underpenetrated, breast tissue can appear

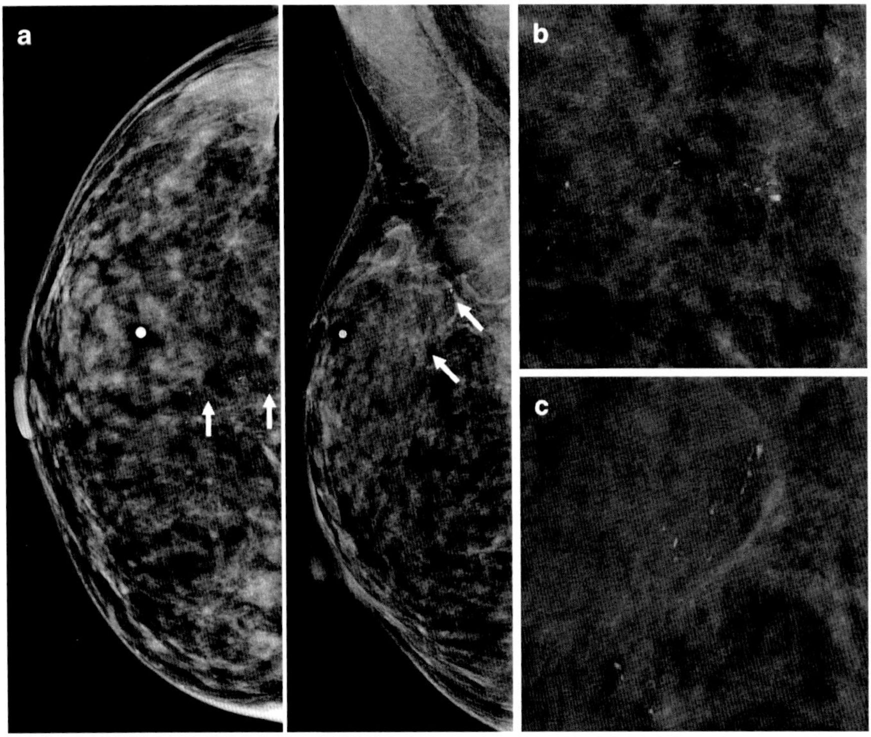

Fig. 1.3 Microcalcifications superimposed on dense breast tissue. (**a**) Standard full paddle CC and MLO views in a 33-year-old patient presenting with a palpable "lump" (marked on the skin with a metallic BB) in the right breast. Calcifications can be seen in the upper central aspect of the breast posteriorly (*arrows*) even on routine views. (**b**) Spot compression magnification CC and (**c**) LM views confirm fine linear calcifications in linear orientation; biopsy showed ductal carcinoma in situ

artificially dense. Making a determination that tissue is dense has serious ramifications for the patient, not the least including anxiety and the possibility of additional tests, and therefore this assessment should be as accurate and reproducible as possible.

Another issue is that breast density does not tend to affect the ability to detect microcalcifications associated with early breast cancer, DCIS, to the same degree as it does for small masses. Calcifications are denser, or "whiter," than dense breast tissue and can therefore still be seen in a background of dense tissue. Therefore, discouraging women from mammography because of dense breast tissue may result in missing the opportunity to find an early-stage intraductal cancer, before it has a chance to progress to invasive disease and form a mass obscured by overlying tissue (Fig. 1.3).

In a similar vein, one of the myths amidst the screening controversies is that mammograms are ineffective in young women because they mostly have dense breast tissue. This is untrue for two reasons. That all young women have dense tissue is a myth; and as indicated above, microcalcifications of DCIS are still apparent in dense tissue.

Women with dense breasts may undergo supplemental screening; however, the trade-off for the increased cancer detection may be increase in false positives, particularly with ultrasound. Perhaps even more of an obstacle is that while breast density notification legislation obligates radiologists to inform patients of their density, in most states, the legislation does not mandate insurance companies to cover supplemental screening tests such as whole-breast ultrasound or MRI, which cost significantly more than screening mammograms. So while we empower patients with information, their ability to act on it may be limited.

Ultrasound

Ultrasound can be used as first line for diagnostic purposes when the risk of even low-dose radiation to the breast tissue outweighs its benefits, mostly when breast tissue is more "active" under strong hormonal influences. This is the case for women under 30, given the continued growth of breast tissue into the 20s, versus the low likelihood of cancer in this age group. Ultrasound is also used preferentially in patients who are or were recently pregnant or breast feeding. Patients who have undergone a mastectomy can also be imaged with ultrasound if presenting with a symptom that requires imaging evaluation.

Otherwise, sonography (ultrasound) should be used as an adjunct to mammography, to further characterize a palpable or radiographic finding and to provide biopsy guidance. Although the utilization of screening ultrasound is increasing with recent breast density notification legislation, even when these are recommended, it is in the setting of concomitant mammography, as the sensitivity and specificity of ultrasound for cancer detection are higher when combined with mammography than when used alone [41, 42]. As mentioned earlier, mammography is not a perfect test; however, we know that some cancers—e.g., intraductal and even some invasive lobular carcinomas—may be occult or at best subtle sonographically. *Mammography is the gold standard for cancer detection, and we would be remiss if we start substituting ultrasound for patients who simply don't want to undergo a mammogram.*

Quality assurance programs similar to those established for mammography are also in place for ultrasound. Though not required by law as for mammography, facilities may participate in the voluntary peer-reviewed ultrasound accreditation process by the ACR, comparable to that required for mammography. This accreditation for ultrasound is mandated by some insurance companies for reimbursement. Similar to mammography, the ultrasound accreditation program, which separates diagnostic ultrasound and ultrasound-guided interventions, assesses issues such as radiologist and technologist qualifications and experience, equipment, image quality, documentation, needle positioning, and radiologic-pathologic concordance and patient outcomes with regard to biopsies and fine needle aspirations.

With regard to day-to-day practice of ultrasound, the ACR has also set practice parameters for image acquisition and annotation. These are not merely boxes to be checked for accreditation, but, when followed, allow for optimum image quality and therefore the best possible visualization and categorization of the finding and subsequent management of the patient. Being mindful of and adjusting technical parameters (such as field of view, focal zone, depth) appropriately must be a part of every patient's scan to obtain accurate diagnostic information. Ensuring that ultrasound findings (with regard to lesion location and imaging characteristics) are concordant with the mammogram is also paramount and is the responsibility of the radiologist even if a sonographer acquires the images. For example, if working up a mammographic finding of a spiculated, solid mass in the upper inner quadrant, a cyst (which is characterized by circumscribed margins and absence of internal echoes) found in the upper outer quadrant would be considered incidental and incongruent with the mammographic finding, which would still need to be identified. Confirmation of findings in perpendicular planes, similar to mammography, is also necessary.

MRI (Magnetic Resonance Imaging)

For breast MRI to be useful in the diagnosis of breast cancer, it must be done with the administration of intravenous gadolinium-based contrast, following which multiple "runs" of repeat imaging are done to provide a dynamic set of images over time. This is because most cancers have avid, rapid influx and outflux of contrast due to increased vascularity and vascular permeability compared with normal tissue, related to tumor angiogenesis [43, 44]. In addition to the visual assessment of lesion morphology and contrast uptake, special software is used to process the kinetic curves of this enhancement. For example, lesions that demonstrate "fast" initial enhancement (>100% signal intensity in the first 2 minutes after contrast injection) and "washout" on delayed images (decrease in signal intensity by >10% from peak enhancement) have the highest likelihood of malignancy.

That being said, hormonal influences can cause (sometimes marked) normal background parenchymal enhancement from which the radiologist must tease out possible lesions (Fig. 1.4). Abnormal findings at MRI may be further worked up with targeted ultrasound and/or biopsy (either sonographically or MRI guided).

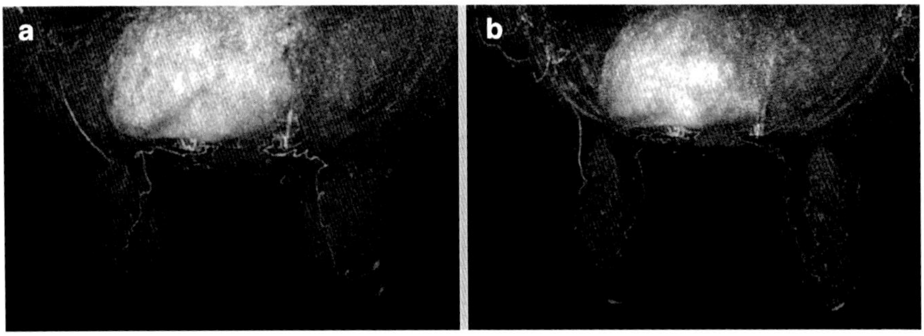

Fig. 1.4 Variations in background parenchymal enhancement related to hormonal changes. These 2 images are from a screening MRI done one year apart in the same patient, at different times in her menstrual cycle. Typically there is less physiologic enhancement during days 7-14, the follicular / proliferative phase, as in (**a**), compared with the luteal/secretory phase as in (**b**)

Although more sensitive than mammography for invasive cancers (88–100%), MRI can be less specific [43, 45, 46]. In addition, *some radiographically apparent low-grade intraductal cancers, and some invasive lobular cancers, may not enhance*. This is why we interpret MRI in conjunction with a recent mammogram; we do not supplant mammography with MRI.

Other "downsides" to MRI include the cost and length of the exam (some protocols are about 35 minutes, although abbreviated protocols are on the horizon) and some of its contraindications that exclude certain patients—e.g., those with pacemakers or other implanted metal and those with renal failure (due to the risk of nephrogenic systemic fibrosis with gadolinium-based contrast, not impairment of renal excretion per se). Claustrophobia is also an issue for many patients.

With regard to quality, facilities that perform and interpret breast MRI may also choose to earn accreditation analogous to that for mammography and ultrasound. Sites that achieve accreditation by the ACR for four breast imaging modalities (mammography, ultrasound, MRI and stereotactic biopsy) are given the designation as a Breast Imaging Center of Excellence.

Screening MRI

The American Cancer Society recommends annual MRI as an adjunct to mammography in women with a >20–25% lifetime risk of breast cancer [21]. This risk may be calculated by one or more of several risk models such as Claus, Tyrer-Cuzick, BRCAPRO, and BOADICEA, the results of which can be discussed with the patient in a larger context of genetic counseling with regard to overall risk assessment and prevention. Patients who are assigned a lifetime risk of >20% include those with a known genetic predisposition; a mutation in one of the many identified genes implicated in breast cancer, such as BRCA1 or BRCA2; those with a first-degree relative with such a mutation but are untested themselves; those who have had mantle (chest) radiation between the ages of 10 and 30 (usually for lymphoma); and those with (or a first-degree relative with) Li-Fraumeni syndrome, Cowden syndrome, or Bannayan-Riley-Ruvalcaba syndrome. With the advancement of genetic testing, more and more mutations are being discovered that may also have a role in increasing risk. For women at high risk, the consensus is to start yearly screening with mammograms and MRIs at 30, but depending on certain risk factors, some may start as early as 25 after discussion with their primary doctors and/or genetic counselors.

In light of the discussion on dense breast tissue above, it is important to note that dense breast tissue alone is currently *not* an indication for screening MRI; nor is a prior history of breast cancer or high-risk lesion. Unless a combination of these and other factors adds up to a >20% lifetime risk, insurance companies may not provide coverage in the United States.

Diagnostic MRI can be used to evaluate the extent of a newly diagnosed breast cancer (including multifocal and multicentric disease, chest wall involvement and axillary lymph nodes), the response to neoadjuvant chemotherapy, and in the setting of axillary node metastatic disease with an unknown primary. Less often, it is used for problem-solving—e.g., to help distinguish between scar versus recurrence—at the discretion of the radiologist. MRI is also helpful in the evaluation of silicone implant integrity, specifically for intracapsular ("internal") rupture.

Imaging Evaluation of the Patient

What is a breast radiologist looking for? Generally speaking, masses, architectural distortion, asymmetries, diffuse changes and calcifications. But, as with everything in medicine, each of these has a differential diagnosis—not everything reported will be a cancer. Actually, the vast majority of findings are benign, and depending on practice variations, some radiologists may not include them in a dictation to prevent cluttering their reports, or confusion or worry on the part of the patient and clinician. For example, normal intramammary and axillary lymph nodes, or skin and vascular calcifications, may not even be mentioned, with preference given to a more general statement such as "no suspicious masses or malignant type calcifications are identified."

So how does the radiologist decide what constitutes a benign finding and what warrants further workup? Therein lies the BI-RADS lexicon (…and experience). Not only does the lexicon allow for clear, consistent reporting, but its focus on feature analysis through specific terminology allows for "triage." When, as an example, through actively looking and engaging in an internal dialogue, the radiologist could describe a mass as oval and fat containing with circumscribed margins in the upper outer quadrant, he/she knows that is defining a normal intramammary lymph node and may decide not to report it at all. If one could report oval, lucent-centered calcifications at the inframammary fold, these are congruent with skin calcifications and can be left alone, even if they are new.

A *mass*, by definition, must occupy space in three dimensions, or on two orthogonal imaging projections. It has convex borders and mammographically is denser centrally than peripherally. Radiologists evaluate masses with regard to shape, margins, radiographic density, internal composition, and other imaging characteristics depending on the modality, such as the effects on surrounding tissue.

Architectural distortion is the disruption of normal tissue planes. Mammographically and on MRI, it appears as straightening of parenchymal lines (Fig. 1.5); normally, the interfaces of intermingled fatty and fibroglandular tissues are gently undulating. Sonographically, the disruption of tissue planes may be more apparent as ligaments seem to stop and start, with interspersed ill-defined, "hazy" parenchyma. While distortion can reflect underlying invasive lobular cancer (Fig. 1.5) or DCIS, benign etiologies such as postsurgical change or trauma need to be considered if consistent with the patient's history and physical exam (i.e., a scar on the skin directly over the area in question on imaging).

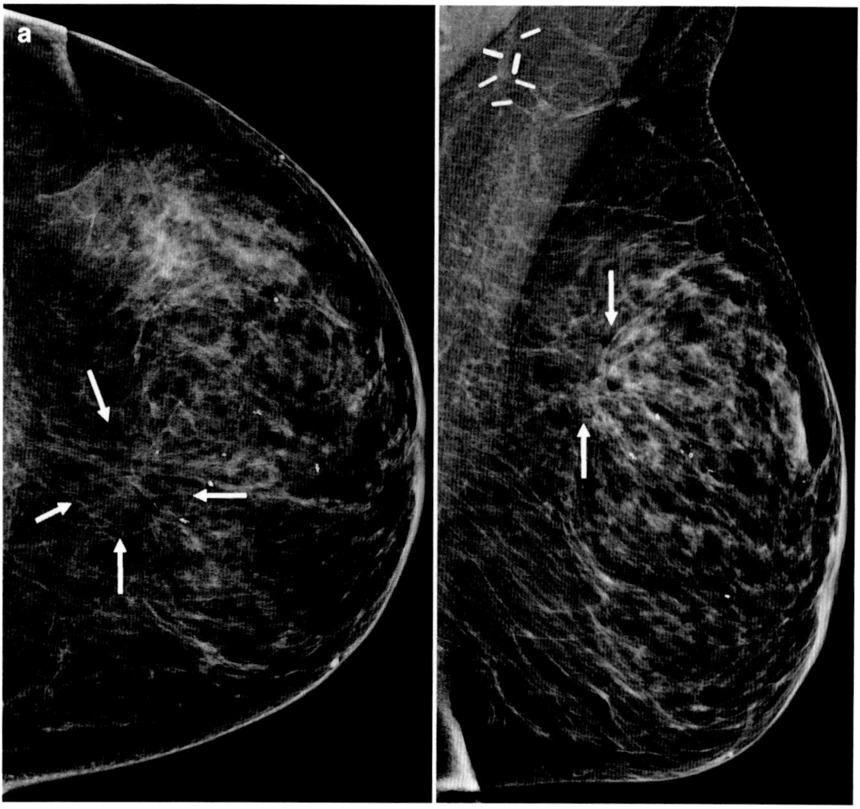

Fig. 1.5 Architectural distortion. (**a**) Screening views of the left breast demonstrate "straightening" of normal parenchymal contours, radiating from a central point in the upper central aspect of the breast posteriorly (*arrows*); this was the sequelae of a prior surgery and unchanged for many years (BI-RADS 2, benign finding). (**b**) Developing distortion (*arrows*) in the absence of prior trauma or surgery resulted in recall of a different patient from screening for spot compression mammographic views; (**c**) targeted ultrasound showed ill-defined hypoechoic tissue with echogenic "peaks" (*arrows*) disrupting normal tissue planes and posterior acoustic shadowing (BI-RADS 5, highly suggestive of malignancy). Biopsy of this showed invasive lobular carcinoma

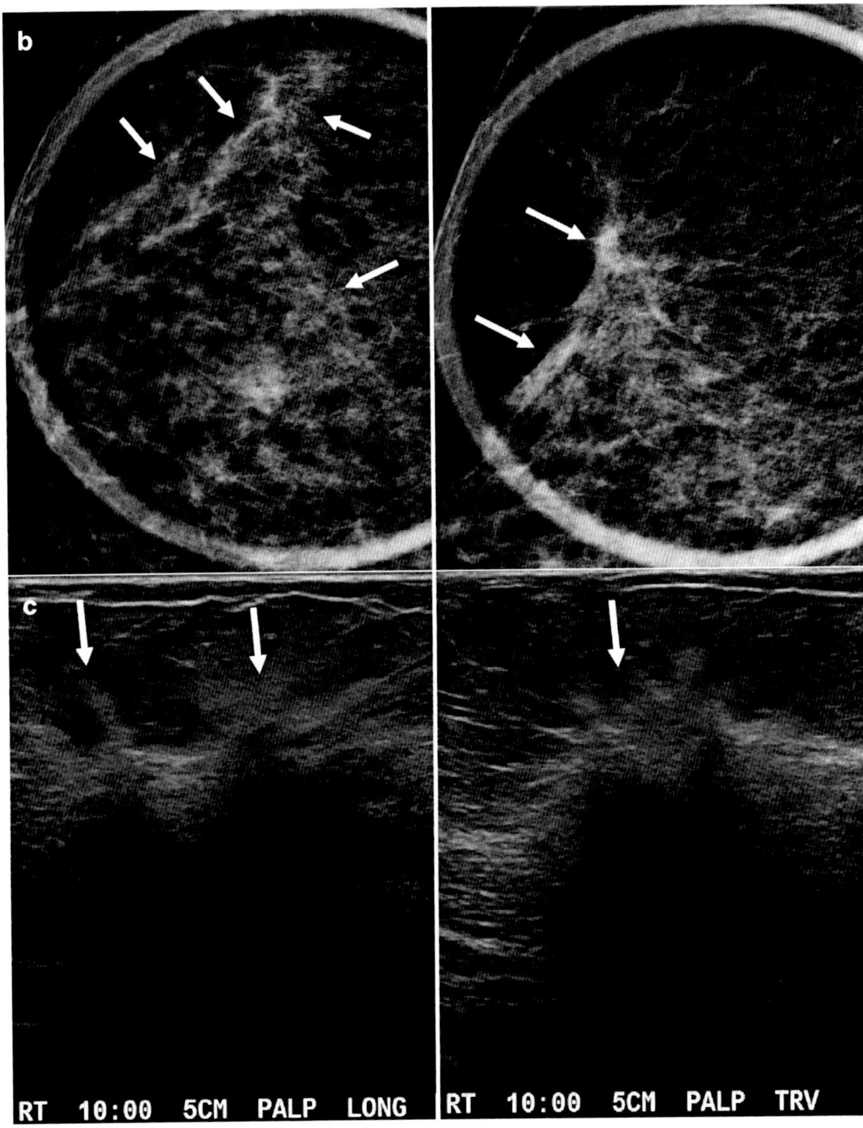

Fig. 1.5 (continued)

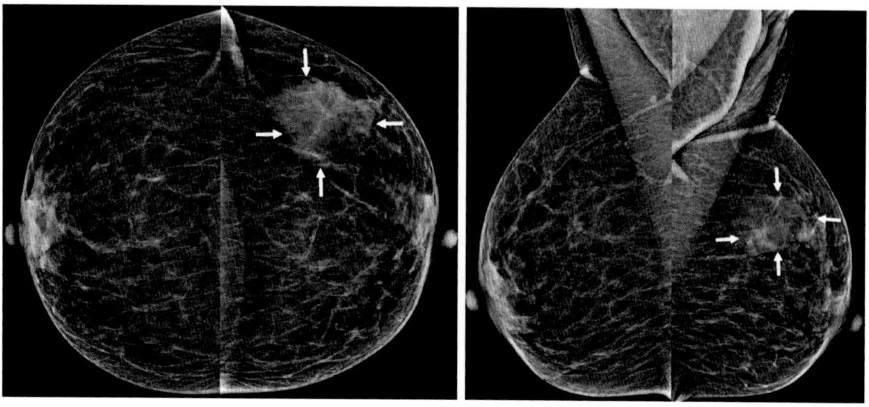

Fig. 1.6 Focal parenchymal asymmetry. An "island" of otherwise normal fibroglandular tissue (*arrows*) that is not mirror imaged in the other breast. As this was unchanged over many annual screenings, it was considered benign (BI-RADS 2, benign finding)

Asymmetry may look like glandular tissue. In fact, more often than not, it *is* normal glandular tissue that is either superimposed on itself such that it stands out in one plane (and may therefore look like a mass); or, simply as it sounds, it can be just an area of tissue that is not "mirror imaged" in the other breast (Fig. 1.6). The latter, which is most often a normal variant (or related to excision of a comparable region on the other side), is termed *focal* asymmetry when it is restricted to one quadrant and *global* when it extends beyond. When stable over time, or in the absence of other suspicious findings, this is benign. As an analogy, one's right foot may be slightly larger than the left foot; aside from making shoe shopping frustrating, this is by no means pathologic. Similarly, having an island of glandular tissue in one breast but not the other is normal for some women and does not increase cancer risk. A *developing* asymmetry, on the other hand, typically warrants a workup, which often includes a biopsy, because, as the name implies, it is a new or increasing finding when compared with prior studies. While some fibrocystic changes and other benign entities such as pseudoangiomatous stromal hyperplasia (PASH) and focal fibrosis may manifest as developing asymmetries in the right clinical setting, malignancy should be considered (Fig. 1.7).

Radiologists must also see the forest through the trees, so to speak. While trained to detect the smallest, most subtle, earliest possible signs of cancer, the "big picture" is also evaluated, for example, with regard to global changes such as altered breast size and edema. Edema manifests as skin and/or trabecular thickening, resulting in a larger or thicker breast that is less compressible. These findings may point to a systemic process if bilateral (such as fluid overload), or a diffuse inflammatory process if unilateral (e.g., mastitis or vascular obstruction). Inflammatory breast cancer is a rare but important cause of unilateral diffuse change, suggested clinically by the rapid (<6 months) onset of swelling, erythema, and peau d'orange change; multiple masses may be seen in the breast and axilla.

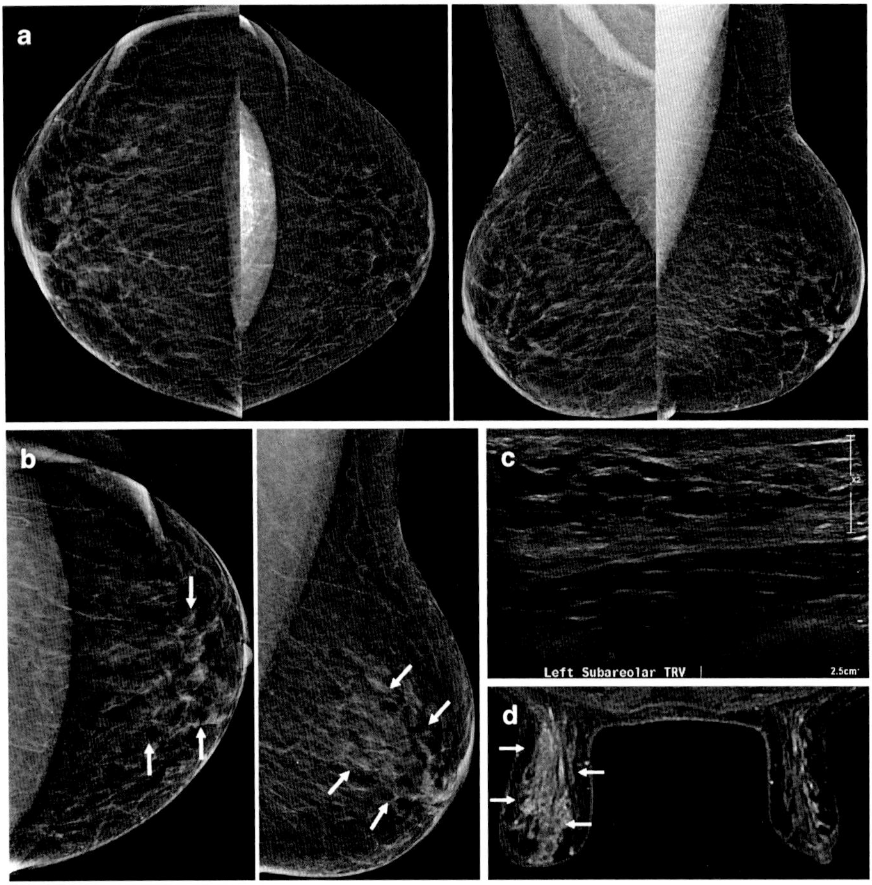

Fig. 1.7 Developing asymmetry. (**a**) Screening mammogram 2 years ago in a 70-year-old woman was normal. (**b**) Screening mammogram 2 years later showed increasing density in a segmental distribution in the left retroareolar region (*arrows*). (**c**) On targeted ultrasound, there were dilated ducts, some with internal echoes and soft tissue that was targeted for biopsy. (**d**) MRI done for biopsy-proven ductal carcinoma in situ, micropapillary type, showed diffusely enhancing ductal structures and tissue extending posteriorly from the left nipple (*arrows*)

Breast Calcifications

Breast calcifications are best seen mammographically. These are most commonly deposits of calcium phosphate; on occasion, the pathologist will find calcium oxalate (often in conjunction with apocrine metaplasia) [47], but radiographically these may not be distinguishable. Calcifications associated with malignancy tend to be small and fine, termed "microcalcifications," at or smaller than 0.5 mm. Again, while there is a differential diagnosis that includes benign and malignant etiologies, their morphology may predict the likelihood of malignancy. For example, classically, fine-linear branching calcifications are associated with DCIS; this makes sense given these calcifications arise amidst intraductal cellular debris and thereby "outline" or "cast" their linear and branching ducts. However, calcifications may have a similar appearance early on in the setting of nascent vascular disease or periductal fibrosis; all calcifications start somewhere and, in their early stages, may mimic cancer.

In fact, most of the calcifications seen on mammography are the result of *benign* processes, such as the wide gamut of fibrocystic and physiologic changes. If these are pathognomonic in appearance, such as in the case of a large, "chunky," or "popcorn-like" calcifications indicative of a hyalinizing fibroadenoma, or the "layering" seen in milk of calcium associated with apocrine metaplasia, these are left alone, and may not even mentioned in a radiology report in an effort to focus on only clinically relevant findings. Table 1.2 lists some of these common benign types of calcifications, listed by their BI-RADS descriptors, and are illustrated in Fig. 1.8.

In contrast, the calcifications hunted and reported by the radiologist are those that may be associated with lesions warranting treatment, for example, high-risk lesions such as atypical ductal hyperplasia (ADH) and the earliest form of breast cancer, ductal carcinoma in situ (DCIS, or intraductal cancer). These are microcalcifications, some smaller than 0.5 mm. The radiographic technique used for mammograms allows for image contrast and resolution that is far superior to other types of x-ray modalities, such as chest x-rays or CT scans, for the detection of these tiny calcifications. In fact, calcifications detected on those modalities are usually the large, dystrophic, coarse ones pathognomonic for benign processes, such as calcifying fat necrosis or hyalinizing fibroadenomas [48]. Not surprisingly, with the advent of routine screening mammography in the United States in the 1980s, the incidence of DCIS skyrocketed (increased by at least 200%)—due in part to the detection of tiny intraductal calcifications that allowed for the diagnosis of breast cancer before its progression to invasive disease felt clinically as a "lump." Because of the earlier detection of breast cancer, the morbidity and mortality from it also plummeted [49, 50].

But as small as they are, microcalcifications are quite variable with regard to morphology, distribution, and density—all features that reflect their origin histologically. These features are best evaluated on special mammographic views—spot compression magnification views—given their higher resolution than even standard views. The BI-RADS lexicon provides an organized approach in classifying calcifications. Along with the lexicon, consideration of patient risk factors, age, and interval change guides the differential diagnosis and determination of an appropriate management plan.

In classifying calcifications, the radiologist considers their size, form or morphology, and distribution. The lexicon is extremely helpful in standardizing this determination and ultimately the report, but one must remember that descriptors are merely that; words should not connote an instant diagnosis or classification of benign versus malignant (a task left up to the pathologist!). For example, "linear and branching" are buzzwords among residents and non-breast imagers for DCIS. But linear and branching calcifications, just using the words as descriptors, can be seen in periductal fibrosis, fibroadenomas, secretory disease, and atherosclerotic disease, all unequivocally benign processes!

Table 1.2 Benign calcifications—descriptors [39]

Skin	Round
Vascular	Rim
Coarse, "popcorn-like"	Dystrophic
Large rodlike	Milk of calcium

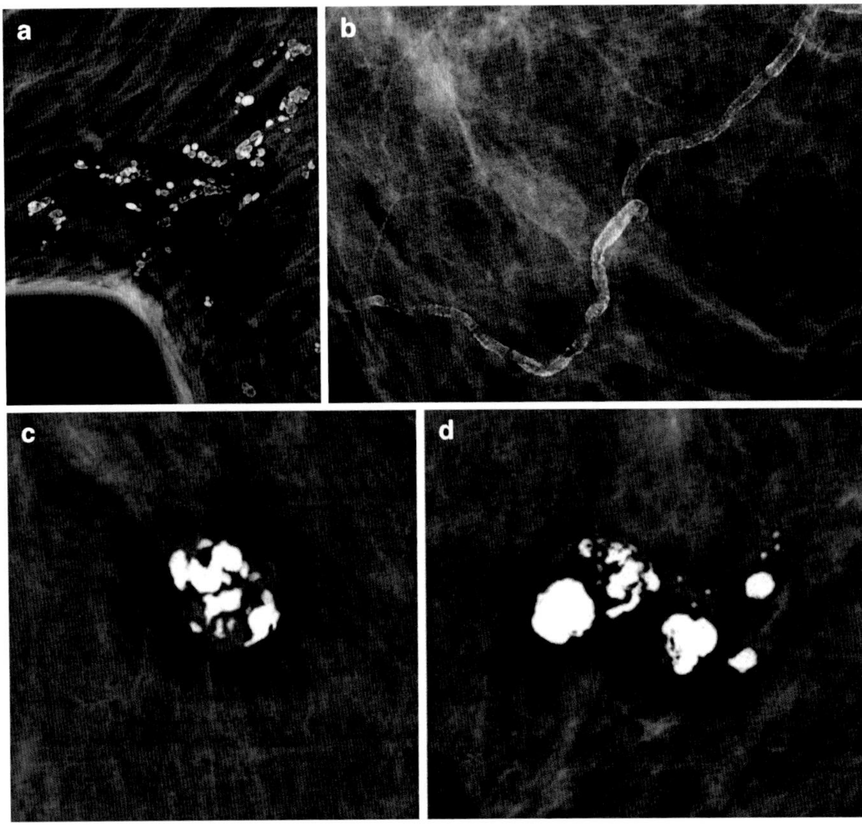

Fig. 1.8 (**a**–**k**) Commonly seen benign-type breast calcifications. (**a**) Skin calcifications are typically round or oval with lucent centers, usually seen in the cleavage, inframammary fold, and along surgical scars. (**b**) Vascular calcifications can sometimes be seen associated with a tubular soft tissue density representing the artery itself; these calcifications line the media and are often referred to as "tram tracking." (**c** and **d**) Coarse "popcorn-like" calcifications are commonly seen in hyalinizing fibroadenomas and can be large enough to be seen on CT scans. (**e** and **f**) Large rodlike calcifications are linear and branching because they are intraductal secretory calcifications; these are distinguished from ductal carcinoma in situ by their larger size, increased density, sharp edges, and "needle" or "cigar" shape and often diffuse distribution. These are associated with duct ectasia. (**g**) Round calcifications may be up to 1 mm in size. (**h**) Rim calcifications are often associated with oil cysts, deposited along the surface of the sphere. (**i**) Dystrophic calcifications can be large (>2–3 mm), "bizarre" shapes, dense, and the result of trauma or radiation or just related to the stroma; in this patient, these are seen at site of remote lumpectomy and radiation. (**j** and **k**) Milk of calcium is calcium in suspension, layered in the bottom of microcysts that are often clustered; the change in configuration of calcifications from round or amorphous ("smudgy") in the craniocaudal view, to curvilinear or linear in the true lateral (90°) projection, is pathognomonic and sometimes called "layering" or a "teacup" appearance

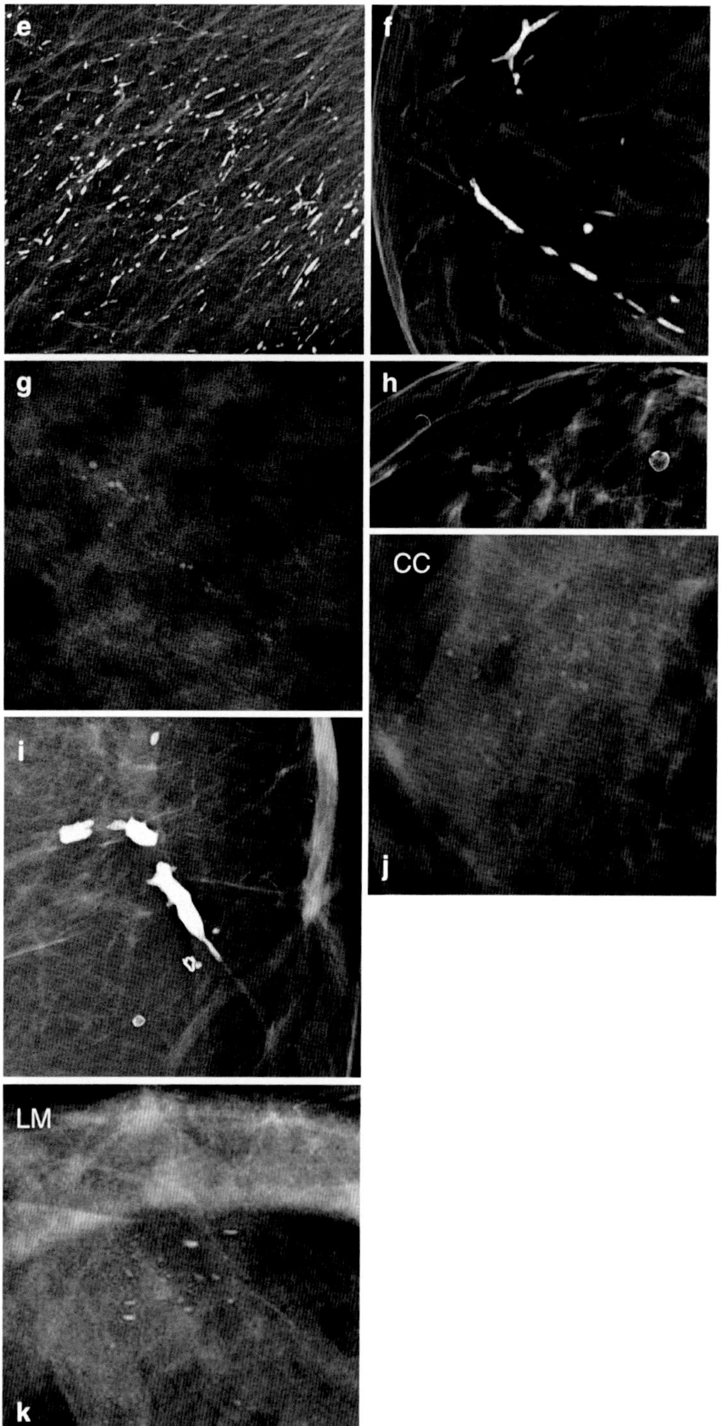

Fig. 1.8 (continued)

Regardless, the likelihood of malignancy with specific morphologies has been studied and is listed in Table 1.3 alongside a list of the BI-RADS descriptors for the morphology of suspicious calcifications [39], with examples in Fig. 1.9.

Table 1.3 Suspicious calcifications: morphology descriptors and likelihood of malignancy [39]

Amorphous	13–26%
Coarse heterogeneous	7–20%
Fine pleomorphic	28–29%
Fine linear or fine-linear branching	53–81%

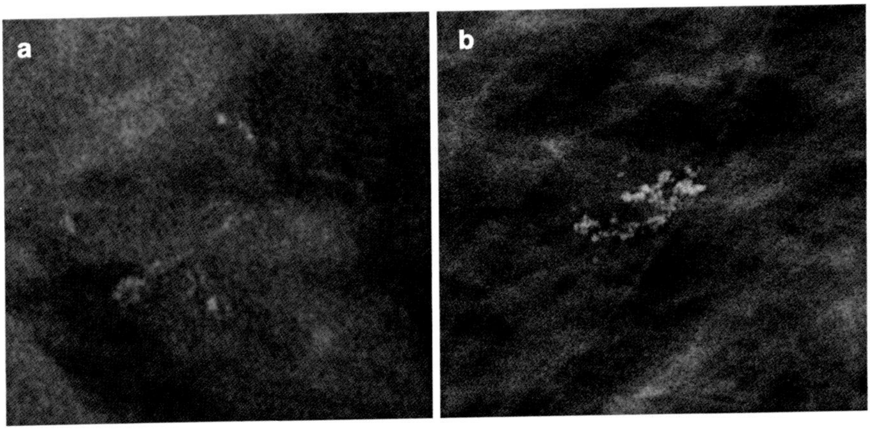

Fig. 1.9 (**a**–**d**) Suspicious morphology calcifications. (**a**) Amorphous calcifications can be thought of as "smudgy" or "indistinct"; the differential diagnosis ranges from fibrocystic changes to atypical lesions to low-nuclear-grade DCIS. If new or an isolated group, biopsy is often done, as in this 53-year-old patient; linear distribution was also suspicious. Histology was benign breast tissue. (**b**) Coarse heterogeneous calcifications may vary in size and density but are more discrete than amorphous or fine forms. Differential diagnosis may include fibroadenoma, papilloma, stromal/periductal fibrosis (as in this 41 year old) or intermediate to high nuclear grade DCIS. (**c**) Fine pleomorphic forms are small and slight; etiology may be benign, for example, "early" forms of popcorn or dystrophic forms, FCC, stromal fibrosis (as in this 40-year-old woman), atypical lesions, or (**d**) DCIS as in this 63 years old. (**e**) Fine linear or fine-linear branching calcifications are the "buzzwords" for DCIS (typically high nuclear grade, with comedonecrosis and resultant "casting" of the ducts, as in these 2 different women. Some benign causes may be congruent on pathology if one is confident of adequate sampling, such as fibroadenoma (**f**; *arrows*, with adjacent vascular calcifications, *arrowheads*), papilloma, fat necrosis, fibrosis—all calcifications start somewhere!

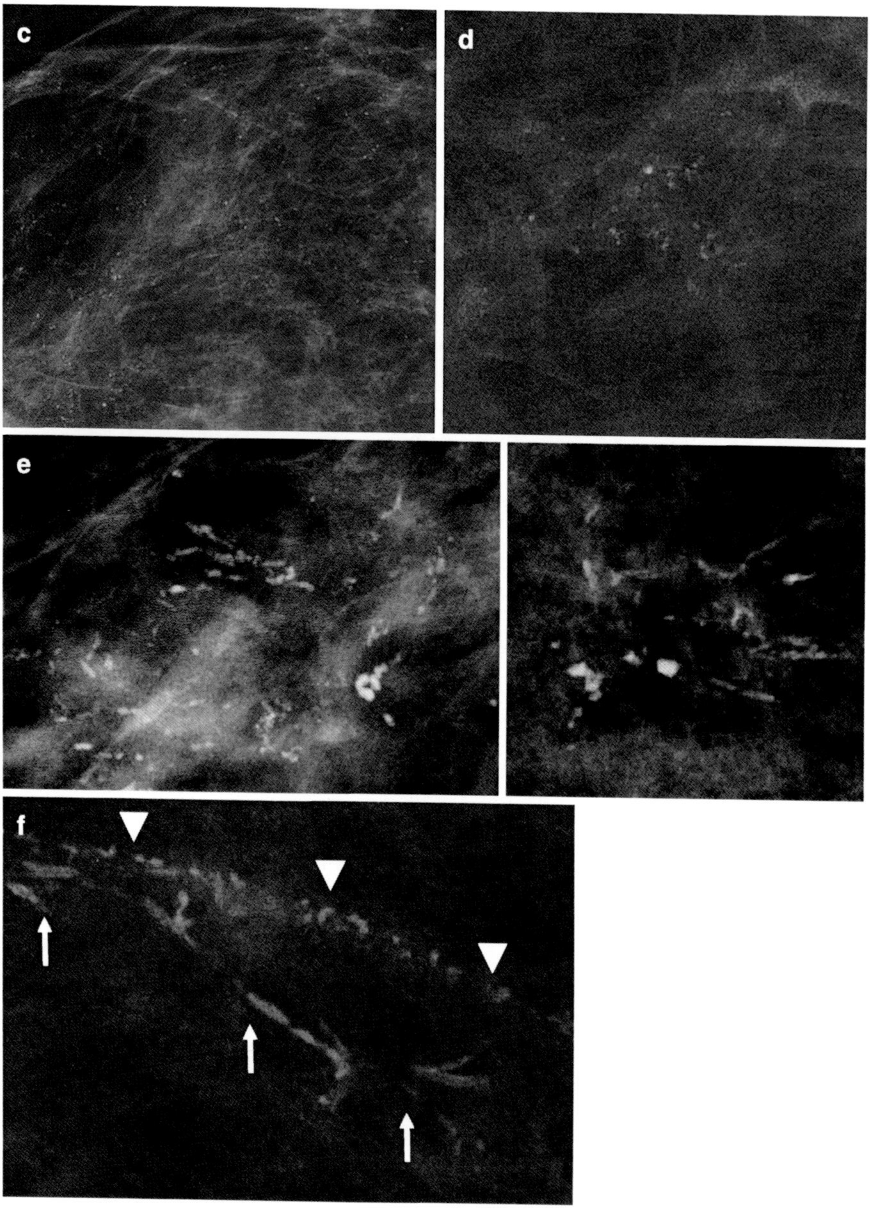

Fig. 1.9 (continued)

With regard to distribution, typically, the more diffuse the calcifications, the more likely they reflect a benign process (however, again, morphology and interval change must also be considered). Linear or segmental calcifications suggest a ductal process, following a ductal distribution (Table 1.4, Fig. 1.10).

It is important to note that although the BI-RADS lexicon is an invaluable guide, the final determination and description of findings, the assessment, and recommendation for management are up to individual radiologist's interpretation. Studies show moderate interobserver disagreement in choice of descriptors for calcifications [6, 7]. Part of this may be related to experience and also to the variability in the calcifications themselves—in practice, they exist in a continuum of shapes and sizes, and so multiple descriptors could be applied. In addition, all calcifications start somewhere. Large, benign calcifications, if imaged in their early stages, may be faint, fine forms that over time "declare themselves" as they evolve into obviously benign findings, but may pose a diagnostic dilemma at that earlier point in time at which they are seen (Fig. 1.11).

After appropriate workup and classification of calcifications, the radiologist may recommend doing nothing (classified as BI-RADS 2, benign finding), short interval (6-month) mammographic follow-up (BI-RADS 3, probably benign finding—this category has a <2% chance of malignancy), or a biopsy (BI-RADS 4 or 5, suspicious or highly suspicious, with at least >2% likelihood of malignancy), similar to the management options in the work up of masses and some asymmetries. A biopsy can be done with a needle under imaging guidance, or surgically with preoperative wire localization. The former is preferred in the majority of cases as it is far less invasive, does not require sedation, costs less, and can allow for appropriate staging and surgical planning prior to definitive treatment if malignant. Moreover, a larger distribution of calcifications may warrant more than one needle biopsy to establish extent of disease as this may have implications for management (e.g., a lumpectomy versus mastectomy).

Since the calcifications are identified mammographically, a core needle biopsy with imaging is most often undertaken with radiographic or, more specifically, *stereotactic guidance* [51]. The patient is positioned in a mammography machine that

Table 1.4 Distribution descriptors for calcifications [39]

Diffuse
Regional
Grouped
Segmental
Linear

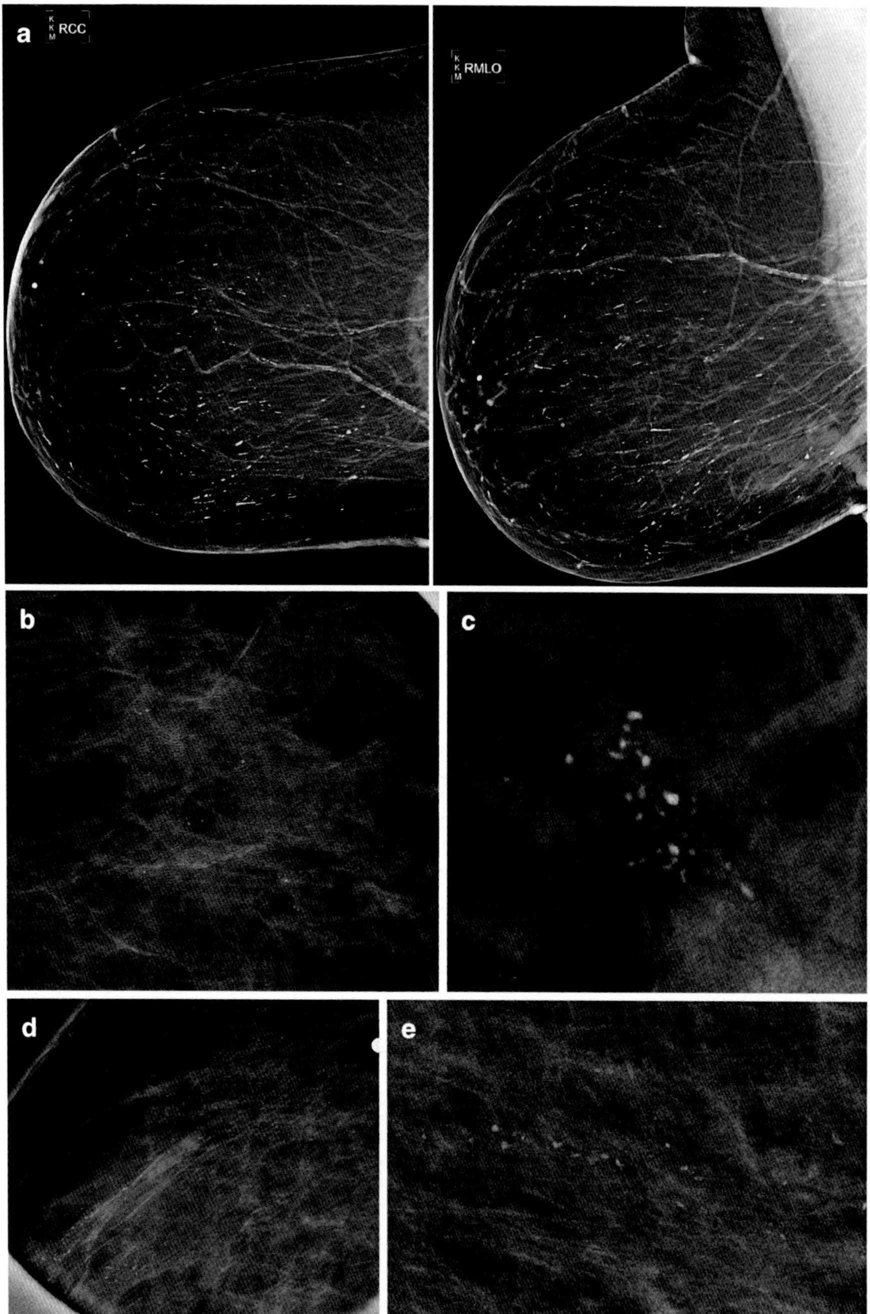

Fig. 1.10 Distribution modifiers for calcifications. (**a**) Diffuse calcifications are seen throughout the breast and are most commonly benign, as are these large rodlike secretory calcifications; vascular calcifications are also seen in this patient. (**b**) Regional calcifications occupy >2 cm of tissue, but are not limited to a ductal distribution. (**c**) Grouped calcifications are typically five or more calcifications that occupy <2 cm of tissue. (**d**) Segmental calcifications follow a ductal distribution; this may follow a "wedge" or "cone" shape toward the nipple. (**e**) Linear calcifications are in a line

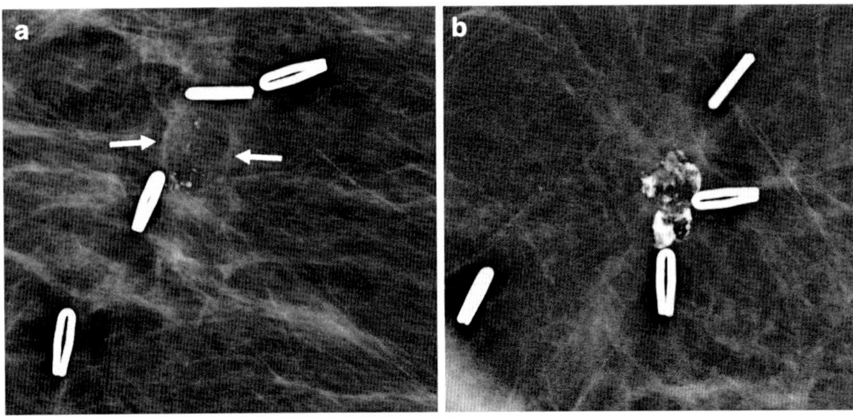

Fig. 1.11 Developing (benign) calcifications. (**a**) Spot compression magnification view of the lumpectomy site in a 77-year-old patient treated for invasive ductal carcinoma 4 years ago. Fine pleomorphic (curvilinear and punctate) calcifications are seen in the background of a fat-containing mass with circumscribed margins (between *arrows*), between surgical clips. Given the background of a fat-containing mass, these were thought most likely reflective of fat necrosis, and short interval follow-up was recommended. (**b**) Comparable view of the lumpectomy site 2.5 years later shows dystrophic and lucent-centered calcifications of fat necrosis. Even large and coarse calcifications start somewhere and may evolve from more suspicious-appearing forms that pose a diagnostic dilemma for the radiologist early on

is specially adapted for this procedure, and a scout image is taken to localize the calcifications. Additional x-rays are then taken "+" and "–" 15° off this midline, and a computer triangulates the location of the calcifications in space with regard to *x*, *y*, and *z* coordinates. Under local anesthesia, the needle is moved to this target, and the operator cuts cores of breast tissue to sample the calcifications. Numerous brands and types of needles exist for this, but these can be generally classified as spring loaded or vacuum assisted. The latter tend to be larger in size (smaller in gauge) and allow for subsequent placement of a metal clip to mark the biopsy site given the possibility of removing all of the calcifications due to the larger needle size and use of suction. Assuming no migration of the clip, the marker acts as a placeholder if surgical excision is later required; otherwise, the marker is considered safe to remain in the breast if no surgical follow-up is needed. As with any procedure involving a needle, risks include bleeding, infection, and tissue damage. The ominous threat of a pneumothorax, listed on virtually every consent form but for which the risk very small, is avoided by keeping the needle parallel to the chest wall. The positioning of the patient and design of the machine ensures this; however, in the case of ultrasound-guided biopsies, the onus of safe needle positioning is on the operator.

After the biopsy of calcifications is taken, it is the standard of care for a radiograph of the cores to be obtained prior to placing a clip or releasing the patient from compression and positioning (Fig. 1.12). Identifying calcifications in the cores confirms a successful biopsy. *There is no set number of calcifications one must extract for the biopsy to be considered a success*; one must take into account the number and type of calcifications to start with and decide if he/she has an adequate sampling of these. If

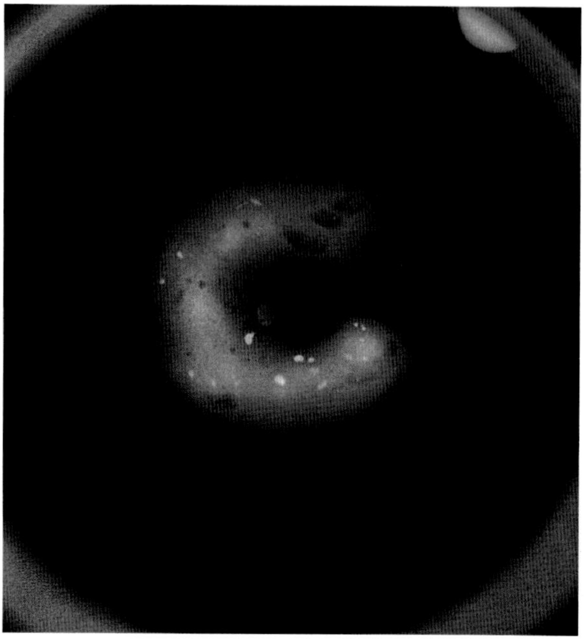

Fig. 1.12 Specimen radiograph of cores from biopsy of calcifications. Multiple calcifications are seen in cores taken from a 14G spring-loaded needle. This was sufficient for diagnosis of ductal carcinoma in situ, nuclear grade 3, with comedonecrosis and calcifications

inadequate, more cores should be taken at that time; troubleshooting maneuvers such as reimaging and retargeting, adjusting needle or patient positioning, and/or changing needles may be undertaken before additional rounds of sampling and repeat specimen radiography [52]. This must be done while being mindful of patient discomfort given that she must remain still with her breast in compression. At some point, the biopsy must stop, and *the samples should still be sent for pathology even if no calcifications are obtained*. If histology reveals no calcifications but a high-risk or malignant disease, and targeting was correct, the patient is still referred for surgical excision. If only benign tissue is reported in the absence of calcifications on histology, another biopsy is advised given that the question of the etiology of the calcifications has not yet been answered. This may be a repeat needle biopsy or, if it is unclear what went wrong the first time, a surgical biopsy with preoperative wire localization. Fortunately, this is a rare occurrence for most radiologists trained in doing these types of biopsies, and re-biopsy rates may be further improved by the use of a vacuum-assisted needle device, the use of which has increased over spring-loaded ones [52, 53].

Assuming a successful biopsy yielding calcifications, if there are residual calcifications in the breast and no question as to which group was targeted, one may consider *not* placing a marker clip; otherwise, a clip must be placed if all of the calcifications have been removed with the biopsy. After clip placement, a two-view full paddle mammogram is done to confirm its deployment and accurate location. If the clip has migrated, this is documented, as it may affect future surgical planning.

The cores may be marked with ink or separated to designate those with calcifications to aid the pathologist. In the event that calcifications are identified on the specimen radiograph, but none are identified at pathology, radiography of the paraffin blocks may be done to further guide the pathologist. Alternatively, the use of polarized light by the pathologist may detect calcium oxalate that is mammographically indistinguishable from calcium phosphate [47, 52]; the latter is more commonly seen.

Establishing radiologic-pathologic concordance is imperative for patient care, and in breast imaging, for the medical audit. At our institution, the breast radiologist assumes this responsibility and communicates directly with the pathologist and the patient, regarding each of his/her biopsy results. Not only is this dialogue helpful in establishing biopsy adequacy and congruence, but it is an effective educational tool for both parties.

Bibliography

1. Cardenosa G. Clinical breast imaging, the essentials. Philadelphia, PA: Wolters Kluwer; 2015.
2. Destout JM, Bassett LW, Yaffe MJ, et al. The ACR's mammography accreditation program: ten years of experience since MQSA. J Am Coll Radiol. 2005;2(7):585–94.
3. https://www.fda.gov/Radiation-EmittingProducts/MammographyQualityStandardsActandProgram/default.htm
4. Burnside E, Sickles EA, Bassett LW, et al. The ACR BI-RADS experience: learning from history. J Am Coll Radiol. 2009;6(12):851–60.
5. D'Orsi CJ, Sickles EA, Mendelson EB, Morris EA, et al. ACR BI-RADS® Atlas breast imaging reporting and data system. Reston, VA: American College of Radiology; 2013.
6. Lee AY, Wisner DJ, Aminololama-Shakeri S, et al. Inter-reader variability in the use of BI-RADS descriptors for suspicious findings on diagnostic mammography: a multi-institution study of 10 academic radiologists. Acad Radiol. 2017;24(1):60–6. Accessed 23 Feb 2017
7. Berg WA, D'Orsi C, Jackson V, et al. Does training in the breast imaging reporting and data system (BI-RADS) improve biopsy recommendations or feature analysis agreement with experienced breast imagers at mammography? Radiology. 2002;224(3):871–80. doi:10.1148/radiol.2243011626. Accessed 25 Feb 2017
8. Blanks RG, Moss SM, Wallis MG. Use of two view mammography compared with one view in the detection of small invasive cancers: further results from the National Health Service breast screening programme. J Med Screen. 1997;4(2):98–101. doi:10.1177/096914139700400206.
9. https://seer.cancer.gov/statfacts/html/breast.html. Accessed 19 Feb 2017.
10. Tabar L, Duffy SW, et al. Breast cancer treatment and natural history: new insights from results of screening. Lancet. 1992;339(8790):412–4.
11. NCI-funded Breast Cancer Surveillance Consortium (HHSN261201100031C). Downloaded 01/09/2017 from the Breast Cancer Surveillance Consortium web site—http://breastscreening.cancer.gov/statistics/benchmarks/screening/2009/tableSensSpec.html
12. Lehman CD, Arao RF, Sprague BL, et al. National performance benchmarks for modern screening digital mammography: update from the Breast Cancer Surveillance Consortium. Radiology. 2017;283(1):49–58. doi:10.1148/radiol.2016161174. Accessed 5 Feb 2017
13. Tabar L, Yen M, Vitak B, et al. Mammography service screening and mortality in breast cancer patients: 20-year follow-up before and after introduction of screening. Lancet. 2003;361:1405–10.
14. Ray KM, Price ER, Joe BN. Evidence to support screening women in their 40s. Radiol Clin N Am. 2017;55(3):429–39. doi:10.1016/j.rcl.2016.12.002. Accessed 5 Feb 2017
15. Tabar L, Faberberg G, Day NE, Holmberg L. What is the optimum interval between mammographic examinations?—an analysis based on the latest results of the Swedish two-county breast cancer screening trial. Br J Cancer. 1987;55:547–51.

16. Hellquist BN, Duffy SW, Abdsaleh S, Björneld L, Bordás P, Tabár L, Viták B, Zackrisson S, Nyström L, Jonsson H. Effectiveness of population-based service screening with mammography for women ages 40–49 years. Cancer. 2011;117(4):714–22.
17. Tabár L, Vitak B, Chen TH-H, Yen AM-F, Cohen A, Tot T, Chiu SY-H, Chen SL-S, Fann JC-Y, Rosell J, Fohlin H, Smith RA, Duffy SW. Swedish two-county trial: impact of mammographic screening on breast cancer mortality during 3 decades. Radiology. 2011;260(3):658–63.
18. Anders CK, Hsu DS, Broadwater G, Acharya CR, Foekens JA, Zhang Y, Wang Y, Kelly Marcom P, Marks JR, Febbo PG, Nevins JR, Potti A, Blackwell KL. Young age at diagnosis correlates with worse prognosis and defines a subset of breast cancers with shared patterns of gene expression. J Clin Oncol. 2008;26(20):3324–30.
19. El Saghir NS, Seoud M, Khalil MK, Charafeddine M, Salem ZK, Geara FB, Shamseddine AI. Effects of young age at presentation on survival in breast cancer. BMC Cancer. 2006;6(1):194. doi:10.1186/1471-2407-6-194.
20. https://www.uspreventiveservicestaskforce.org
21. https://www.cancer.org/cancer/breast-cancer/screening-tests-and-early-detection/american-cancer-society-recommendations-for-the-early-detection-of-breast-cancer.html
22. US Preventive Services Task Force. Screening for breast cancer: U.S. preventive services task force recommendation statement. Ann Intern Med. 2009;151(10):716.
23. Tosteson AN, Fryback DG, Hammond CS. Consequences of false-positive screening mammograms. JAMA. 2014;174(6):954–61.
24. Brodersen J, Siersma VD. Long-term psychosocial consequences of false-positive screening mammography. Ann Fam Med. 2013;11(2):106–15.
25. Lee J, Hardesty LA, Kunzler NM, Rosenkrantz AB. Direct interactive public education by breast radiologists about screening mammography: impact on anxiety and empowerment. J Am Coll Radiol. 2016;13(1):12–20.
26. Hislop TG, Harris SR, Jackson J, Thorne SE, Rousseau EJ, Coldman AJ, Vestrup JA, Wright CJ, Olivotto IA. Satisfaction and anxiety for women during investigation of an abnormal screening mammogram. Breast Cancer Res Treat. 2002;76(3):245–54.
27. Hauge IHR, Pedersen K, Olerud HM, Hole EO, Hofvind S. The risk of radiation-induced breast cancers due to biennial mammographic screening in women aged 50–69 years is minimal. Acta Radiol. 2014;55(10):1174–9.
28. Skaane P. Dose hysteria and concern about radiation exposure should not prevent women from undergoing life-saving mammography screening. Acta Radiol. 2014;55(10):1155–6.
29. Hendrick RE. Radiation doses and cancer risks from breast imaging studies. Radiology. 2010;257:246–53. doi:10.1148/radiol.10100570. Accessed 26 Feb 2017
30. Linver MN, Paster SB, Rosenberg RD, Key CR, Stidley CA, King WV. Improvement in mammography interpretation skills in a community radiology practice after dedicated teaching courses: 2-year medical audit of 38,633 cases. Radiology. 1992;184(1):39–43. doi:10.1148/radiology.184.1.1609100. Accessed 13 Aug 2017
31. https://www.acr.org/~/media/ACR/Documents/PDF/Annual%20Meeting/Abstracts/2016/16079/16079_Rabinovich.pdf. Accessed 30 May 2017.
32. Harvey SC, Geller B, Oppenheimer RG, Pinet M, Riddell L, Garra B. Increase in cancer detection and recall rates with independent double interpretation of screening mammography. Am J Roentgenol. 2003;180(5):1461–7.
33. Sharpe RE, Venkataraman S, Phillips J, Dialani V, Fein-Zachary VJ, Prakash S, Slanetz PJ, Mehta TS. Increased cancer detection rate and variations in the recall rate resulting from implementation of 3D digital breast tomosynthesis into a population-based screening program. Radiology. 2016;278(3):698–706.
34. Rafferty EA, Park JM, Philpotts LE, Poplack SP, Sumkin JH, Halpern EF, Niklason LT. Diagnostic accuracy and recall rates for digital mammography and digital mammography combined with one-view and two-view tomosynthesis: results of an enriched reader study. Am J Roentgenol. 2014;202(2):273–81.
35. Skaane P, Bandos AI, Gullien R, Eben EB, Ekseth U, Haakenaasen U, Izadi M, Jebsen IN, Jahr G, Krager M, Niklason LT, Hofvind S, Gur D. Comparison of digital mammography

alone and digital mammography plus tomosynthesis in a population-based screening program. Radiology. 2013;267(1):47–56.
36. Comparative effectiveness of core-needle and open surgical biopsy for the diagnosis of breast lesions—executive summary. https://effectivehealthcare.ahrq.gov/ehc/products/17/372/exec-summforposting.pdf. Accessed 23 Jan 2017.
37. Somerville P, Seifert PJ, Destounis SV, et al. Anticoagulation and bleeding risk after core needle biopsy. AJR Am J Roentgenol. 2008;191:1194–7.
38. Harvey JA, Bovbjerg V. Quantitative assessment of mammographic breast density: relationship with breast cancer risk. Radiology. 2004;230:29–41.
39. Sickles EA, D'Orsi CJ, Bassett LW, et al. ACR BI-RADS® mammography. In: ACR BI-RADS® Atlas, editor. Breast imaging reporting and data system. Reston, VA: American College of Radiology; 2013.
40. Gard CC, Aiello Bowles EJ, Miglioretti DL, Taplin SH, Rutter CM. Misclassification of Breast Imaging Reporting and Data System (BI-RADS) mammographic density and implications for breast density reporting legislation. Breast J. 2015;21(5):481–9.
41. Berg WA, Blume JD, Cormack JB. Combined screening with ultrasound and mammography vs mammography alone in women at elevated risk of breast cancer. JAMA. 2008;299(18): 2151–63.
42. Brem RF, Lenihan MJ, Lieberman J, et al. Screening breast ultrasound: past, present, and future. AJR Am J Roentgenol. 2015;204:234–40.
43. Bartella L, Dershaw DD. Magnetic resonance imaging of the invasive breast carcinoma. In: Morris E, Liberman L, editors. Breast MRI: diagnosis and intervention. New York, NY: Springer; 2005.
44. Morris EA, Comstock CE, Lee CH, et al. ACR BI-RADS® magnetic resonance imaging. In: ACR BI-RADS® Atlas, editor. Breast imaging reporting and data system. Reston, VA: American College of Radiology; 2013.
45. Orel SG, Schnall MD. MR imaging of the breast for the detection, diagnosis, and staging of breast cancer. Radiology. 2001;220(1):13–30.
46. Liu PF, Debatin JF, Caduff RF, Kacl G, Garzoli E, Krestin GP. Improved diagnostic accuracy in dynamic contrast enhanced MRI of the breast by combined quantitative and qualitative analysis. Br J Radiol. 1998;71(845):501–9.
47. Surratt JT, Monsees BS, Mazoujian G. Calcium oxalate microcalcifications in the breast. Radiology. 1991;181:141–2. doi:10.1148/radiology.181.1.1887023. Accessed 26 Feb 2017
48. Harish MG, Konda SD, MacMahon G, Newstead GM. Breast lesions incidentally detected with CT: what the general radiologist needs to know. Radiographics. 2007;27(1):S37–51. doi:10.1148/rg.27si075510. Accessed 25 Feb 2017
49. Ernster VL, Barclay MS, Kerlikowske K, et al. Incidence of and treatment for ductal carcinoma of the breast. JAMA. 1996;275(12):913–8. doi:10.1001/jama.1996.03530360023033. Accessed 26 Feb 2017
50. Ernster VL, Barclay J. Increases in ductal carcinoma in situ (DCIS) of the breast in relation to mammography: a dilemma. J Natl Cancer Inst Monogr. 1996;22:151–6. Accessed 25 Feb 2017
51. Bolmgren J, Jacobson B, Nordenström B. Stereotaxic instrument for needle biopsy of the mamma. AJR Am J Roentgenol. 1977;129(1):121–5. doi:10.2214/ajr.129.1.121. Accessed 26 Feb 2017
52. Lewin J. Breast biopsy: beyond the basics; Part I: getting the tissue. Presentation slides ACR society of breast imaging symposium; 2016. https://www.sbi-online.org/Portals/0/Breast%20Imaging%20Symposium%202016/Final%20Presentations/312C%20Lewin-Flowers%20-%20Breast%20Biopsy%20Beyond%20the%20Basics.pdf. Accessed 29 Jan 2017.
53. Philpotts LE, Shaheen NA, Carter D, Lange RC, Lee CH. Comparison of rebiopsy rates after stereotactic core needle biopsy of the breast with 11-gauge vacuum suction probe versus 14-gauge needle and automatic gun. AJR Am J Roentgenol. 1999;172:683–7. doi:10.2214/ajr.172.3.10063860. Accessed 26 Feb 2017

2

Overview of Pathology Evaluation of Breast Lesions and Quality Assurance

Michael O. Idowu, Jaime A. Singh, and Margaret M. Grimes

Masses/Densities/Distortions: General Considerations

Radiologic evaluation of breast masses or architectural distortion generally requires assessment of shape, margin, density, orientation, echogenicity pattern, asymmetry, and enhancements, as defined by Breast Imaging-Reporting and Data System (BI-RADS), depending on the imaging modalities used (mammogram, ultrasound, or magnetic resonance imaging [MRI]). Both benign and malignant breast conditions may present as masses, densities or distortions with or without associated calcifications. Progressive asymmetry of the breast, so-called shrinking breast, may be seen in association with invasive lobular carcinoma. Radiologically identified lesions require biopsies for pathologic evaluation.

Core needle biopsy performed with ultrasound or with stereotactic guidance is often the first approach to tissue diagnosis. While palpable lesions lend themselves to diagnosis by means of fine needle aspiration (FNA) biopsy, core needle biopsy is preferred for primary breast lesions, because the intact tissue specimen and generally larger sample obtained via core needle biopsy usually allows for a more definitive diagnosis compared with FNA biopsy. In the case of invasive carcinoma, a core needle biopsy more often allows for ancillary testing, such as, estrogen receptor (ER), progesterone receptor (PGR commonly known as PR) and human epidermal growth factor receptor 2/erb-b2 receptor tyrosine kinase 2 (ERBB2 commonly known as HER2). While FNA was a component of the original "triple approach" (physical examination, mammography, and FNA) for initial

M.O. Idowu, MD, MPH (✉) • J.A. Singh, MD • M.M. Grimes, MD, MEd
Department of Pathology, Virginia Commonwealth University Health (VCU HEALTH), Richmond, VA, USA
e-mail: michael.idowu@vcuhealth.org; margaret.grimes@vcuhealth.org; jaime.singh@vcuhealth.org

M.O. Idowu et al. (eds.), *Diagnosis and Management of Breast Tumors*,
DOI 10.1007/978-3-319-57726-5_2

diagnosis of breast masses, it is currently less commonly used for this purpose in the United States [1–3]. However, when core needle or surgical specimens are not available, cytology specimens are acceptable especially in cases of metastasis [4, 5].

From a pathology standpoint, it is critical to ensure that the radiographically targeted lesion can be explained by the histologic findings [6]. Of utmost importance in assessing core needle biopsies of breast lesions is correlation of the mammographic or clinical findings with the pathology. The pathologist should communicate with the radiologist or clinician if there is apparent radiologic–pathologic discordance, and the pathology report should include a comment to that effect. In cases where clinical/radiologic information is not available to the pathologist, the determination of radiologic–pathologic concordance becomes challenging, and such correlation will depend solely on the radiologists or clinicians. Discordant radiologic–pathologic correlation on core needle biopsies should trigger additional evaluation, re-biopsy, or an excision. For example, a spiculated mass on breast imaging (BI-RADS 4 or 5) diagnosed as benign breast tissue with no specific lesion on histopathology (discordant findings) requires additional evaluation, re-biopsy, or excision to ensure that the targeted lesion has been adequately sampled (Fig. 2.1). The negative discordant findings on histology may be due to sampling or technical difficulties with the biopsy. While the importance of radiologic–pathologic

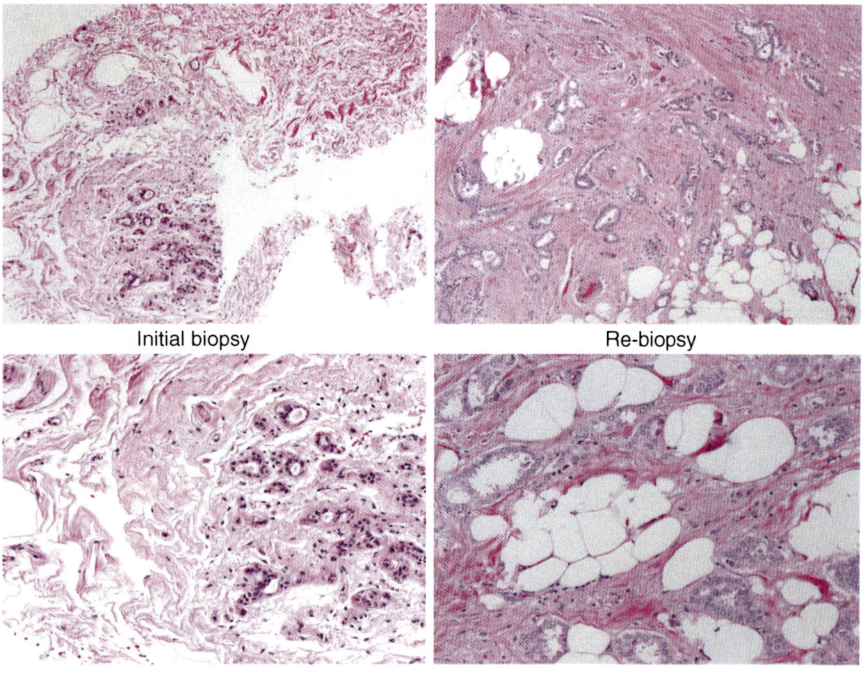

Fig. 2.1 Spiculated mass with only benign breast tissue on initial biopsy (*left images*). Re-biopsy performed because of radiologic–pathologic discordance showed invasive ductal carcinoma (*right images*)

correlation cannot be overemphasized, it must be pointed out that correlation and accuracy are not synonymous.

Widely acceptable pathologic diagnostic criteria should be strictly applied to minimize suboptimal management. Accurate assessment of pathologic changes seen in core biopsies performed for mass lesions or distortions requires not only knowledge of pathologic criteria required for diagnosis, but also of the potential pitfalls related to sampling. False-positive and false-negative histologic diagnoses could lead to suboptimal management. Equivocal diagnoses, although occasionally unavoidable, should be minimized [7]. For example, a large, centrally located papilloma will be sampled only partially by a core needle biopsy; absence of atypical ductal hyperplasia (ADH) or ductal carcinoma in situ (DCIS) involving the papilloma on core needle biopsy cannot exclude these possibilities on surgically excisied specimens. Similarly, it is possible for only DCIS to be present on core needle biopsy, but for invasive carcinoma to be associated with the DCIS on surgical excision. Therefore, optimal management often depends not only on the pathological diagnoses on biopsies but also on clinical and imaging considerations.

The probability of having invasive carcinoma on surgical specimens after a diagnosis of DCIS in core needle biopsies may inform the decision to perform sentinel lymph node sampling. Although controversial, performance of sentinel lymph node(s) samplings following a diagnosis of DCIS on core needle biopsies may eliminate the need for second surgery should invasive carcinoma be identified on surgical excision specimens. Higher probability of invasive carcinoma on surgical excision (with only DCIS on core needle biopsies) may be associated with any one of the following [8]:

1. Extensive calcifications on imaging
2. Palpable mass or solid mass on imaging
3. Lesion larger than 25 mm on imaging
4. High-grade DCIS on histology

Sentinel lymph node mapping is significantly affected following total mastectomy. In view of this, sentinel lymph node sampling is often performed in the setting of total mastectomy, even if the diagnosis on core needle biopsy is DCIS. Currently, sentinel lymph node sampling following DCIS diagnosed on needle core biopsy in the setting of breast conservation surgery is controversial and discouraged, given the potential complications [8, 9].

While there are several breast lesions that may present as masses, distortion, or densities, some of the more common lesions with potential diagnostic challenges and pitfalls will be considered in this chapter.

Fibroepithelial Lesions: Fibroadenoma and Phyllodes Tumor

Fibroepithelial tumors are biphasic tumors characterized by both epithelial (ductal) and mesenchymal (stromal) components and consist predominantly of fibroadenoma and phyllodes tumor. Fibroadenoma is more commonly seen in adolescent or young adult women, but may be seen in older or postmenopausal women as well. The stromal component of fibroadenoma can be highly collagenized, myxoid or cellular, but generally appears homogenous in any given case. In older women, the stroma may be sclerotic and calcified. The stromal component typically compresses the ducts to slit-like "intracanalicular" structures or open and rounded "pericanalicular" structures. There is no evidence that these patterns have biological significance.

Fibroadenomas are generally mobile lesions with smooth, well circumscribed borders on physical examination. However, they may also present as nodular densities or calcified lesions on breast imaging. Fibroadenomas are benign tumors and excision is usually curative. Rarely incomplete excision of a fibroadenoma may be followed by recurrence. Diagnosis of fibroadenoma on core needle biopsy usually is straightforward because of the classic appearance of a biphasic tumor with an intracanalicular or less likely pericanalicular patterns (Fig. 2.2). If the edge of the fibroadenoma is present in the core biopsy, there is a distinct tissue plane (circumscribed) between the lesion and the adjacent normal breast tissue; in the event that the lesional tissue appears to be infiltrating the adjacent breast or adipose tissue, the possibility of phyllodes tumor should be entertained. Fibrocystic changes including papillary apocrine metaplasia, sclerosing adenosis, cystic spaces and epithelial calcifications may be present within the lesion (Fig. 2.3). Sometimes the term "complex fibroadenoma" is applied to fibroadenomas having these changes [10]. The ductal epithelium of a fibroadenoma in the majority of cases is completely benign. However there are exceptions, and the pathologist must evaluate the epithelium of a fibroadenoma with the same criteria used in any breast biopsy. Rarely, atypical hyperplasia or ductal or lobular carcinoma in situ may be found within a fibroadenoma (Fig. 2.4); even more rarely, invasive carcinoma may be present.

Stromal cellularity and atypia are evaluated in fibroepithelial lesions. While such assessment is somewhat subjective, it has been suggested that the stroma of adjacent uninvolved breast lobules be used to determine degree of cellularity and atypia in a fibroepithelial lesion to minimize subjectivity (Table 2.1). One of the diagnostic difficulties facing pathologists in evaluation of core needle biopsies in fibroepithelial lesions is interpretations of lesions with apparently increased stromal cellularity. Young women may have fibroadenomas that are more cellular than those found in older women. There is overlap between so-called cellular fibroadenoma and low-grade (histologically benign) phyllodes tumor on core needle biopsy [11–13], and differentiating between these two can be challenging. The major criterion

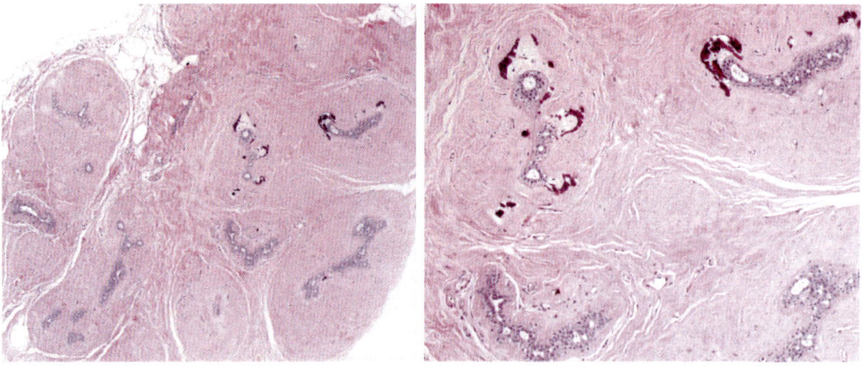

Fig. 2.2 Fibroadenoma. The stroma is sclerotic or collagenized and the ducts are compressed. Calcifications are sometimes associated with fibroadenoma

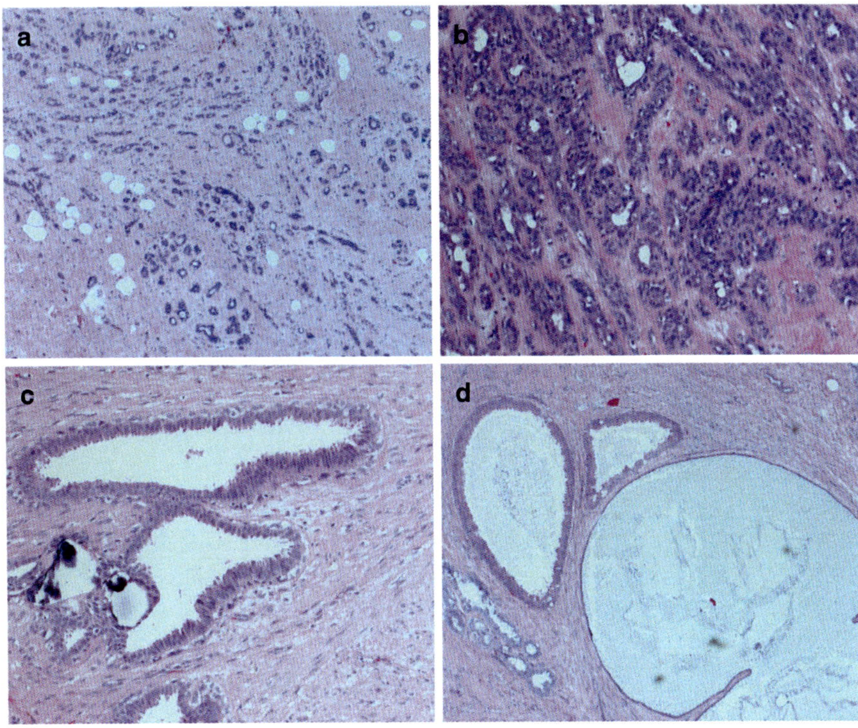

Fig. 2.3 So-called complex fibroadenoma. A fibroadenoma having the following: (**a**, **b**) sclerosing adenosis, (**c**) epithelial calcifications, (**d**) apocrine metaplasia and cyst

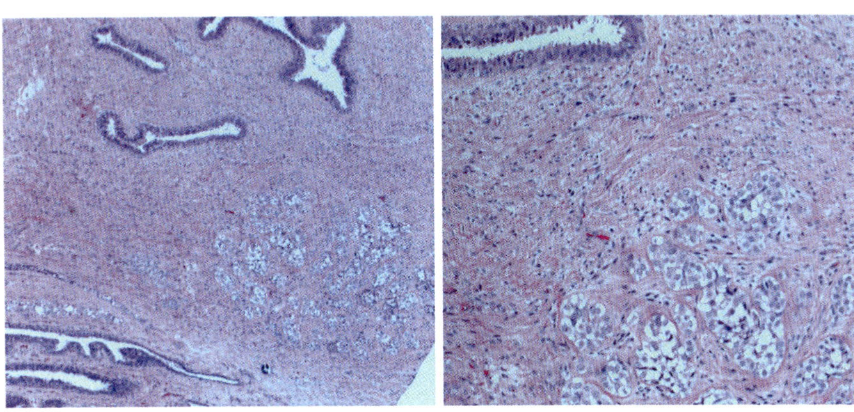

Fig. 2.4 Fibroadenoma with lobular neoplasia

differentiating phyllodes tumor from fibroadenoma is the degree of stromal cellularity and stroma atypia. Table 2.2 highlights some clinical, radiologic, and pathologic features requiring evaluation in fibroepithelial lesions [14–16]. The diagnosis of phyllodes tumor (Fig. 2.5) requires a constellation of features to be present, as no single feature is entirely specific.

Table 2.1 Suggested criteria for evaluating stroma cellularity and atypia in fibroepithelial lesions focusing on the most cellular zones of the tumor compared to normal perilobular stroma if available [14–16]

Grade	Cellularity (compared to normal perilobular stroma)	Atypia
Mild	Slight increase (up to twice that of normal perilobular stroma) of evenly spaced nuclei with no overlap or touching	Nuclei with smooth nuclear contours and little variation in size similar to normal perilobular stroma
Moderate	Intermediate findings with some overlapping nuclei	Some variation in nuclear size with wrinkled nuclear membrane
Marked	Confluent areas of densely overlapping nuclei	Marked variation in nuclear size, coarse chromatin/hyperchromasia, and irregular nuclear membranes with discernible nucleoli at 10× objective and 10× eyepiece (100×)

Table 2.2 Features of fibroadenoma and phyllodes tumor

Clinical, pathology, and imaging features	Fibroadenoma	Phyllodes tumor
Mass	Palpable lesion or mammographic density	Typically palpable
Age	Usually <30 years; may be seen in older women	Typically 40 years or older, premenopausal, uncommon in young adults
Shape	Rounded, circumscribed	Circumscribed or infiltrative
Size	Usually ≤3 cm; pediatric cases may be larger	Variable but typically large (>3 cm)
Growth rate	Slow (over months to years)	Typically rapid (over weeks to months)
Epithelial pattern	Intracanalicular or pericanalicular	Exaggerated intracanalicular pattern is typical
Stromal cellularity	Typically low; stromal cells do not overlap	Moderate to high; stromal cells overlap in higher grades Heterologous differentiation may be present in malignant phyllodes tumors
Stromal mitoses (mitoses are counted at 40× objective and 10× eye-piece; that is, 400× high power field [hpf])	Absent or rare	Benign: ≤4/10 hpf Borderline: 5–9/10 hpf Malignant: 10 or more/10 hpf [5]
Stromal overgrowth (stroma without epithelium in at least one 40× low power field, i.e. 4× objective and 10× eye-piece)	No	No, in benign and borderline; yes, in malignant
Stromal heterogeneity	Usually not	Variable
Tissue fragmentation on core biopsy	No	Typical but not observed in all cases
Tumor margin	Circumscribed	Circumscribed or infiltrative into adjacent fat or breast tissue
Recurrence	Not usual	Benign: 10–15% Borderline: 20–25% Malignant: 25–30% [17]

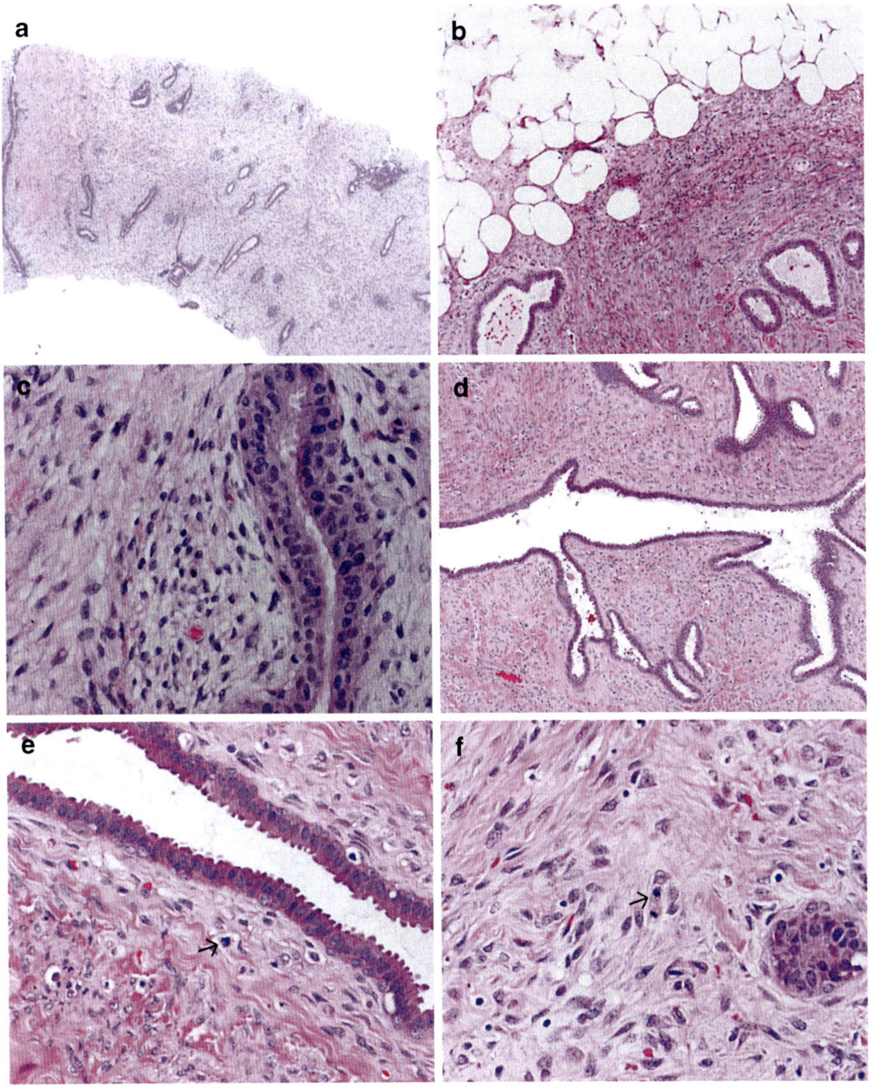

Fig. 2.5 Phyllodes tumor with (**a**) increase stroma cellularity, (**b**) invasion into surrounding adipose tissue, (**c**) periductal cuffing, (**d**) clover leaf appearance/exaggerated intracanalicular pattern, (**e**, **f**) increased mitosis (*arrows*)

In phyllodes tumor, there is increased cellularity with increased stroma cells around ductal epithelium (referred to as periductal condensation/accentuation), but this pattern is not observed in all cases or may not be evident in a core biopsy. Complicating the assessment of stromal cellularity is the variable degree and distribution of cellularity that may exist within a single phyllodes tumor (stromal heterogeneity). The stroma heterogeneity contributes to the difficulty encountered in making a definitive diagnosis or grading of a phyllodes tumor on core needle biopsy [17].

Aside from the degree of cellularity, the presence of increased mitotic activity in the stroma, and stromal cell nuclear atypia, may allow the diagnosis of phyllodes tumor on core needle biopsy. An additional feature that has been noted is the tendency for some phyllodes tumors to fragment on core needle biopsy, a feature related to the exaggerated ductal lumens typically seen in these tumors [11]. While some low-grade (benign) phyllodes tumors can be identified with confidence on core needle biopsy, cases that are equivocal are often called "cellular fibroepithelial lesion (or tumor)," a term intended to convey the uncertainty in excluding phyllodes tumor. High-grade (malignant) phyllodes tumors (Fig. 2.6) have a very high degree of cellularity, marked nuclear atypia, and mitotic activity, and in some cases histologically sarcomatous and heterologous stroma. The diagnosis of high grade phyllodes is usually not challenging on core needle biopsy as long as the epithelial component (in a typical exaggerated intracanalicular pattern) is also present. When the ductal component is not present in the biopsy, the differential diagnosis of high-grade (malignant) phyllodes tumor will include metaplastic carcinoma (mesenchymal type) or the rare stromal sarcoma of the breast, potentially leading to immunohistochemistry work-up. In both metaplastic carcinoma or stromal sarcoma, normal breast ducts may become surrounded or entrapped by the tumor; this should not be mistaken for evidence of a biphasic neoplasm. Metaplastic carcinoma in many cases can be excluded by the absence of diffuse staining with

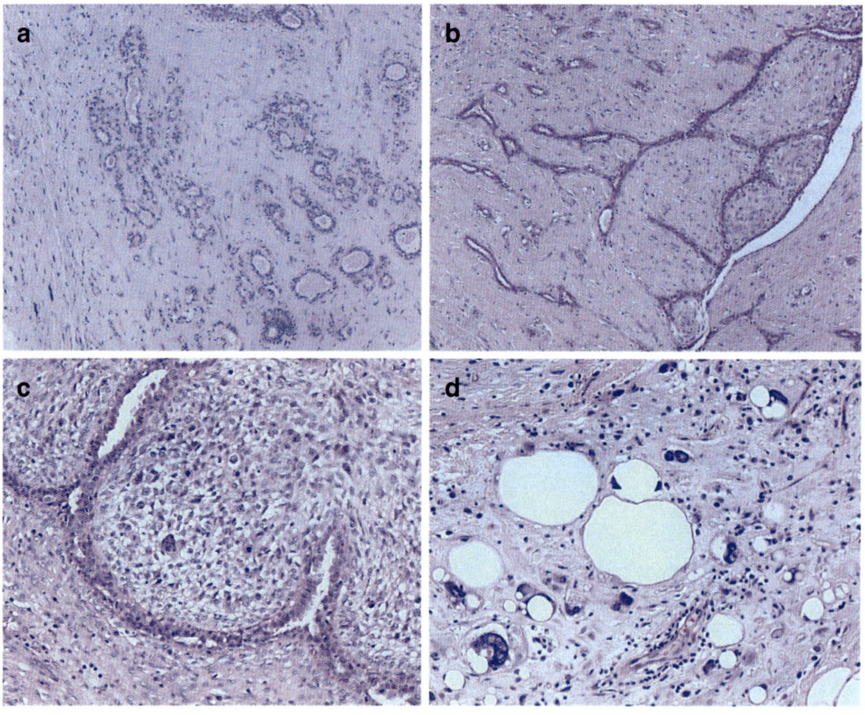

Fig. 2.6 Malignant phyllodes. The same tumor showing stroma heterogeneity. Less cellular (**a**, **b**) and more cellular area with malignant cells having liposarcomatous differentiation (**c**, **d**)

antibodies to cytokeratin; exclusion of stromal sarcoma may require examination of the excised lesion. If a diagnosis of phyllodes tumor is made on core needle biopsy, the lesion should be excised with a margin of normal tissue, since recurrence of incompletely excised phyllodes tumor may occur. Recurrence in low-grade (benign) lesions has been reported in as many as 10–15% compared to 30% or more for malignant cases [15, 17, 18]. Recurrent phyllodes tumors are sometimes higher grade than the original lesion; it is uncertain whether this is due to progression or to heterogeneity in the tumor [15, 19]. Metastases may occur in cases of phyllodes tumors; the majority of these occur in cases of histologically malignant phyllodes tumors, but rarely metastasis of borderline and, even more rarely, of histologically benign phyllodes tumors has been reported [17].

Once diagnosed, a phyllodes tumor is graded (low versus high) or categorized as benign, borderline, or malignant, based on histological parameters. A recent consensus statement outlines the grading scheme: benign phyllodes tumors have minimal nuclear atypia, pushing borders, and four or fewer mitoses per ten high-power fields (hpf); malignant phyllodes tumors have marked stromal cellularity and atypia, infiltrative margins, and ten or more mitoses per ten hpf and usually have areas of *stromal overgrowth* (stroma without epithelium in at least one 40× microscopic field: 4× objective and 10× eye-piece); borderline phyllodes tumors have features intermediate between benign and malignant [5].

In some cases, definitive classification of a fibroepithelial lesion into fibroadenoma or phyllodes tumor may require examination of surgically excised nodule or mass, which would allow assessment of overall architecture, stromal cellularity, nuclear features, and mitotic activity. In addition to stromal hypercellularity, the typical phyllodes tumor has an exaggerated intracanalicular pattern producing "leaf-like" invaginations, a pattern that may not be evident on core needle biopsy.

Fibroepithelial tumors are rare in the male breast because these tumors arise from intralobular stroma; lobules are normally absent or rare in the male breast. Fibroadenomas may however be seen in males taking androgen suppression therapy, estrogen hormonal treatments, or male-to-female transsexual [20–22].

Papillary Neoplasms

Papillary lesions or neoplasms of the breast consist of a spectrum of entities which include, papillary hyperplasia, juvenile papillomatosis, nipple adenoma (florid papillomatosis of the nipple), intraductal papilloma, sclerosing papilloma, "atypical papilloma" (ADH or DCIS involving papilloma), encapsulated papillary carcinoma, solid papillary carcinoma, papillary DCIS, and invasive papillary carcinoma. A comprehensive review [23–26] of these entities is beyond the scope of this text. The approach to interpretation and the pitfalls in the evaluation of selected papillary lesions will be highlighted. Intraductal papillomas (Fig. 2.7a, b) are lesions composed of epithelial proliferations supported by fibrovascular cores (papillary architecture), and confined to a duct; they may be single or multiple. Solitary papillomas usually occur in the large central (subareolar) ducts, while multiple papillomas typically are located in terminal ductal lobular units (TDLU) of the peripheral breast.

Papillomas range in size from microscopic to macroscopic; the larger lesions may be identified on mammography as a density or mass. Papillomas may occasionally be described on ultrasound as a mass that disappears after the first biopsy; this radiologic description may also be associated with apocrine metaplasia. For a partially cystic mass/lesion, it is often prudent to drain the fluid before biopsy of the solid component, if any. Microscopic papillomas almost always are incidental findings in biopsies or excisions performed for other reasons. Occasionally, however, papillomas, even microscopic ones, become sclerosed and calcified and are identified on the basis of mammographic calcifications.

The epithelial component of a papilloma may be nonproliferative or proliferative. The same histologic criteria used to evaluate non-papillary proliferative ductal epithelial lesions are used to assess papillomas. Papillomas may exhibit varying degrees of usual ductal hyperplasia (UDH), atypical ductal hyperplasia (ADH) and ductal

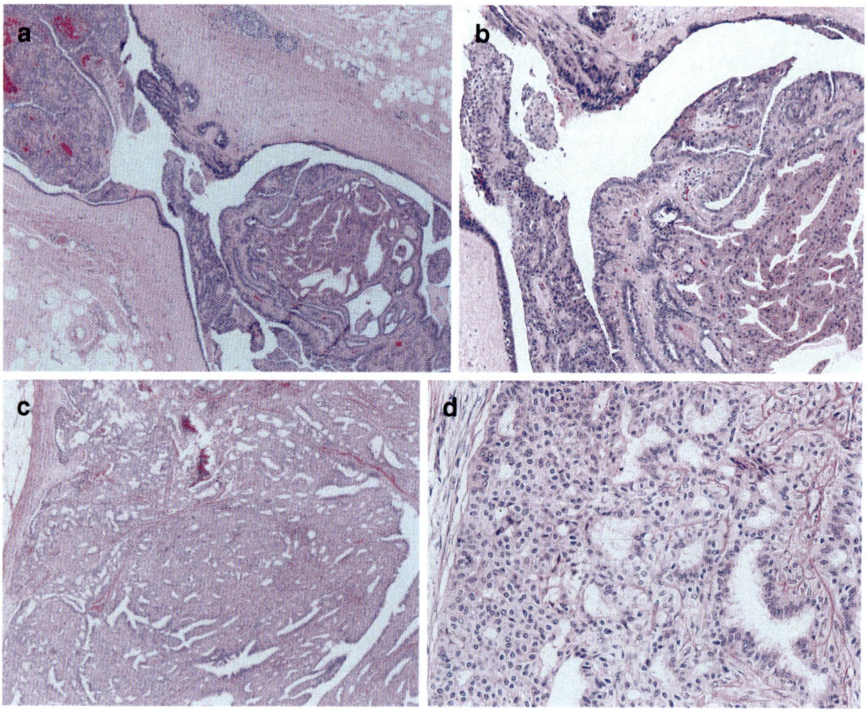

Fig. 2.7 Papillary lesions. (**a**, **b**) Intraductal papilloma. Notice the growth of the tumor in the duct. The duct has broad papillary fronds and apocrine metaplasia. (**c**, **d**) Intraductal papilloma with atypical ductal hyperplasia (aka atypical papilloma). (**e**, **f**) Intraductal papillary carcinoma. Note the monomorphic population of neoplastic cells consisting of one or more layers of hyperchromatic columnar cells surrounding fibrovascular stalk with no myoepithelial cells. (**g**, **h**) Intraductal papillary carcinoma - cribriform architectural pattern. Intraductal papillary carcinoma may also have cribriform, solid, or micropapillary architectural pattern, obscuring the spaces between the fibrovascular or papillary fronds. Myoepithelial cells are absent. Myoepithelial markers may be useful to highlight the absence of myoepithelial cells

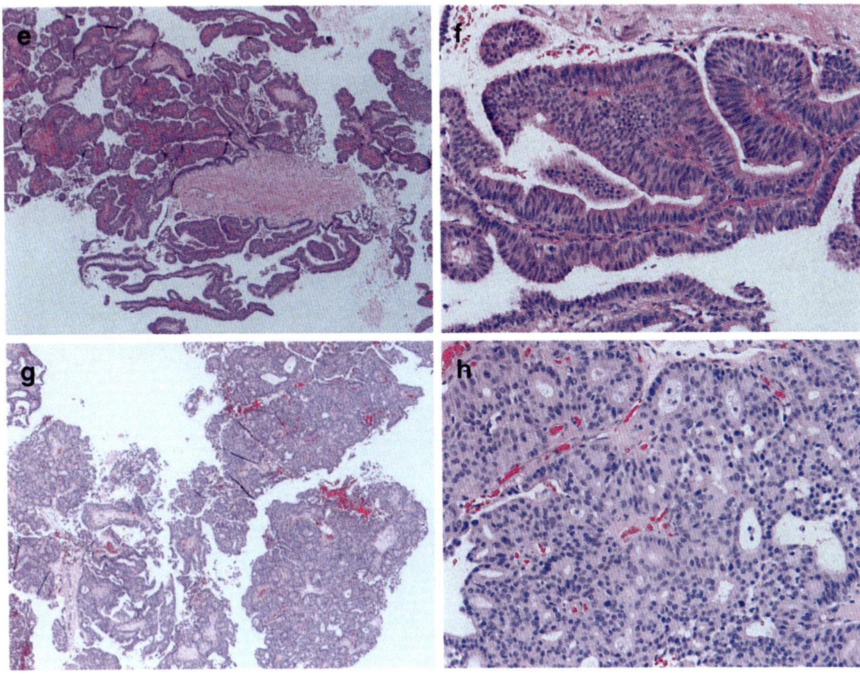

Fig. 2.7 (continued)

carcinoma in situ (DCIS). The term "atypical papilloma" is often used for papillomas in which a portion of the epithelial component is consistent with atypical ductal hyperplasia (ADH) or low-grade DCIS (Fig. 2.7c, d). The 2012 WHO categorization of papillomas recommended the use of the terms "papilloma with atypical ductal hyperplasia (ADH)" and "papilloma with ductal carcinoma in situ (DCIS)" instead of atypical papilloma in the context of low-grade lesions. High-grade DCIS in a papilloma is diagnosed as such regardless of the extent of involvement of the papilloma [27]. According to the WHO, papilloma with ADH and papilloma with DCIS are defined as a papilloma with a monotonous population of low-grade cells with architectural and cytologic features of ADH (<3 mm) or DCIS (3 mm or more), respectively [5, 23, 27]. Note that the size or extent cutoff of 3 mm is different from the cutoff used for de novo (i.e., non-papillary) ADH and DCIS which has a cutoff of 2 mm. It must also be pointed out that the current WHO size criteria for ADH and DCIS in papilloma is slightly different from the original criteria proposed by Page et al., whose criteria were: ≤3 mm for ADH in papilloma and >3 mm for DCIS in papilloma [28]. The use of CK5/6, CK14, and estrogen receptor (ER) may be useful in distinguishing ADH from hyperplasia without atypia (or UDH), with ER having strong homogenous positivity in ADH/DCIS in papilloma and heterogeneous positivity or outright negativity in papilloma without atypia; CK5/6 and CK14 have opposite staining pattern to ER-they are positive in UDH in papilloma but negative or weakly positive in ADH/DCIS in papilloma [5, 23, 27]. The management of non-atypical papillary lesions on core needle biopsy is controversial. Risk assessment of association with carcinoma should probably inform the decision to surgically excise or not. For example, a central papilloma is associated with a twofold increase in the risk of subsequent carcinoma [29, 30], which is similar to the risk of de novo UDH [5, 31, 32]. While atypical papilloma (ADH/DCIS in papilloma) is associated with a risk of associated invasive carcinoma ranging from 5 to 7.5 [28, 30]; this is slightly higher than the risk associated with de novo ADH [5, 31, 32]. It is generally accepted that atypical papillomas and papillary DCIS on core needle biopsies should be surgically excised [25]. However, there are ongoing controversies on the management of central papilloma on core needle biopsy [33–39]. We do not subscribe to "a one-size-fits-all approach" and believe that a prudent approach should involve optimal radiologic–pathologic correlation and clinical presentation. For example microscopic papillomas with no evidence of atypia that are completely encompassed in a core needle biopsy, especially in young patients, probably do not need to be excised [39]. On the other hand, central papilloma may need to be excised to ease patient's symptoms.

Papillomas may undergo sclerosis, with marked alteration of the papillary architecture; epithelial cells that are "pinched off" by the sclerosis may be present in stroma adjacent to the involved duct. Care should be taken not to mistake entrapped epithelium for invasive carcinoma. Clues include the low-power histologic pattern and the cytologic features. Entrapped epithelium usually is directly adjacent to the involved duct within fibroblastic or sclerotic connective tissue. At high magnification, attention to the cytologic features and the presence of myoepithelial cells (identified on H&E or immunohistochemical stain) is helpful in the distinction from invasive carcinoma.

Papillary Carcinomas

Intraductal papillary carcinoma (also known as papillary ductal carcinoma in situ or noninvasive papillary carcinoma) is an in situ carcinoma with no evidence of underlying benign papilloma. It may present as blood-stained nipple discharge, a mass, or mammographic calcifications. The neoplastic cells (usually low to intermediate nuclear grade, rarely high nuclear grade) are arranged as one or more columnar epithelium lining a fibrovascular stalk (Fig. 2.7e, f). Intraductal papillary carcinoma may also have micropapillary, solid, or cribriform architectural patterns (Fig. 2.7g, h). Myoepithelial cells are absent in the papillary fronds within the duct but present in the periphery of the main duct with the papillary growth. Often multiple ducts are involved. Adjacent stroma should be assessed for evidence of invasive carcinoma. *The main differentiating feature of intraductal papillary carcinoma and papilloma with DCIS is that the entire lesion in intraductal papillary carcinoma is comprised of monotonous neoplastic cell population, while in papilloma with DCIS, there is a background of nonneoplastic cells with focal areas of low grade DCIS.*

Encapsulated papillary carcinoma, a variant of papillary carcinoma, usually presents as a circumscribed mass with or without nipple discharge. The "encapsulated" nomenclature is apparently due to a thick fibrous capsule or wall surrounding the mass, which consists of histologic features similar to those of intraductal papillary carcinoma. However, encapsulated papillary carcinoma generally has cribriform or solid architectural patterns. The controversies surrounding encapsulated papillary carcinoma revolve around the fact that it usually lacks myoepithelial cells within and at the periphery of the tumor. This has led to the notion that encapsulated papillary carcinoma may in fact be a low-grade indolent invasive papillary carcinoma. Rarely, metastasis has been reported in encapsulated papillary carcinoma [40, 41]. While this absence of myoepithelial cells raises the possibility of an invasive process histologically, encapsulated papillary carcinoma typically behaves in an indolent fashion and should probably be managed like DCIS [24]. We stage pure encapsulated papillary carcinoma as an in situ carcinoma (Tis), unless there is frank invasion. The size of the invasive component is used for staging, not the size of entire encapsulated papillary carcinoma. DCIS may be present in adjacent breast tissue with potential higher risk of recurrence.

Solid papillary carcinoma usually presents histologically at low power as one or more well-defined *solid* nests of cells. *At higher magnification, the presence of fine fibrovascular cores can be identified among the solid rounded or geographic duct-like structure, which usually are of low or intermediate grade.* Neuroendocrine differentiation and mucinous features may be present. Myoepithelial cells usually are absent within and at the periphery of the lesion. When they are present focally in lesions of low nuclear grade, distinction from intraductal papilloma with epithelial hyperplasia may be difficult. In such cases, immunohistochemical staining may be helpful: solid papillary carcinoma should be negative for high molecular weight cytokeratin and positive for estrogen receptor (ER). Similar to encapsulated papillary carcinoma, these tumors are typically indolent, and are treated as DCIS, unless there is definitive evidence of frank invasion. Although it may be difficult to determine in situ and invasive components, it has been suggested that irregular/jagged areas lacking myoepithelial cells be considered invasive carcinoma; we subscribe to this notion.

Invasive papillary carcinoma, generally, refers to an invasive carcinoma, in which >90% of the tumor is papillary. This is rare and difficult to diagnose because of its resemblance to nests of solid papillary carcinoma. The tumor has an irregular crowded papillary architecture with invasive or infiltrating borders. Metastatic papillary carcinoma from extramammary sites, especially the ovary and lung, should be considered and excluded. The invasive component of solid papillary carcinoma and encapsulated papillary carcinoma is by convention not invasive papillary carcinoma.

Invasive papillary carcinoma also should be distinguished from ***invasive micropapillary carcinoma***, which has an entirely different morphology, namely, small clusters of tumor cells with absent fibrovascular cores and in empty spaces (retraction artifact). *Invasive micropapillary carcinoma has reverse polarity (so-called inside-out pattern), which can be demonstrated by epithelial membrane antigen (EMA) staining on the periphery rather than the lumen.*

Adenomyoepithelioma

Adenomyoepithelioma is a biphasic tumor comprised of myoepithelial cells and ductal/luminal cells. There is usually proliferation of the myoepithelial cells around small ductal epithelium-lined spaces (Fig. 2.8). Adenomyoepithelioma can occur at any age, but more frequently in postmenopausal women. It may rarely be seen in men. It usually presents as a solitary centrally located mass

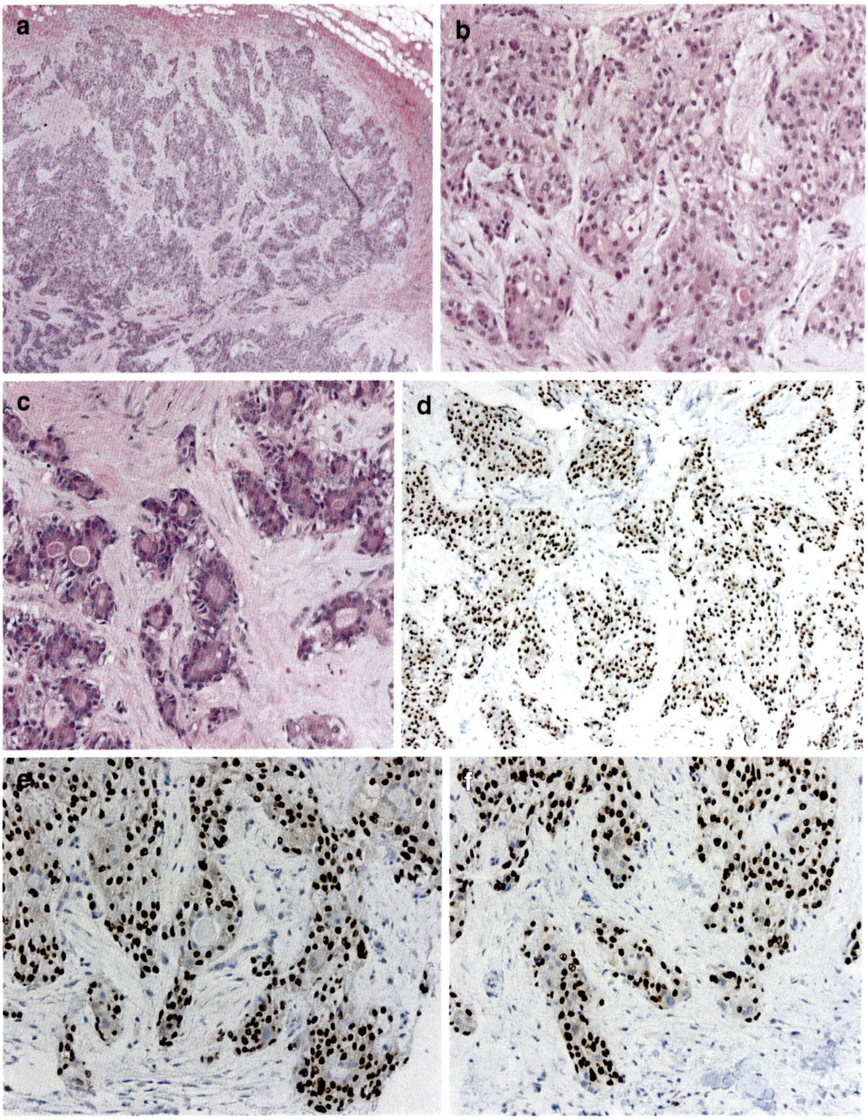

Fig. 2.8 Adenomyoepithelioma. Note the proliferation of the myoepithelial cells around small ductal epithelium lined spaces (**a**–**c**), myoepithelial cells highlighted by p63 (**d**–**f**)

lesion with or without calcifications. It is often considered to be a variant of papillary neoplasms. The myoepithelial component may be spindled, epithelioid, plasmacytoid, or myoid, sometimes with clear cytoplasm, forming nests or sheets of cells. The myoepithelial component which stains with normal myoepithelial markers (p63, calponin, smooth muscle myosin heavy chain, smooth muscle actin, and CD10) may sometimes compress and obscure luminal epithelium. There have been reports of malignant transformation [42–44] and excision is the recommended management [5].

Fat Necrosis

Fat necrosis (Fig. 2.9) is a common incidental finding in the breast, most often evidence of a biopsy that preceded excision of a target lesion. Fat necrosis may present as a palpable lump or mammographic density.

Fat necrosis may also be secondary to blunt trauma, a ruptured cyst or ectatic duct, breast infection, anticoagulation, hyperparathyroidism, and connective tissue disorders (e.g., polyarteritis nodosa, Weber-Christian disease, granulomatous angiopanniculitis). In some cases the etiology is unknown.

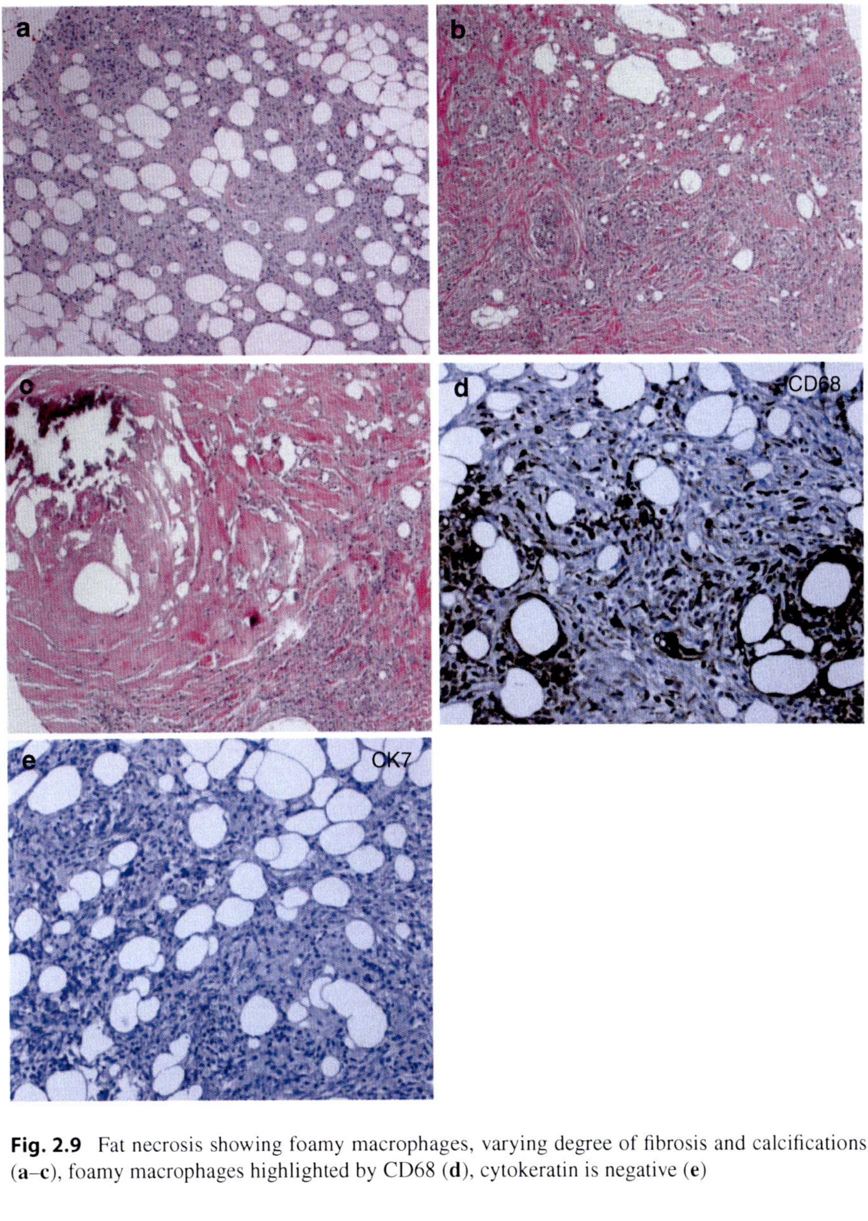

Fig. 2.9 Fat necrosis showing foamy macrophages, varying degree of fibrosis and calcifications (**a–c**), foamy macrophages highlighted by CD68 (**d**), cytokeratin is negative (**e**)

Necrotic adipocytes and lipid-laden histiocytes may elicit fibrosis, making areas of fat necrosis firm to palpation. These lesions are nonencapsulated, and the mammographic and gross appearance may be suspicious for carcinoma. On imaging, fat necrosis may present as spiculated mass, mixed density mass, distortion, or calcifications (some of these calcifications may be linear with linear orientation). Histologically, there are necrotic adipocytes with foamy macrophages infiltration and varying degree of calcifications and fibrosis. The presence of histiocytes infiltrating fat rarely may be mistaken for infiltrating carcinoma on histologic examination, but careful analysis of the cytologic features and the absence of cytokeratin staining for epithelial cells and positive CD68 staining for histiocytes by immunohistochemistry should help in making the diagnosis.

Radial Scar

Radial scars (Fig. 2.10) may be small incidental findings or larger lesions that are detected mammographically. Larger lesions are sometimes termed "complex sclerosing lesion." Radial scars are nonencapsulated proliferations of ductal structures in and around a central zone of fibrosis/sclerosis and elastosis. Typically the centrally located ductal structures are small and compressed, while the outermost ducts are dilated and hyperplastic, lending a "radial" appearance on histologic examination at low magnification. A radial configuration may not be evident in the larger complex sclerosing lesions. Within the central sclerotic zone, the entrapped ducts may mimic invasive carcinoma. Careful attention to the presence of an outer layer of myoepithelial cells around these structures assists in differentiating them from carcinoma. However, radial scars may be associated with carcinoma, either in situ or invasive. The hyperplastic ducts in the peripheral zones should be examined for evidence of architectural and cytologic atypia. Invasive carcinoma may be present in the outer zones or periphery of the lesion. Conversely, some cases of invasive carcinoma may mimic a pattern of radial scar. For these reasons, the finding of radial scar on core needle biopsy often triggers surgical excision to exclude the presence of carcinoma.

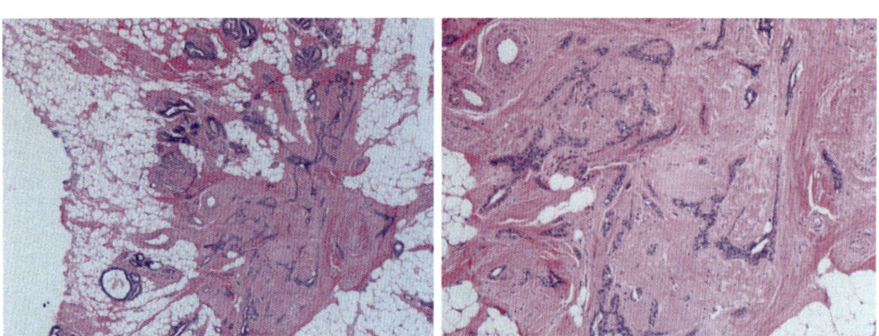

Fig. 2.10 Radial scar. Note the central elastotic stroma with compressed ducts in the center and more dilated ducts at the periphery. It is important to ensure that the compressed duct has myoepithelial cells

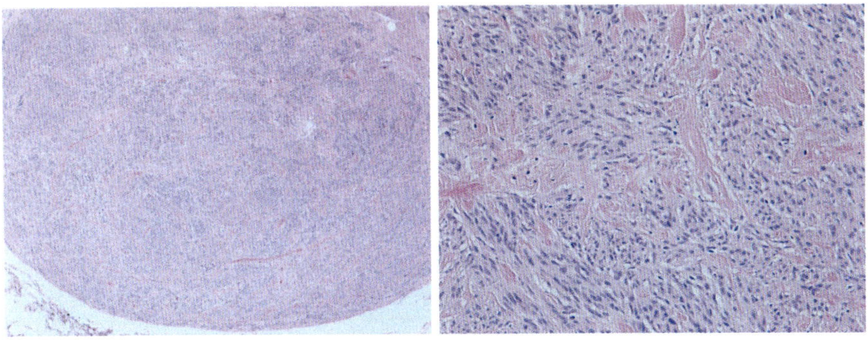

Fig. 2.11 Myofibroblastoma. Note the bland spindle cells arranged in short, haphazard fascicles or nests separated by eosinophilic keloid-like fibers

Hamartoma

Hamartoma of the breast is a mass lesion, usually circumscribed or encapsulated, composed of benign breast ducts and lobules, connective tissue stroma, and adipose tissue, without an organized architecture [45]. A palpable hamartoma may be mistaken clinically for fibroadenoma. Fibrocystic changes may be present in the hamartoma and, rarely, carcinoma may be present. Because of the histologic resemblance of hamartoma to normal breast tissue, diagnosis on core needle biopsy may be difficult and requires close correlation with the mammographic findings and the targeted lesion. Recurrence after excision is rare.

Myofibroblastoma

Myofibroblastic proliferations in the breast range from incidental foci of pseudoangiomatous hyperplasia (PASH) to mass lesions known as myofibroblastoma (Fig. 2.11). Myofibroblastomas may be seen at any age, but are more commonly seen in postmenopausal women. Classically myofibroblastomas are circumscribed but nonencapsulated tumors with pushing borders. Myofibroblastoma consists of bland spindle cells arranged in short, haphazard fascicles or nests separated by eosinophilic keloid-like fibers. However, several histologic variants have been described, including epithelioid variant which may mimic invasive lobular carcinoma [46, 47]. Familiarity with these variants will minimize misdiagnosis as invasive carcinoma. The myofibroblasts are identified by positive immunohistochemical staining for desmin, CD34, and vimentin; smooth muscle actin, BCL2, CD99, CD10, ER, and PR are variably positive. Cytokeratins, EMA, S100, HMB45, and CD117 (ckit) are consistently negative.

Invasive Breast Carcinomas

Invasive breast carcinomas are the most common carcinomas in women accounting for almost a quarter of all breast cancers in women. Invasive breast carcinomas (Fig. 2.12) denote primary malignant epithelial neoplasm in the breast with

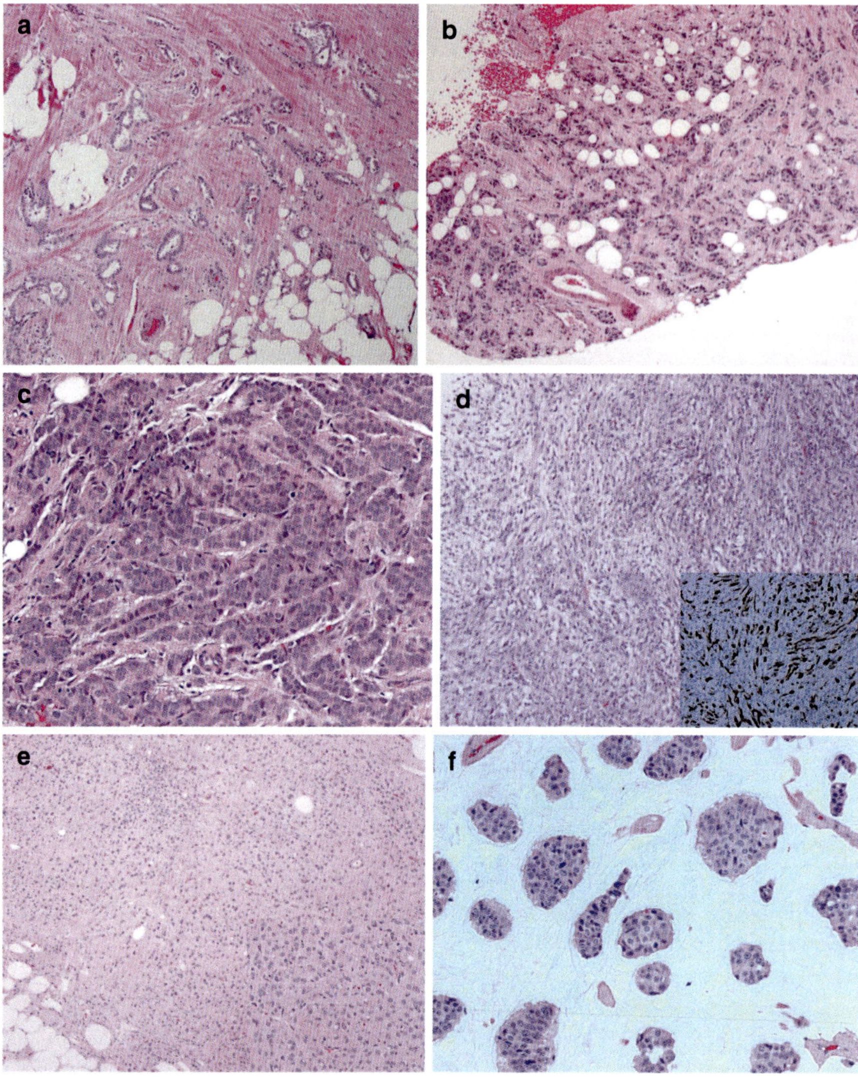

Fig. 2.12 Invasive carcinomas. (**a–c**) Invasive carcinoma NOS (invasive ductal carcinoma), (**d**) metaplastic carcinoma (inset shows cytokeratin positivity in spindle cells), (**e**) invasive lobular carcinoma (inset shows higher power), and (**f**) mucinous carcinoma

stromal invasion. Vascular invasion, useful when present, is not required for a diagnosis of invasive carcinoma. Morphologically, invasive carcinoma may have apparent glandular differentiation, single-cell infiltration, targetoid features, or other morphologic types. Invasive carcinomas are heterogeneous and consist of different histologic types. The most common type (40–75% of mammary carcinomas) used to be called *invasive/infiltrating "ductal" carcinoma* because it was originally thought to arise from the ductal rather than the terminal ductal lobular unit (TDLU) which was thought to be the origin of invasive lobular carcinoma.

TDLU is now known as the entity where all breast carcinomas originates, not just invasive lobular carcinoma [48]. In view of this, the WHO recommends a preferred term *invasive carcinoma of no special type* instead of invasive ductal carcinoma [5]. In addition to *invasive carcinoma of no special type*, the other subtypes of invasive breast carcinoma include, but are not limited to the following: invasive lobular carcinoma, tubular carcinoma, cribriform carcinoma, carcinoma with medullary features, metaplastic carcinoma, invasive papillary carcinoma, invasive micropapillary carcinoma, adenoid cystic carcinoma, secretory carcinoma, and others.

Of note, it is important to exclude *metaplastic carcinoma* when a spindle cell neoplasm is encountered in the breast whether atypical or fibromatosis-like spindle cells. Non-spindle cell histomorphology may also be seen in metaplastic carcinoma including low-grade adenosquamous and squamous cell carcinoma. Metaplastic carcinoma may occasionally have mesenchymal differentiation (osseous, chondroid, rhabdomyoid, and even neuroglial) mixed with the carcinoma component [5].

There are well-known criteria to help differentiate the different subtypes. Table 2.3 highlights some features of invasive carcinomas. However, comprehensive discussion of the different histologic criteria of the different subtypes of invasive breast carcinomas is beyond the scope of this text.

Table 2.3 Histologic features of common invasive breast carcinomas

Type of invasive carcinoma	Epidemiology	Histologic features
Invasive carcinoma of no special type (aka invasive ductal carcinoma, invasive carcinoma not otherwise specified, or infiltrating ductal carcinoma)	Most common invasive breast carcinoma (40–75%)	Diagnosed when other types of breast carcinoma have been excluded. There is stromal invasion and a variety of architectural patterns ranging from solid, glandular, to single-cell infiltrates with variable cytoplasm. It may be mixed with other types of invasive carcinoma
Invasive lobular carcinoma	5–15% of invasive breast cancer	Classic variant consists of proliferation of non-cohesive small neoplastic cells with invasion into the stroma in single file or in a concentric pattern around normal ducts. There is generally no desmoplastic stromal reaction. There is often associated intracytoplasmic lumen. Other histologic variants include solid, alveolar, pleomorphic, and tubulolobular variant. Generally negative for E-cadherin *Invasive lobular carcinoma more frequently metastasizes to the gastrointestinal tract, uterus, ovary, meninges, and bone*, compared to invasive carcinoma of no special type, which frequently metastasizes to the lung
Tubular carcinoma	~2%	Characteristically consists of tubules with oval/rounded and angulated shape haphazardly arranged (>90% of the tumor). The nuclei are generally low grade (high nuclear grade would argue against tubular carcinoma). Apical snouts may be present, but are not required for diagnosis

(continued)

Table 2.3 (continued)

Type of invasive carcinoma	Epidemiology	Histologic features
Mucinous carcinoma (aka colloid carcinoma)	~2%	Characterized by nests of tumor cells floating in mucin in >90% of the tumor for pure mucinous carcinoma. It may however be mixed with other carcinoma especially invasive carcinoma of no special type, in which case "mucinous features" is commonly used
Carcinoma with medullary features (aka medullary carcinoma, atypical medullary carcinoma, invasive carcinoma with medullary features)	<1%	The tumor shows some or all of the following criteria: syncytial architecture (>75% of tumor mass), pushing margins, no tubular differentiation, pleomorphic tumor cells with vesicular nuclei, and at least one nucleolus, prominent and diffuse lymphoplasmacytic stroma. Most are triple negative. Relatively good outcome, possibly due to prominent lymphoplasmacytic infiltrate
Metaplastic carcinoma	0.2–0.5%	Heterogeneous morphology, namely, *adenosquamous* (tubuloglandular architecture admixed with squamous cells), *fibromatosis-like* (bland spindle cells arranged in fascicles infiltrating breast parenchyma, reminiscent of fibromatosis, positive for cytokeratins) *Squamous cell carcinoma* (like squamous cell carcinoma in other parts of the body) *Spindle cell carcinoma* (atypical spindle cells arranged in variable architectural patterns [which are positive for high molecular weight cytokeratins] often admixed with inflammatory cells) *Metaplastic carcinoma with mesenchymal differentiation* (metaplastic carcinoma having osseous, chondroid, rhabdomyoid, etc. components which may appear bland or overtly malignant) *Mixed metaplastic carcinoma* (mixture of the different metaplastic carcinoma morphology) The rule of thumb is that metaplastic carcinoma must be excluded in any spindle cell lesion in the breast. Often triple negative

Surgical Excision of Mass Lesion/Density/Distortion

It is important for the pathologist to describe carefully and in detail the gross measurements of the specimen and the location of the imaged target lesion. Information on the presence or absence of biopsy clips is important. Attention should be paid to the margins of the specimen; it is common to use ink to identify the surgical margin on histologic sections. The use of different colors of ink to correspond to different margins may be helpful. To minimize the possibility of ink tracking in the fatty crevices, thereby complicating margin evaluation, attention to the following steps is important: ensure that the specimen is dry by patting with paper towels; gently and carefully apply the ink(s) on the specimen's margin(s); gently pat the specimen to remove excessive ink; allow the specimen to dry for about 30 s; and apply 5% acetic acid (vinegar) as mordant [49]; some use Bouin solution as mordant. The pathologist or other qualified personnel should then serially section the tissue and record the presence of any gross lesions, including the size and distance from the surgical margins.

In some cases, the gross measurements are different from measurements made on histologic examination of the tissue sections. Nonneoplastic changes such as fibrosis- or biopsy-related changes may not be distinguishable from invasive carcinoma at the macroscopic level. Conversely, microscopic areas of invasive carcinoma may extend beyond the limits of the lesion identified grossly. In both circumstances, the histologic measurement supersedes the gross impression and is the basis for pathologic tumor staging (pT). Similarly, the grossly measured distance of lesion from margins must be compared with the histologic findings, and the latter should take precedence.

It may be difficult to accurately assess margins in breast excision specimens due to the following [50]:

1. Artifactual narrowing after extirpation due to lack of supporting tissue normally present in vivo.
2. The artifactual narrowing is further compounded by radiologic manipulation of surgical specimens. Specimens excised with wire localization usually are imaged prior to receipt in the pathology laboratory, and the compression of the specimen may distort the tissue planes and the suture-designated margins.
3. Ink that is used in the pathology laboratory to mark the margins, if not properly fixed to the tissue and dried prior to sectioning the specimen, often tracks into the deeper portion of tissue making assessment of the true inked margin difficult on histology.
4. Generally, only a portion of the whole specimen or margin is examined histologically.
5. Inadequate pathologic sampling of the closest margin.
6. Perpendicular versus en face margin evaluation may have different margin status.

Uncommonly, inadequate markings by the surgeon may make accurate orientation of margins impossible; in such cases assistance of the surgeon(s) to orient the specimen should be sought.

Further complicating the issue is the question of what constitutes a "clear" margin for in situ and invasive carcinomas [51–53]. Perpendicular versus "en face" (pathology radial shaved margin) evaluation of margin introduces variability in margin assessment. It has been reported that pathologic en face margins may overestimate positive margins [50, 54] as positive en face margin may still have a clearance of up to 2 mm to inked margin depending on the thickness of the sections. Perpendicular inked margin is more commonly used in the pathologic evaluation of margins for breast-conserving surgery specimen. Recent consensus guidelines for invasive carcinoma and DCIS in patients undergoing breast-conserving surgery with whole-breast irradiation indicated that "ink on tumor" is considered a positive margin [50, 55] and that clinical judgment should be used in determining whether a negative margin of less than 1.0 mm requires re-excision; re-excision should not be routinely performed for "no ink on tumor." Factors to consider on whether to re-excise or not include residual calcifications on post-excision mammography and extent of DCIS in proximity to the margin [55]. In view of these, our practice is to take sections of margins perpendicular to the edge of the lesion, and we report both the distance of tumor from excision margins and the extent of disease closest to the margin(s), when less than 1.0 mm to the margin(s).

Lymph Nodes

Excision of biopsy-proven invasive carcinoma is usually accompanied by sentinel lymph nodes. In some cases, excision of pure DCIS diagnosed on core needle biopsy may be accompanied by sentinel lymph node biopsy, especially in the setting of total mastectomy. There are controversies on the performance of sentinel lymph node biopsy for pure DCIS on needle core biopsy, in the setting of breast-conserving surgery as indicated earlier in this chapter [8, 9].

Sentinel and non-sentinel lymph node(s) should be sectioned at 2 mm intervals and entirely submitted, unless there is gross evidence of metastatic carcinoma in the node, in which case a single representative section is appropriate. Since metastatic tumor deposits can vary in size and macrometastasis is metastasis greater than 2.0 mm, cutting the node at 2 mm intervals theoretically should allow identification of small foci that might escape detection with only partial submission of the node or thicker sectioning of the node. There are controversies regarding the number of histologic hematoxylin and eosin (H&E)-stained sections and whether nodes that are negative on H&E should be further examined with immunohistochemical staining for cytokeratin. Since isolated tumor cells in a lymph node do not impact nodal status for pathologic staging, the benefit of this additional testing appears to be of little value; therefore, it has been suggested that routine cytokeratin immunohistochemistry should be discouraged [56]. We subscribe to this practice, if the sentinel lymph nodes are sectioned at 2.0 mm intervals. However, this cannot always be assumed. Furthermore, invasive lobular carcinoma may sometimes be particularly difficult to identify in the lymph nodes. In these particular instances, we believe that the use of cytokeratin immunohistochemistry in the evaluation of sentinel lymph nodes is not unreasonable. Size of nodal metastasis have implications on whether axillary dissection is performed or not. Contiguous tumor deposit less than 0.2 mm or less than 200 tumor cells in a lymph node is referred to as isolated tumor cells (ITC); contiguous tumor deposit between 0.2 mm and 2.0 mm is referred to as micrometastasis; while contiguous tumor deposit with at least one nodal metastasis greater than 2.0 mm is referred to as macrometastasis. Nodes with ITC are not counted as positive nodes, even if there is another lymph node with macrometastasis. Axillary dissection is generally performed for macrometastasis.

Prognostic and Predictive Markers in Invasive Carcinoma

Estrogen and Progesterone Receptors

Testing for estrogen receptor (ER) and progesterone receptor (PR) status and for HER2 (ERBB2) overexpression or amplification is standard in the pathologic assessment of invasive breast carcinoma. These tests are generally performed on formalin-fixed, paraffin-embedded tissue sections of biopsies or of excision specimens. Patients with invasive carcinomas that express ER and/or PR are candidates for antihormonal therapies. ER and PR are assessed by immunohistochemical staining. The proportion of positive tumor cells and the intensity of staining typically are reported. Assessment of positive staining may be performed manually (semiquantitative assessment) or quantified via image analysis. Certain caveats pertain to hormone receptor testing. The College of

American Pathologists (CAP) in collaboration with other professional societies, has determined that the minimum length of formalin fixation time for tissues stained for ER and PR (and for HER2) is 6 h. Additionally, cold ischemic time (length of time between removal of the tissue from the patient and placement in formalin) should be 1 h or less. Prolonged cold ischemic time or inadequate formalin fixation may produce false results. Fixation for more than 72 h may also interfere with the staining reaction. Cases falling outside these guidelines and in which negative results are obtained should prompt repeat testing on a subsequent specimen (repeat biopsy or excision specimen). The recommended scoring guidelines should be strictly followed [57–59].

Proliferative Index

It is increasingly of clinical interest to determine the proliferation rate of the malignant cells in invasive carcinomas. This typically is performed by immunohistochemical staining for a proliferation antigen such as Ki-67. The percentage of positive malignant cells can be assessed either manually (semiquantitative estimation of percent positive cells) or with automated quantitative measurement. High and low proliferation rates portend, respectively, a more or less aggressive potential behavior of a carcinoma and may factor into clinical decision-making. Specific guidelines for assigning low, intermediate, or high proliferation ranges have not yet been determined.

HER2

HER2 (ERBB2, human epidermal growth factor receptor) is a tyrosine kinase protein that is encoded by the *HER2 (ERBB2)* gene. The overexpression of the protein, and/or the amplification of the gene, in invasive breast carcinoma, is associated with poor prognosis but also identifies patients who are candidates for HER2 targeted therapy. HER2-positive invasive carcinomas (which comprise approximately 15–20% of all invasive breast carcinomas) tend to respond well, to anti-HER2-targeted therapies, providing considerable survival benefit. The effectiveness of this treatment makes identification of such cases of paramount importance. HER2 protein overexpression is determined by immunohistochemical staining; *positive HER2 status is based on more than 10% of tumor cells staining with intense, complete membranous staining. Less complete staining, weak staining, or intense staining of less than 10% of cells is considered equivocal.* Amplification of the *HER2* gene typically is determined by in situ hybridization, either fluorescent (FISH) or chromogenic (CISH). *In testing that uses a control probe, amplification is based on a HER2 to control signal ratio of >2 or a HER2 copy number of 6 or greater (even if the ratio is less than 2). Cases with a ratio less than 2 and an average HER2 copy number of at least 4 but less than 6 are considered equivocal.* Because of the clinical importance of identifying HER2-positive cases, equivocal results in either testing modality (immunohistochemistry or ISH) should trigger reflex or repeat testing, either by the alternate modality (ISH or immunohistochemistry) or using a different or subsequent tissue sample because of tumor heterogeneity [57]. *It is critical, however, to use the most current HER2 scoring guidelines because these guidelines undergo periodic review and update.* If a tumor

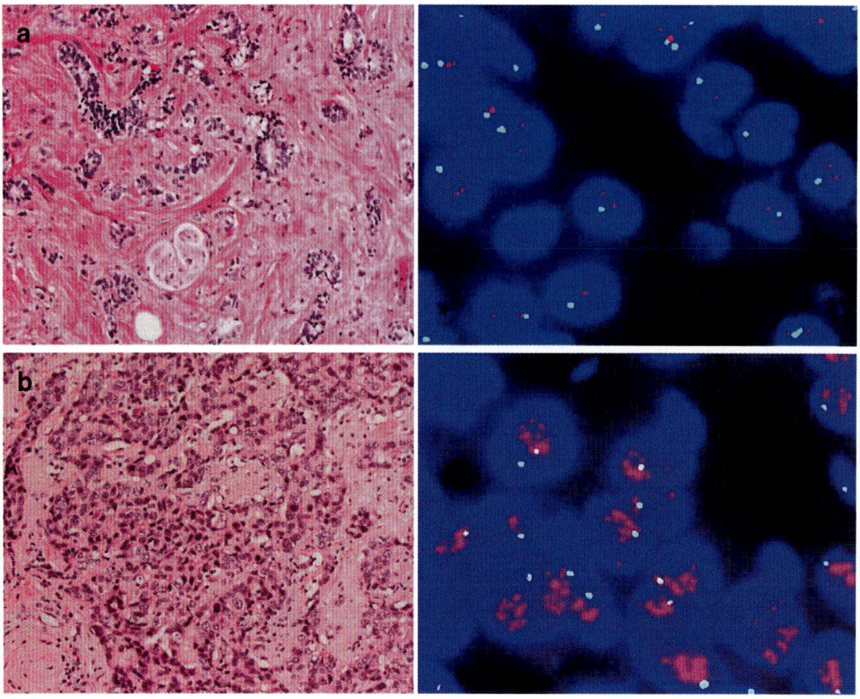

Fig. 2.13 Two masses in the same breast. (**a**) H&E of mass 1 invasive carcinoma NOS, low nuclear grade, and corresponding non-amplified HER2 FISH. (**b**) Mass 2 H&E of invasive carcinoma NOS, high nuclear grade, and corresponding amplified HER2 FISH, same patient as in Fig. 2.13a

has morphologically different areas, it may be prudent to perform HER2 on the different tumors in view of tumor heterogeneity, because one morphologic type may be negative, while the other may be positive (Fig. 2.13a, b).

Reporting

Use of a synoptic reporting template in cases of surgically excised breast carcinomas and DCIS is a requirement for laboratory accreditation by the College of American Pathologists (CAP). The CAP has deemed status with the Centers for Medicare and Medicaid Service (CMS), so that accreditation by the CAP qualifies a laboratory for payment for pathology services through Medicare and Medicaid. In the case of invasive carcinomas, the elements of the template include the specimen site, type of procedure, histologic type of carcinoma, histologic scoring and grading, size of the carcinoma, margin status, lymph node status, and hormone receptor and HER2 status, followed by the pathologic TNM staging. Synoptic reporting ensures the reporting of elements that are important for clinical management. The use of synoptic report also ensures that the required elements in the quality category of the merit-based incentive payment system (MIPS), previously known as physician quality reporting system (PQRS), are always included in breast cancer reports.

Breast Calcifications

Breast calcifications are not created equal. Some radiologic calcifications are more commonly associated with benign processes than others. The evaluation of breast calcifications in radiology and pathology is distinctly different but converges with the overarching goal of detecting precursor lesions (e.g., ductal carcinoma in situ [DCIS]) that are potentially curable. Radiology determines which calcifications require biopsy and further histological evaluation. Pathology on the other hand identify the radiologically targeted calcifications in histology specimens and determine the histologic association of such calcifications.

The initial evaluations of breast calcifications fall on the breast radiologist. At least half of the biopsies performed for non-palpable breast abnormalities are due to mammographically detected calcifications, and about half of these may have ductal carcinoma in situ (DCIS). The evaluations of breast calcifications by radiologists, which have evolved over time, are to identify, characterize (morphology and distribution patterns, location), and determine which calcifications or groups of calcifications may be associated with a precursor lesion or cancer and therefore require biopsy. The reporting of such evaluation by the radiologists has now been standardized by the BI-RADS (Breast Imaging Reporting and Data System). *BI-RADS categories generally divide calcifications into typically benign or suspicious morphology*; the BI-RADS categories are discussed further in the radiologic section of this text [60–68].

The pathogenesis of these calcifications is unclear [69]. There are controversies on whether such calcifications are formed by cellular degeneration, an active cell-mediated process or both [68, 69]. It has been suggested that it may be secondary to membrane-bound vesicles (extracellular/intracellular) of degenerating cells, extracellular matrix, apoptotic bodies, or from the mitochondria of dying cells that have lost their ability to regulate intracellular calcium [68, 70]. Regardless of the mechanism or pathogenesis, *from a pathology standpoint, breast calcifications are mostly dystrophic*, forming in an abnormal local environment rather than calcifications secondary to systemic metabolic derangements like hypercalcemia, which is referred to as metastatic calcifications in pathology [70].

It is worth mentioning that "dystrophic calcifications" as described mammographically have different connotation from the dystrophic type calcifications in pathology. Mammographically, dystrophic calcifications are coarse, irregularly shaped calcifications, which are variable in size, shape, and densities because they do not form in preformed spaces; they may be bilateral. Bilaterally significantly increased radiologic dystrophic calcifications may raise the possibility of metabolic disorders like renal disease, autoimmune disorders, chest wall trauma, or burns. From a radiology standpoint, mammographically detected "dystrophic calcifications" are considered "typically benign" in BI-RADS lexicon and are generally not biopsied [62, 71]. Clinically, pathogenesis of calcifications is not important; the significance lies in whether the detected calcifications are associated with lesion(s) that require surgical intervention to prevent or at least minimize the future occurrence of invasive carcinoma.

Breast calcifications detected on histology may be morphologically different (Fig. 2.14a–p). The morphologic differences though interesting are of no clinical significance; pathologists evaluate breast biopsies performed for calcifications to

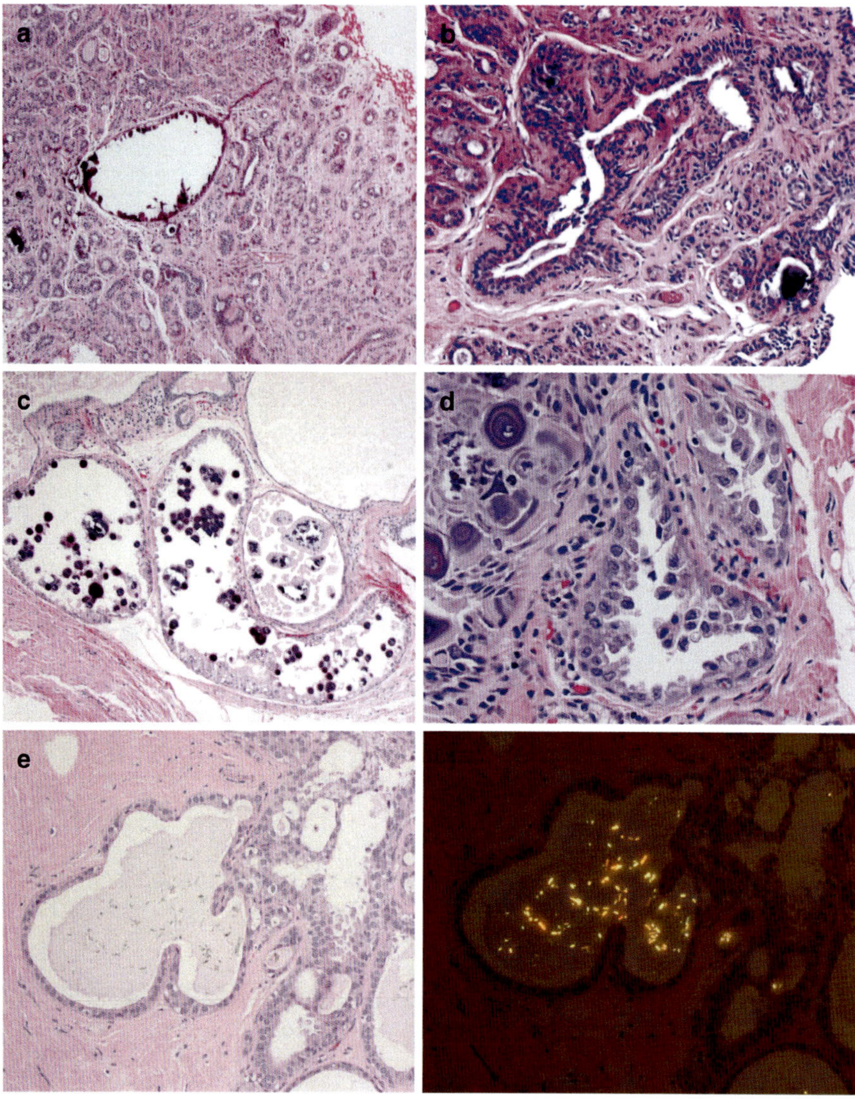

Fig. 2.14 Calcifications and associated lesions. Calcifications associated with benign adenosis (**a**) and intraductal papilloma (**b**). Calcifications (psammomatous calcifications with round and laminated calcifications) associated with cystic hypersecretory hyperplasia (**c**) and cystic hypersecretory carcinoma (**d**). Calcifications (calcium oxalate) associated with apocrine metaplasia (**e**), best seen with polarization (**f**). Calcifications associated with ductal carcinoma in situ (DCIS) with comedonecrosis (**g**, **h**). Calcifications associated with lobular carcinoma in situ (LCIS), though uncommon may be seen. Inset shows negative E-cadherin immunohistochemical stain (**i**, **j**). Calcifications associated with fibroadenoma (**k**, **l**). Stromal calcifications. (**m**, **n**). Calcifications associated with fat necrosis (**o**) and benign ductal epithelium (**p**)

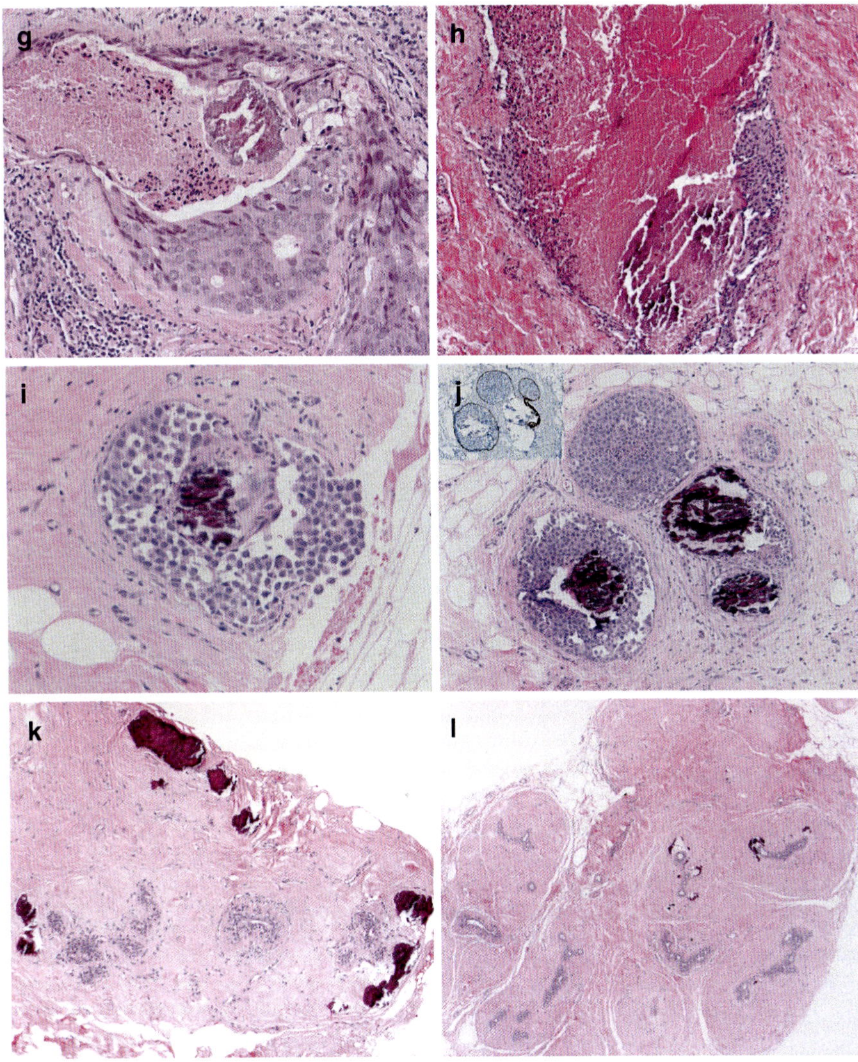

Fig. 2.14 (continued)

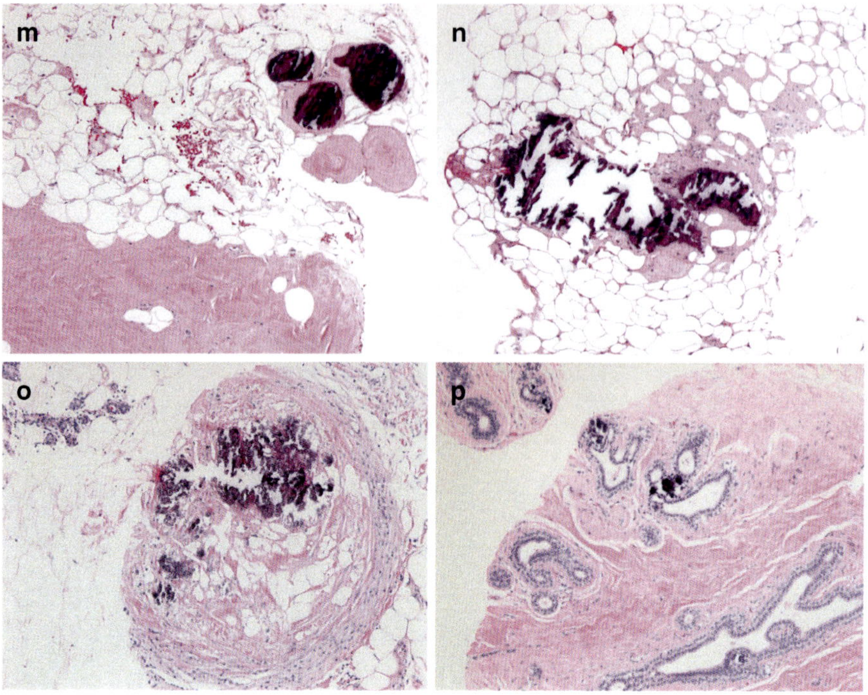

Fig. 2.14 (continued)

determine the presence or absence of calcifications and more importantly its associations—benign or malignant lesions or lesions with higher relative risk of malignancy [72]. It is useful for pathologists to have a basic understanding of radiologic evaluation and description of calcifications to foster meaningful radiologic–pathologic correlation and minimize false-negative diagnosis due to sampling which may lead to delayed diagnosis [73–75]. To facilitate such correlation, it is necessary for pathologists to have appropriate information regarding the distribution or types of calcifications and the specimen/biopsy radiographs [76]. However, in most cases needle core biopsy specimens are often not accompanied by specimen radiographs, and the requisition sheets often simply indicates "calcifications" without describing the type or distribution of such calcifications, essentially leaving the responsibility for such correlation to radiologists. Although the radiologic–pathologic correlation should ideally be performed by the radiologist who obtain the biopsy, it is important for pathologists to attempt such correlation to minimize cases "falling through the cracks."

It cannot always be assumed that radiologic–pathologic correlation is performed by radiologists because of the following: (a) radiologists' workload, (b) *a radiologist different* from the one who performed the initial radiologic interpretation and biopsy may get the pathology report, (c) lack of specific regulatory requirement for such correlation, (d) breast biopsies for calcifications may be performed by surgeons (not radiologists), and (e) breast biopsy pathology reports may end up with the primary care physicians or surgeons, some of whom may rely solely on the pathology report without radiologic–pathologic correlation, especially for negative histology. Given that there may be up to 8% radiologic–pathologic discordance of breast biopsies and almost a quarter of these discordant cases may harbor carcinoma, the need for radiologic–pathologic correlation for optimal patient care cannot be overemphasized [77]. Hence, *pathologists should attempt to determine whether the pathologic findings provide reasonable and acceptable explanation of the breast imaging findings* from an optimal patient care standpoint.

Adequate Evaluation of Breast Calcifications by Pathologists

For biopsies performed for calcifications, there is at least some radiologic suspicion of a premalignant or malignant lesion. Ideally x-rays of the biopsied tissues are performed by breast radiologists to ensure that the biopsies indeed contain the targeted calcifications [76]. It has been suggested that separation of the cores with and without calcifications by radiologists enhances identifications of calcification histologically; others do not find this practice necessary [6, 78, 79]. We have not found such separation particularly useful in our practice.

Pathologic evaluation of breast calcifications can be considered adequate as long as the following questions are appropriately considered and addressed:

(a) *If there are calcifications:*

What is the estimated size of the largest calcifications? Are these the calcifications targeted by the radiologists?

What types of calcifications are there?

What are the calcifications associated with?

(b) *If there are no calcifications:*

Is there a lesion (e.g. DCIS or invasive carcinoma) than can be treated?

Is there a standard institutional approach to search for calcifications?

Are deeper levels obtained? Fixed number of levels or cutting through the block?

Are x-rays obtained? Have steps been taken to ensure exhaustive search for calcifications?

If there are calcifications, the following should be considered:

Size of calcifications: The resolution of mammography matters in determination of calcifications seen on histology. The resolution of full-field digital mammography is 50 to 100 microns [80, 81]. This means that digital mammography (tomosynthesis) can detect calcifications as small as 50 microns or approximately the size of seven red blood cells. It is likely that the resolutions may significantly improve in the future. Currently, histopathologic evaluation of calcifications must be informed by the resolution of mammography to ensure that the calcifications seen on histology are indeed what was targeted. Tiny speck(s) of calcifications the size of one (7–8 microns) or two red blood cells are unlikely to be seen with the current resolution of mammogram and may not be the calcifications targeted on mammography, especially if a precursor lesion is not seen. This knowledge should help determine whether to pursue additional steps to search for more calcifications (e.g., deeper levels, leveling through the block or x-ray of the paraffin tissue block), if no specific lesion is found.

Type of calcifications: Subtyping calcifications seen histologically is usually not necessary in pathology since the importance of such calcifications in the breast is the associated lesions. However, it is generally known that there are two types of breast microcalcifications [67]: type I (composed of calcium oxalate) and type II (composed of calcium phosphate, mainly hydroxyapatite); most breast calcifications are calcium phosphates/hydroxyapatite. Therefore, breast evaluation for calcifications is not complete unless the possibility of calcium oxalate, which is often associated with apocrine lesions, is considered and addressed [68, 82].

Calcification and associated lesions: Indicating the location or associations of calcifications was recommended by the joint task force of the American College of Radiology (ACR), American College of Surgeons (ACS), and College of American Pathologists (CAP) in 1997 [76] and is therefore a good pathology practice. For example, certain lesions are more commonly associated with some calcifications (e.g., high-grade DCIS is often associated with linear or pleomorphic calcifications with linear or segmental orientation) and must therefore be excluded [66]. *However, different lesions may be associated with similar types of radiologic calcifications.* Similarly, different types of calcifications may be associated with the same lesion. For example, fat necrosis may rarely be associated with pleomorphic or linear calcifications; linear calcifications may also be associated with sutures especially in the context of postsurgical evaluation of residual or recurrent disease; and filarial calcifications may be linear and should be considered in patients who are living in, who have visited, or who have emigrated from endemic areas [66, 83]. The identification of radiologically targeted calcifications is critical histologically in order to provide satisfactory explanation for the radiologic findings (correlation/congruence).

The mechanisms of some of the associated lesions are mostly of academic not clinical or management interests. For example, mammary apocrine changes is similar to normal apocrine glands of axillary, areolar, or perineal apocrine cells with similar histochemical or immunohistochemical staining reaction (positive for PASD, cytokeratins 8 and 18, AR [Androgen Receptor], and GCDFP15 [Gross Cystic Disease Fluid Protein 15; also known as BRST2], but negative for ER and PR) and secretion [84, 85]. Apocrine change in the breast is generally regarded as metaplastic as the gradual change from normal cuboidal epithelium to apocrine cells can be seen in breast sections (Fig. 2.15), however, this position is controversial [84]. Apocrine change in the breast is considered a benign lesion.

Table 2.4 highlights common lesions associated with calcifications in the breast.

If there are no calcifications on initial evaluation and no precursor lesion is identified: Additional efforts should be made to identify the radiologically targeted calcifications. The joint task force of the ACR (American College of Radiology), ACS (American College of Surgeons), and CAP (College of American Pathologists) recommended that deeper levels beyond the initial sections should be examined if no calcifications are identified on the initial sections but calcifications are present in the specimen radiograph. The task force also recommended that radiograph of the paraffin blocks may be obtained and the specimen should be examined for calcium oxalate by polarizing [76]. The task force did not indicate the minimum number of levels. Hence, to find a balance between optimal patient management and cost containment,

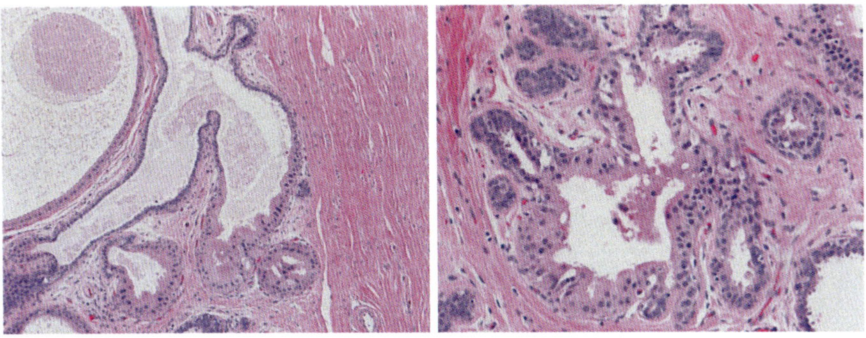

Fig. 2.15 Apocrine metaplasia developing in native duct, supporting a metaplastic rather than de novo lesion

Table 2.4 Summary of diagnostic criteria for common lesions associated with various calcifications [5, 31, 32]

Common breast lesions associated with calcifications	Diagnostic criteria	Mimics
Ductal carcinoma in situ (DCIS), high grade	Proliferation of pleomorphic, poorly polarized cells with irregular contours, coarse, clumped chromatin and prominent nucleoli. Single-cell layer of similar cells is sufficient for a diagnosis of high-grade DCIS. Mitoses and comedonecrosis (though often associated) are not required for diagnosis. No quantitative criteria needed for high-grade DCIS—any high-grade DCIS should be considered DCIS High-grade DCIS is generally surgically excised with or without sentinel lymph node sampling	DCIS involving lobules or sclerosing adenosis may mimic invasive carcinoma. Myoepithelial markers are useful in such cases
Ductal carcinoma in situ (DCIS), low grade	Uniform size or monomorphic, round (i.e., atypical), evenly spaced cell population with distinct cell borders. May be solid, cribriform, papillary, or micropapillary in architecture. If cribriform, the spaces/hole should be almost cookie cutter in appearance (not slit-like or irregular). Risk for development of invasive carcinoma is 8–10 times that of the reference population. Quantitative criteria: at least 2.0 mm or involving at least two ducts/spaces (controversial) Low-grade DCIS is generally surgically excised	Invasive carcinoma (when involving sclerosing adenosis), invasive cribriform carcinoma, LCIS, atypical ductal hyperplasia, usual ductal hyperplasia, collagenous spherulosis

(continued)

Table 2.4 (continued)

Common breast lesions associated with calcifications	Diagnostic criteria	Mimics
Atypical ductal hyperplasia (ADH)	The proliferation in ADH as in low-grade DCIS is monotonous; however, in ADH there may be a second population of cells admixed with the monotonous population or only partially involving the TDLU spaces. Quantitative criteria are useful in distinction of ADH and DCIS. Two common quantitative criteria are involvement of at least two membrane-bound spaces or a size >2.0 mm for low grade DCIS Risk for development of invasive carcinoma is 3–5 times that of the reference population The risk applies to either breast. ADH is generally surgically excised	Collagenous spherulosis usual ductal hyperplasia, low grade DCIS
Flat epithelial atypia (FEA)	While the cells may be cuboidal/columnar, the nuclei (similar to low-grade DCIS or ADH) are round, uniform with inconspicuous nucleoli. The involved acini are variably distended with smooth contours having secretory materials and calcifications. Associated with coexistence of ALH, LCIS, ADH, DCIS, and invasive carcinoma. FEA is not equivalent to ADH or ALH in spite of "atypia" in the name. Radiologic-pathologic correlation to determine whether all targeted calcifications have been removed, in which case close follow-up rather than excision, is recommended	Fibrocystic change, columnar cell change
Columnar cell change and columnar cell hyperplasia	Variably dilated acini lined by columnar cells with oval nuclei with inconspicuous nucleoli. Lesions with one or two cell layers of columnar cell change; those with more than two cell layers are referred to as columnar cell hyperplasia. May be associated with other lesions including ALH and LCIS. Relative risk of 1.5 for subsequent development of cancer No surgical excision necessary for pure columnar cell change/hyperplasia in the absence of concomitant proliferative lesions	FEA
Ductal hyperplasia without atypia (or usual ductal hyperplasia)	Filling and distension of spaces with haphazardly oriented epithelial cells with variability in shape which may occasionally show streaming or syncytial growth in the center of the involved spaces and slit-like unevenly distributed fenestrations at the periphery in contrast to rigid ridges in ADH and DCIS. Risk for developing invasive carcinoma is 1.5–2 times that of reference population. Risk conferred on either breast No surgical excision necessary for ductal hyperplasia without atypia in the absence of concomitant proliferative lesions	ADH

a good starting point should probably be ensuring that there are indeed calcifications in the specimen radiographs. Such radiographs may not be readily available to pathologists, but efforts should be made to at least review the radiology report or have a discussion with the radiologist. Some obtain an *initial 3–5 deeper levels and obtain more levels if the initial levels still show no calcifications; others simply exhaust the block to minimize turnaround time*; while others x-ray the paraffin blocks before deciding whether further evaluation is needed, as the calcifications may have been dislodged and fallen out of the tissue [6]. It is important to point out that exhaustive search for calcifications has been associated with low yield and high cost [86]. Therefore, each institution should determine appropriate protocol with emphasis on adequate and effective communications between pathologists and radiologists.

If there are no calcifications on initial evaluation and a precursor lesion is identified: If no calcifications are identified, but there is a specific diagnosis of a potentially treatable or precursor lesion, the question as to whether to embark on an exhaustive search of calcifications in this case will depend on the type of lesions. For example, if the lesion identified is DCIS or ADH, even in the absence of calcifications, it is probably unnecessary to continue to look for calcifications, since the purpose of the mammographic screening and biopsy has been achieved, namely, identification and management of treatable precursor lesions. Further search for calcifications in this scenario is likely an academic exercise which may not be cost-effective. On the other hand, if the lesion identified is the so-called flat epithelial atypia (FEA) in the absence of calcifications, it may be prudent to search for calcifications by obtaining deeper levels, since it would be useful to determine if there is a worse lesion, namely, ADH or DCIS. In the absence of lesions worse than FEA, the current recommendation is to closely watch the patient rather than excise pure FEA, especially if there are no residual calcifications on breast imaging, given the low positive predictive value of FEA for malignancy [87–90]. Additionally, if the only lesion identified is atypical lobular hyperplasia (ALH) or lobular carcinoma in situ (LCIS), which is not commonly associated with calcifications, it may be prudent to search for additional lesions known to be commonly associated with calcifications.

Finally, in the event that it is determined that the histologic findings do not provide satisfactory explanation of the breast imaging findings, further actions need to be taken for optimal patient care. Such actions include, but are not limited to: re-biopsy, recommendation of excision based on level of radiologic suspicion, or closer follow-up. Having a system in place for routine correlation of radiologic and pathologic findings, and for open communication with other members of the breast health team is critical.

References

1. Steinberg JL, Trudeau ME, Ryder DE, Fishell E, Chapman JA, McCready DR, et al. Combined fine-needle aspiration, physical examination and mammography in the diagnosis of palpable breast masses: their relation to outcome for women with primary breast cancer. Can J Surg. 1996;39(4):302–11.
2. Morris A, Pommier RF, Schmidt WA, Shih RL, Alexander PW, Vetto JT. Accurate evaluation of palpable breast masses by the triple test score. Arch Surg. 1998;133(9):930–4.

3. Kaufman Z, Shpitz B, Shapiro M, Rona R, Lew S, Dinbar A. Triple approach in the diagnosis of dominant breast masses: combined physical examination, mammography, and fine-needle aspiration. J Surg Oncol. 1994;56(4):254–7.
4. Kocjan G, Bourgain C, Fassina A, Hagmar B, Herbert A, Kapila K, et al. The role of breast FNAC in diagnosis and clinical management: a survey of current practice. Cytopathology. 2008;19(5):271–8.
5. WHO classification of tumours of the breast. 4th ed. Lyon: International Agency for Research on Cancer; 2012.
6. Idowu MO, Hardy LB, Souers RJ, Nakhleh RE. Pathologic diagnostic correlation with breast imaging findings: a College of American Pathologists Q-Probes study of 48 institutions. Arch Pathol Lab Med. 2012;136(1):53–60.
7. Idowu MO, Wiles A, Wan W, Wilkinson DS, Powers CN. Equivocal or ambiguous terminologies in pathology: focus of continuous quality improvement? Am J Surg Pathol. 2013;37(11):1722–7.
8. van Roozendaal LM, Goorts B, Klinkert M, Keymeulen KB, De Vries B, Strobbe LJ, et al. Sentinel lymph node biopsy can be omitted in DCIS patients treated with breast conserving therapy. Breast Cancer Res Treat. 2016;156(3):517–25.
9. Coromilas EJ, Wright JD, Huang Y, Feldman S, Neugut AI, Hillyer GC, et al. Axillary evaluation and lymphedema in women with ductal carcinoma in situ. Breast Cancer Res Treat. 2016;158(2):373–84.
10. Dupont WD, Page DL, Parl FF, Vnencak-Jones CL, Plummer WD Jr, Rados MS, et al. Long-term risk of breast cancer in women with fibroadenoma. N Engl J Med. 1994;331(1):10–5.
11. Bandyopadhyay S, Barak S, Hayek K, Thomas S, Saeed H, Beydoun R, et al. Can problematic fibroepithelial lesions be accurately classified on core needle biopsies? Hum Pathol. 2016;47(1):38–44.
12. Tsang AK, Chan SK, Lam CC, Lui PC, Chau HH, Tan PH, et al. Phyllodes tumours of the breast – differentiating features in core needle biopsy. Histopathology. 2011;59(4):600–8.
13. Lawton TJ, Acs G, Argani P, Farshid G, Gilcrease M, Goldstein N, et al. Interobserver variability by pathologists in the distinction between cellular fibroadenomas and phyllodes tumors. Int J Surg Pathol. 2014;22(8):695–8.
14. Jacobs TW, Chen YY, Guinee DG Jr, Holden JA, Cha I, Bauermeister DE, et al. Fibroepithelial lesions with cellular stroma on breast core needle biopsy: are there predictors of outcome on surgical excision? Am J Clin Pathol. 2005;124(3):342–54.
15. Tan BY, Acs G, Apple SK, Badve S, Bleiweiss IJ, Brogi E, et al. Phyllodes tumours of the breast: a consensus review. Histopathology. 2016;68(1):5–21.
16. Jara-Lazaro AR, Akhilesh M, Thike AA, Lui PC, Tse GM, Tan PH. Predictors of phyllodes tumours on core biopsy specimens of fibroepithelial neoplasms. Histopathology. 2010;57(2):220–32.
17. Giri D. Recurrent challenges in the evaluation of fibroepithelial lesions. Arch Pathol Lab Med. 2009;133(5):713–21.
18. Cowan ML, Argani P, Cimino-Mathews A. Benign and low-grade fibroepithelial neoplasms of the breast have low recurrence rate after positive surgical margins. Mod Pathol. 2016;29(3):259–65.
19. Grimes MM. Cystosarcoma phyllodes of the breast: histologic features, flow cytometric analysis, and clinical correlations. Mod Pathol. 1992;5(3):232–9.
20. Kanhai RC, Hage JJ, Bloemena E, van Diest PJ, Karim RB. Mammary fibroadenoma in a male-to-female transsexual. Histopathology. 1999;35(2):183–5.
21. Lemmo G, Garcea N, Corsello S, Tarquini E, Palladino T, Ardito G, et al. Breast fibroadenoma in a male-to-female transsexual patient after hormonal treatment. Eur J Surg Suppl. 2003;588:69–71.
22. Karihtala P, Rissanen T, Tuominen H. Male malignant phyllodes breast tumor after prophylactic breast radiotherapy and bicalutamide treatment: a case report. Anticancer Res. 2016;36(7):3433–6.
23. Agoumi M, Giambattista J, Hayes MM. Practical considerations in breast papillary lesions: a review of the literature. Arch Pathol Lab Med. 2016;140(8):770–90.

24. Wei S. Papillary lesions of the breast: an update. Arch Pathol Lab Med. 2016;140(7):628–43.
25. Collins LC, Schnitt SJ. Papillary lesions of the breast: selected diagnostic and management issues. Histopathology. 2008;52(1):20–9.
26. Ueng SH, Mezzetti T, Tavassoli FA. Papillary neoplasms of the breast: a review. Arch Pathol Lab Med. 2009;133(6):893–907.
27. Tan PH, Schnitt SJ, van de Vijver MJ, Ellis IO, Lakhani SR. Papillary and neuroendocrine breast lesions: the WHO stance. Histopathology. 2015;66(6):761–70.
28. Page DL, Salhany KE, Jensen RA, Dupont WD. Subsequent breast carcinoma risk after biopsy with atypia in a breast papilloma. Cancer. 1996;78(2):258–66.
29. Dupont WD, Page DL. Risk factors for breast cancer in women with proliferative breast disease. N Engl J Med. 1985;312(3):146–51.
30. Lewis JT, Hartmann LC, Vierkant RA, Maloney SD, Shane Pankratz V, Allers TM, et al. An analysis of breast cancer risk in women with single, multiple, and atypical papilloma. Am J Surg Pathol. 2006;30(6):665–72.
31. Page DL, Dupont WD. Benign breast disease: indicators of increased breast cancer risk. Cancer Detect Prev. 1992;16(2):93–7.
32. Jensen RA, Dupont WD, Page DL. Diagnostic criteria and cancer risk of proliferative breast lesions. J Cell Biochem Suppl. 1993;17G:59–64.
33. Laval M, Delangle R, Ndoye A, Sylvestre E, Laviolle B, Lavoue V, et al. The role of percutaneous biopsy and prognostic factors of malignancy in solitary breast papilloma: a retrospective multicenter study of 259 cases. Anticancer Res. 2015;35(12):6881–6.
34. Wyss P, Varga Z, Rossle M, Rageth CJ. Papillary lesions of the breast: outcomes of 156 patients managed without excisional biopsy. Breast J. 2014;20(4):394–401.
35. Yamaguchi R, Tanaka M, Tse GM, Yamaguchi M, Terasaki H, Hirai Y, et al. Management of breast papillary lesions diagnosed in ultrasound-guided vacuum-assisted and core needle biopsies. Histopathology. 2015;66(4):565–76.
36. Shamonki J, Chung A, Huynh KT, Sim MS, Kinnaird M, Giuliano A. Management of papillary lesions of the breast: can larger core needle biopsy samples identify patients who may avoid surgical excision? Ann Surg Oncol. 2013;20(13):4137–44.
37. Fu CY, Chen TW, Hong ZJ, Chan DC, Young CY, Chen CJ, et al. Papillary breast lesions diagnosed by core biopsy require complete excision. Eur J Surg Oncol. 2012;38(11):1029–35.
38. Tseng HS, Chen YL, Chen ST, Wu YC, Kuo SJ, Chen LS, et al. The management of papillary lesion of the breast by core needle biopsy. Eur J Surg Oncol. 2009;35(1):21–4.
39. McGhan LJ, Pockaj BA, Wasif N, Giurescu ME, McCullough AE, Gray RJ. Papillary lesions on core breast biopsy: excisional biopsy for all patients? Am Surg. 2013;79(12):1238–42.
40. Rakha EA, Gandhi N, Climent F, van Deurzen CH, Haider SA, Dunk L, et al. Encapsulated papillary carcinoma of the breast: an invasive tumor with excellent prognosis. Am J Surg Pathol. 2011;35(8):1093–103.
41. Mulligan AM, O'Malley FP. Metastatic potential of encapsulated (intracystic) papillary carcinoma of the breast: a report of 2 cases with axillary lymph node micrometastases. Inter J Surg Pathol. 2007;15(2):143–7.
42. Hayes MM. Adenomyoepithelioma of the breast: a review stressing its propensity for malignant transformation. J Clin Pathol. 2011;64(6):477–84.
43. McLaren BK, Smith J, Schuyler PA, Dupont WD, Page DL. Adenomyoepithelioma: clinical, histologic, and immunohistologic evaluation of a series of related lesions. Am J Surg Pathol. 2005;29(10):1294–9.
44. Yoon JY, Chitale D. Adenomyoepithelioma of the breast: a brief diagnostic review. Arch Pathol Lab Med. 2013;137(5):725–9.
45. Wahner-Roedler DL, Sebo TJ, Gisvold JJ. Hamartomas of the breast: clinical, radiologic, and pathologic manifestations. Breast J. 2001;7(2):101–5.
46. Magro G. Mammary myofibroblastoma: an update with emphasis on the most diagnostically challenging variants. Histol Histopathol. 2016;31(1):1–23.
47. Magro G. Mammary myofibroblastoma: a tumor with a wide morphologic spectrum. Arch Pathol Lab Med. 2008;132(11):1813–20.

48. Wellings SR, Jensen HM, Marcum RG. An atlas of subgross pathology of the human breast with special reference to possible precancerous lesions. J Natl Cancer Inst. 1975;55(2):231–73.
49. Williams AS, Hache KD. Recognition and discrimination of tissue-marking dye color by surgical pathologists: recommendations to avoid errors in margin assessment. Am J Clin Pathol. 2014;142(3):355–61.
50. Moran MS, Schnitt SJ, Giuliano AE, Harris JR, Khan SA, Horton J, et al. Society of Surgical Oncology-American Society for Radiation Oncology consensus guideline on margins for breast-conserving surgery with whole-breast irradiation in stages I and II invasive breast cancer. J Clin Oncol. 2014;32(14):1507–15.
51. Sigal-Zafrani B, Lewis JS, Clough KB, Vincent-Salomon A, Fourquet A, Meunier M, et al. Histological margin assessment for breast ductal carcinoma in situ: precision and implications. Mod Pathol. 2004;17(1):81–8.
52. Silverstein MJ, Lagios MD, Groshen S, Waisman JR, Lewinsky BS, Martino S, et al. The influence of margin width on local control of ductal carcinoma in situ of the breast. N Engl J Med. 1999;340(19):1455–61.
53. Dunne C, Burke JP, Morrow M, Kell MR. Effect of margin status on local recurrence after breast conservation and radiation therapy for ductal carcinoma in situ. J Clin Oncol. 2009;27(10):1615–20.
54. Wright MJ, Park J, Fey JV, Park A, O'Neill A, Tan LK, et al. Perpendicular inked versus tangential shaved margins in breast-conserving surgery: does the method matter? J Am Coll Surg. 2007;204(4):541–9.
55. Morrow M, Van Zee KJ, Solin LJ, Houssami N, Chavez-MacGregor M, Harris JR, et al. Society of Surgical Oncology-American Society for Radiation Oncology-American Society of Clinical Oncology consensus guideline on margins for breast-conserving surgery with whole-breast irradiation in ductal carcinoma in situ. Ann Surg Oncol. 2016;23(12):3801–10.
56. Weaver DL. Pathology evaluation of sentinel lymph nodes in breast cancer: protocol recommendations and rationale. Mod Pathol. 2010;23(Suppl 2):S26–32.
57. Wolff AC, Hammond ME, Hicks DG, Dowsett M, McShane LM, Allison KH, et al. Recommendations for human epidermal growth factor receptor 2 testing in breast cancer: American Society of Clinical Oncology/College of American Pathologists clinical practice guideline update. Arch Pathol Lab Med. 2014;138(2):241–56.
58. Fitzgibbons PL, Murphy DA, Hammond ME, Allred DC, Valenstein PN. Recommendations for validating estrogen and progesterone receptor immunohistochemistry assays. Arch Pathol Lab Med. 2010;134(6):930–5.
59. Hammond ME, Hayes DF, Dowsett M, Allred DC, Hagerty KL, Badve S, et al. American Society of Clinical Oncology/College of American Pathologists guideline recommendations for immunohistochemical testing of estrogen and progesterone receptors in breast cancer (unabridged version). Arch Pathol Lab Med. 2010;134(7):e48–72.
60. Bassett LW. Mammographic analysis of calcifications. Radiol Clin North Am. 1992;30(1):93–105.
61. Monsees BS. Evaluation of breast microcalcifications. Radiol Clin North Am. 1995;33(6):1109–21.
62. Lazarus E, Mainiero MB, Schepps B, Koelliker SL, Livingston LS. BI-RADS lexicon for US and mammography: interobserver variability and positive predictive value. Radiology. 2006;239(2):385–91.
63. Gallagher R, Schafer G, Redick M, Inciradi M, Smith W, Fan F, et al. Microcalcifications of the breast: a mammographic-histologic correlation study using a newly designed path/rad tissue tray. Ann Diagn Pathol. 2012;16(3):196–201.
64. Hofvind S, Iversen BF, Eriksen L, Styr BM, Kjellevold K, Kurz KD. Mammographic morphology and distribution of calcifications in ductal carcinoma in situ diagnosed in organized screening. Acta Radiol. 2011;52(5):481–7.
65. Kopans D, Gavenonis S, Halpern E, Moore R. Calcifications in the breast and digital breast tomosynthesis. Breast J. 2011;17(6):638–44.

66. Demetri-Lewis A, Slanetz PJ, Eisenberg RL. Breast calcifications: the focal group. AJR Am J Roentgenol. 2012;198(4):W325–43.
67. Scimeca M, Giannini E, Antonacci C, Pistolese CA, Spagnoli LG, Bonanno E. Microcalcifications in breast cancer: an active phenomenon mediated by epithelial cells with mesenchymal characteristics. BMC Cancer. 2014;14:286.
68. Cox RF, Morgan MP. Microcalcifications in breast cancer: lessons from physiological mineralization. Bone. 2013;53(2):437–50.
69. Morgan MP, Cooke MM, McCarthy GM. Microcalcifications associated with breast cancer: an epiphenomenon or biologically significant feature of selected tumors? J Mammary Gland Biol Neoplasia. 2005;10(2):181–7.
70. Tse GM, Tan PH, Cheung HS, Chu WC, Lam WW. Intermediate to highly suspicious calcification in breast lesions: a radio-pathologic correlation. Breast Cancer Res Treat. 2008;110(1):1–7.
71. Michaels AY, Birdwell RL, Chung CS, Frost EP, Giess CS. Assessment and management of challenging BI-RADS category 3 mammographic lesions. Radiographics. 2016;36(5):1261–72.
72. Page DL, Dupont WD. Anatomic markers of human premalignancy and risk of breast cancer. Cancer. 1990;66(Suppl 6):1326–35.
73. Dahlstrom JE, Sutton S, Jain S. Histologic-radiologic correlation of mammographically detected microcalcification in stereotactic core biopsies. Am J Surg Pathol. 1998;22(2):256–9.
74. Dahlstrom JE, Jain S. Histological correlation of mammographically detected microcalcifications in stereotactic core biopsies. Pathology. 2001;33(4):444–8.
75. Tse GM, Tan PH, Pang AL, Tang AP, Cheung HS. Calcification in breast lesions: pathologists' perspective. J Clin Pathol. 2008;61(2):145–51.
76. Bassett L, Winchester DP, Caplan RB, Dershaw DD, Dowlatshahi K, Evans WP 3rd, , et al. Stereotactic core-needle biopsy of the breast: a report of the Joint Task Force of the American College of Radiology, American College of Surgeons, and College of American Pathologists. CA Cancer J Clin 1997;47(3):171–190.
77. Liberman L, Menell JH. Breast imaging reporting and data system (BI-RADS). Radiol Clin North Am. 2002;40(3):409–30, v.
78. Margolin FR, Kaufman L, Jacobs RP, Denny SR, Schrumpf JD. Stereotactic core breast biopsy of malignant calcifications: diagnostic yield of cores with and cores without calcifications on specimen radiographs. Radiology. 2004;233(1):251–4.
79. Easley S, Abdul-Karim FW, Klein N, Wang N. Segregation of radiographic calcifications in stereotactic core biopsies of breast: is it necessary? Breast J. 2007;13(5):486–9.
80. Pisano ED, Zuley M, Baum JK, Marques HS. Issues to consider in converting to digital mammography. Radiol Clin North Am. 2007;45(5):813–30, vi.
81. Pagliari CM, Hoang T, Reddy M, Wilkinson LS, Poloniecki JD, Given-Wilson RM. Diagnostic quality of 50 and 100 mum computed radiography compared with screen-film mammography in operative breast specimens. Br J Radiol. 2012;85(1015):910–6.
82. Tornos C, Silva E, el-Naggar A, Pritzker KP. Calcium oxalate crystals in breast biopsies. The missing microcalcifications. Am J Surg Pathol. 1990;14(10):961–8.
83. Lai KC, Slanetz PJ, Eisenberg RL. Linear breast calcifications. AJR Am J Roentgenol. 2012;199(2):W151–7.
84. Wells CA, El-Ayat GA. Non-operative breast pathology: apocrine lesions. J Clin Pathol. 2007;60(12):1313–20.
85. Zagorianakou P, Zagorianakou N, Stefanou D, Makrydimas G, Agnantis NJ. The enigmatic nature of apocrine breast lesions. Virchows Arch. 2006;448(5):525–31.
86. Grimes MM, Karageorge LS, Hogge JP. Does exhaustive search for microcalcifications improve diagnostic yield in stereotactic core needle breast biopsies? Mod Pathol. 2001;14(4):350–3.
87. Dialani V, Venkataraman S, Frieling G, Schnitt SJ, Mehta TS. Does isolated flat epithelial atypia on vacuum-assisted breast core biopsy require surgical excision? Breast J. 2014;20(6):606–14.
88. Calhoun BC, Sobel A, White RL, Gromet M, Flippo T, Sarantou T, et al. Management of flat epithelial atypia on breast core biopsy may be individualized based on correlation with imaging studies. Mod Pathol. 2015;28(5):670–6.

89. Maeda I, Kanemaki Y, Tozaki M, Koizumi H, Oana Y, Okanami Y, et al. Positive predictive value for malignancy of pure flat epithelial atypia diagnosis by percutaneous needle biopsy of the breast: management of FEA in ultrasonography. Breast Cancer. 2015;22(6):634–40.
90. Said SM, Visscher DW, Nassar A, Frank RD, Vierkant RA, Frost MH, et al. Flat epithelial atypia and risk of breast cancer: a Mayo cohort study. Cancer. 2015;121(10):1548–55.

3 Surgical Oncology Evaluation and Management of Breast Diseases

Harry D. Bear

History and Physical Examination

For women with breast complaints/symptoms, key questions, aside from general questions about medical history, that need to be addressed include: masses on self-exam, pain, nipple discharge (including whether it is grossly bloody and spontaneous or elicited by pressure), how long a mass or other symptom has been present, skin changes, enlarged axillary nodes, arm pain or arm swelling, bone pain, cough, or other symptoms that might indicate distant metastatic disease. Family history of breast or ovarian cancer is important for determining whether the patient may carry a heritable mutation increasing the risk of cancer, but absence of positive family history should not affect clinical suspicion of cancer, since most breast cancers are not the result of a germline mutation.

Physical examination focused on breast issues, aside from routine elements, should begin with inspection of the breasts with the patient sitting upright, with hand by her sides, then raised over her head, and then hands pressing against her waist. If the patient reports that she can only feel a mass when she is sitting up, palpation of the breasts in this position can be useful. These positions can accentuate tethering or dimpling of the skin overlying a cancer. Lymphatic examination should include palpation for cervical, supraclavicular, and axillary adenopathy. The last is best accomplished with the patient upright, holding the weight of the arm in the examiner's same hand (right arm, right hand) and rolling the axillary tissue between the examiner's hand and the chest wall (Fig. 3.1). Examining the axilla after the patient is supine may miss even large pathologic lymph nodes that can fall back out of reach in that position.

H.D. Bear, MD, PhD
Division of Surgical Oncology, Department of Surgery,
Virginia Commonwealth University Health (VCU HEALTH), Richmond, VA, USA
e-mail: harry.bear@vcuhealth.org

M.O. Idowu et al. (eds.), *Diagnosis and Management of Breast Tumors*,
DOI 10.1007/978-3-319-57726-5_3

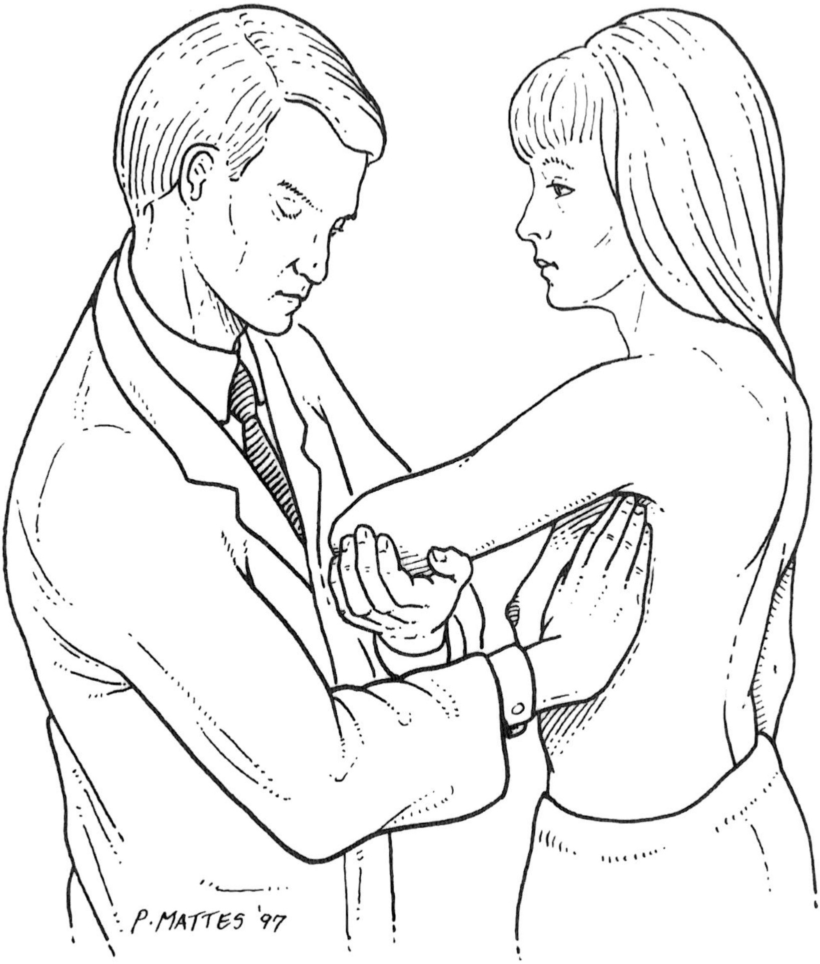

Fig. 3.1 Cartoon illustrating technique for examination of the axilla

With the patient supine, all of the breast tissue should be palpated in a systematic way, including the retroareolar area and the axillary tail of the breast. It is useful to use two hands together, with one hand feeling more superficially and the other more deeply. The pads of the fingers, around the distal interphalangeal joint, not the tips of the fingers, are most sensitive for detection of masses. The location, size (measured with a ruler or caliper and not estimated), discreteness, and texture (soft, hard, rubbery, possibly fluid filled, etc.) of any masses need to be carefully recorded. It is helpful to make the description somewhat redundant (e.g., upper inner quadrant of the left breast, at 10 o'clock, 6 cm from the nipple, deep in the breast) so that the finding can be used to guide focused breast imaging or another exam by a different examiner or the same examiner at a later time.

Evaluation of Breast Symptoms and Findings

Masses

As noted above, careful physical examination and documentation of findings is an important first step in the evaluation of a mass found by the patient or a physician. Breast imaging is also a critical component for most patients, especially those over 30 years of age. For some patients, the characteristics of the mass on exam may be typical for a cystic mass. If so and the mass is symptomatic (i.e., painful), the most expeditious management may be to aspirate the cyst with a syringe and needle in the clinic, guided by palpation. For indeterminate masses, breast imaging, especially ultrasound (US), can distinguish between solid and cystic masses. Asymptomatic simple cysts can be followed without intervention; complex cysts (e.g., with internal echoes or nodules) and solid masses will most often need to be biopsied, usually a needle biopsy with imaging guidance.

Mobile, lobulated masses in young women (teens and 20s) are usually fibroadenomas (FA; see below under benign disease). If there is uncertainty, the US or a needle biopsy can be used to confirm this.

Nipple Discharge

Perhaps the most important point to make about evaluation of nipple discharges is that non-spontaneous nipple discharges (i.e., elicited by pressure on the breast tissue) are *not* pathologic and should not lead to any evaluation whatsoever. Spontaneous nipple discharges, on the other hand, are reason for concern, either because they may indicate significant pathology or because they may be bothersome to the patient. Nipple discharge fluid that most often indicates a neoplastic process, in addition to being spontaneous, is either visibly bloody or clear and copious in amounts. However, testing for occult blood using testing kits that are intended for fecal material should be discouraged. This is not the intended purpose of these tests and often leads to unnecessary testing and/or surgery. Furthermore, sending nipple fluid for cytological examination is also fraught with hazard; false-negative and false-positive tests are both frequent, and this will generally not resolve the diagnosis [1, 2]. The use of ductograms (or galactograms) is controversial but may delineate a mass lesion in a duct system and may localize a lesion that might be missed by "blind" excision of the central ducts leading to the orifice from which the discharge was observed [3]. Excision of the central ducts behind the nipple may well result in stopping the discharge but could leave a peripheral malignant or premalignant lesion in place. Some have advocated duct endoscopy to evaluate nipple discharges [4–6]. Nipple discharges are usually caused by duct ectasia, by intraductal papillomas, and, rarely, by ductal carcinoma in situ (DCIS) or invasive ductal cancer (IDC). Duct ectasia usually causes clear, yellowish, greenish, or brown discharge, and excision of dilated or ectatic ducts usually only has the benefit of resolving the annoying symptom. Management of papillary lesions, especially when diagnosed by core needle biopsy, is controversial, but papillomas with atypia have about a 30% chance of being malignant on excision [7–14]. And like atypical ductal hyperplasia (ADH) or atypical lobular hyperplasia (ALH), atypia associated with a papillary lesion increases the risk of developing breast cancer long term.

Breast Pain

Breast pain, whether generalized or localized, is rarely the presenting symptom of a cancer, but about 10% of patients with a new cancer may have associated pain. Most breast pain is attributable to a "wastebasket" of diagnoses under the heading of fibrocystic change. The first responsibility of the surgeon evaluating a patient for breast pain is to rule out cancer or other serious diseases. This can be done by careful physical exam and routine imaging, mammography, and/or US, depending on the age of the patient. Rarely is a "blind" biopsy going to be productive. Recommendations for pain relief are mostly empiric and include non-steroidal anti-inflammatory drugs (NSAIDs), ice packs, local heat, good support, and reassurance. Anecdotally, severe pain from fibrocystic disease (FCD) has been ameliorated by treatment with selective estrogen receptor modulators (SERMs, e.g., tamoxifen), bromocriptine, or danazol [15–17]. However, because of the potential side effects, we would only rarely resort to these measures unless the patient was also at increased risk for breast cancer and over the age of 35. Pain can also be caused by breast cysts, and these can be aspirated with almost instant relief. Mastitis and breast abscesses (see below) can also cause severe acute breast pain.

Changes of Nipple

Scaling lesions of the nipple may be a manifestation of eczema or a form of ductal carcinoma in situ known as Paget's disease. Essentially, Paget's represents DCIS emerging from the nipple milk ducts into the epidermis of the nipple (intraepidermal adenocarcinoma). It generally presents with a scaly crusted appearance that may spread out onto the surrounding areola. Evaluation should include thorough physical examination and mammography for associated masses. The only reliable way to make this diagnosis and distinguish it from more benign conditions is to biopsy the nipple. Generally, a small wedge of nipple tissue can be excised under local anesthesia and closed with a few small sutures. Foci of invasive cancer or DCIS in the breast parenchyma are associated with Paget's in a majority of cases [18–20]. This may have a profound effect on treatment decisions. For isolated Paget's of the nipple, excision of the nipple with a small amount of underlying breast tissue is generally sufficient for breast conservation treatment (BCT). Whether or not to add radiation therapy will depend on patient age, margins, and grade, similar to DCIS in general (see below) [21]. For those patients with additional sites of cancer within the breast parenchyma, total mastectomy with lymph node sampling is usually recommended, unless the focus of invasion is directly under the nipple. However, just as in patients with two separate sites of cancer and depending on breast size, two segmental resections may be feasible and acceptable.

Use of Breast Imaging Modalities

Low radiation dose mammography is the mainstay of breast evaluation and screening. Although screening guidelines from various organizations have changed over the past few decades, not without significant controversy, current guidelines vary between annual and biannual mammograms for women over 50, with more controversy about the role of screening mammograms in women between 40 and 50 years of age [22, 23]. Newer modalities that may increase the sensitivity and specificity of screening include tomosynthesis (3D) mammograms, whole breast ultrasound, and magnetic resonance imaging (MRI), but the roles of these methods for routine population-based screening have not been clearly established [24–28]. MRI is currently recommended for women with germline genetic mutations or family history that puts them at >20–25% lifetime risk for developing breast cancer [29]. Whole breast ultrasound, tomosynthesis, and rapid MRI scanning have been proposed as additional tests for women with dense breast tissue, who are at increased risk of breast cancer and in whom detection of small breast cancers can be difficult [24–28, 30, 31].

For women with a breast mass or symptoms who have not had a screening mammogram in the past 3–6 months, diagnostic mammograms should be ordered, and ultrasound may also help to delineate the nature and extent of any lesion that is palpated or seen on mammogram. US may also be used to guide needle biopsy or aspiration of fluid, if indicated. Other modalities that have been proposed for additional screening or to assess mammographic or clinically detectable abnormalities include breast-specific molecular imaging of radiotracer uptake, such as PET-mammograms using F^{18}-labeled glucose or gamma imaging of Tc^{99}-sesatmibi uptake, and are used in a number of centers, but have not yet become mainstream routine modalities for breast imaging.

Biopsy Methods and Key Information

Needle Biopsy

The most important "take-away" from this section is that all palpable and imaging-detected abnormalities that require biopsy should first be considered for a needle biopsy, either fine-needle aspiration (FNA) or core needle biopsy (preferred) rather than surgical, incisional, or excisional biopsy. This is considered a quality indicator and is recommended by the Commission on Cancer as part of the "Choosing Wisely" program of the American Board of Internal Medicine Foundation [32–35]. Needle biopsy usually establishes a definitive diagnosis with the least morbidity, avoids excision with positive margins requiring reoperation, and also avoids the need for a second surgical procedure for nodal staging. Core needle biopsy is more likely to distinguish invasive cancer from in situ cancer than FNA and also provides more tissue for breast biomarkers, including estrogen receptors, progesterone receptors, human epidermal growth factor receptor 2 (ER, PR, HER-2), and Ki67 or other ancillary testing. This information should be provided by pathology for any needle biopsy showing invasive cancer, since these may be important for decisions about which patients may need adjuvant or neoadjuvant systemic therapy (more on this later). For core biopsies showing DCIS, we do not generally ask for these markers, since the phenotype of an invasive cancer, if present, in the definitive surgical resection has greater significance [36]. We therefore only perform biomarkers in cases of pure DCIS on surgical specimens, not on needle core biopsy. The exception to this would be patients who, for reasons of comorbidity or on a clinical trial, might be considered for primary or neoadjuvant hormonal therapy as initial treatment.

Surgical Biopsy

When Is This Appropriate?

Some situations call for surgical biopsy rather than needle biopsy. These include very thin breasts that compress to a width that is less than the "throw" distance of a biopsy needle. Some consider the presence of augmentation implants a relative contraindication to needle biopsy, but with ultrasound guidance, this can usually be accomplished safely without violation of the implant. Surgical biopsy may be indicated for a number of reasons, but as noted above, needle biopsy should always be considered first. Probably the most common reason for surgical excisional biopsy today is a "borderline" diagnosis on core needle biopsy. These include lobular carcinoma in situ (LCIS), ADH, ALH, or papillary lesions with atypia, for which excisional biopsy may find invasive cancer or DCIS in up to 30% of cases [37]. More controversial are papillary lesions without atypia and radial scar. Most reports, including a review of our own experience, have found that excision of lesions that are papillomas *without* atypia will find cancer with a low frequency, 5–10% [9–11, 38]. Radial scar is also unsettled but is particularly worrisome when the mammographic appearance is suspicious for cancer. For any needle biopsy result that is considered discordant with the imaging appearance, surgical excision should be considered [39–42].

Methods for Localizing the Target Lesion

When surgical excision of an occult (non-palpable) lesion of the breast is indicated, a number of different methods can be used to guide the surgical approach. The classic approach is mammographic or ultrasound-guided insertion of a wire in the breast. The surgeon can then use this, along with the films showing the relationship of the wire to the target lesion or marker clip placed at the time of needle biopsy, to find the target lesion. Although many illustrations show making an incision near the entry point of the wire, this is most often not the most direct or cosmetically optimal approach. Based on the localization films and the measurements provided by the radiologist, a more direct approach can be determined.

Other methods of localization have been described in recent years. A number of these have the advantage of avoiding the need for a mammographic procedure on the morning of surgery, facilitating surgery scheduling. For surgeons who are comfortable with breast ultrasound, intraoperative guidance using this modality is very helpful. This can be used for lesions that are solid masses that can be "seen" with US or if the lesion has been marked with a clip that is detectable on US. Recently, a number of institutions have been using a radioactive seed of ^{125}I that can be located with the same gamma detection devices that are used to find sentinel nodes mapped with radiotracer. This has been reported to be highly successful, and some data suggest that smaller volumes of tissue and higher rates of negative margins are achieved with this method than with needle localization [43–46]. However, it does require a good deal of preparation and compliance with complex regulatory measures to ensure against loss of the radioactive seed. A significant advantage of this approach is that the localization procedure can be performed several days before the surgery. Similarly, new devices have recently been approved for this use, including the Savi Scout, which depends on transmission of a radiofrequency signal from a tiny transmitter in the breast that can be detected with a probe [47]. Insertion of a ferromagnetic marker (Magseed) that can be detected with a specially designed probe can also be used to localize breast lesions for later excision.

The lesion should be approached either directly over the lesion or, if possible without tunneling through too much breast tissue, can be removed through a circumareolar incision. The latter may provide a well-hidden incision but, if the lesion is peripheral, may result in tunneling through more breast tissue than is desirable. This may lead to difficulty if re-excision is needed for positive margins or if oncoplastic rearrangement of tissue is needed to optimize the cosmetic result. Moreover, if the lesion is malignant and the margins are positive, then it may be difficult to identify the margins to re-excise. If a cancer is located close to the skin, it may be useful to remove a segment of the skin overlying the lesion. This helps to ensure a negative anterior or superficial margin and also avoids closing a thin layer of the skin over a cavity that may become a seroma.

Management of Benign Breast Conditions

Fibrocystic Changes/Breast Pain

The so-called fibrocystic change really refers to a clinical entity characterized by intermittent breast pain and nodularity or dense breast tissue without a definite or discrete mass. This is not really a disease, since it is so common and is associated with a variety of histopathologic findings if biopsied. This most commonly occurs in late pre- and perimenopausal women. Pain may be cyclical or constant. In general, surgery is not indicated for this complaint, unless associated with a definite imaging abnormality or a palpable discrete mass. This can make it difficult to detect breast cancer and may cause significant patient anxiety. Recommendations for relief of symptoms include local ice, heat, or NSAIDS. Although many recommend avoidance of caffeine for these patients, there is little evidence that this is a causative agent [48–51].

Cysts

In contrast to fibrocystic change, which may include collections of small cysts, larger cysts may present as discrete masses detected on palpation or on mammogram. These may be painful or asymptomatic. If cysts are painful, the most expeditious management is aspiration with a needle (20 gauge is usually sufficient), under either ultrasound guidance or by palpation ("digital" guidance). If there is uncertainty as to whether a mass detected by palpation or mammography is cystic, ultrasound can be used to distinguish solid from cystic lesions. If the cyst is "simple" (no internal echoes or mural nodules) and not symptomatic, nothing further needs to be done. If it is painful or "complex" by ultrasound, then aspiration or biopsy should be undertaken to rule out a neoplasm. If the aspirated fluid is not bloody, then it does NOT need to be sent for any testing (e.g., cytology), as this will rarely yield a malignant diagnosis and is expensive. If the cyst does not recur, then nothing further needs to be done. If the cyst recurs, it should be managed according to symptoms. Cysts can be aspirated again if symptomatic or excised if repeated aspirations do not resolve the patient's concerns.

Papillary Lesions

Papillary lesions of the lactiferous ducts may present as a nipple discharge, sometimes bloody or blood tinged, or as a mass found on imaging or physical exam. These are usually centrally located, but can be some distance from the nipple-areolar complex. For this reason, many advocate galactograms as part of the workup for nipple discharge, but this is controversial [3]. Excision, possibly with guidance from the galactogram, is usually indicated for ductal lesions with nipple discharge. If a papillary lesion is diagnosed on needle biopsy, the question of whether to surgically excise the lesion depends on whether or not there is associated atypia on pathology. A number of reports indicate that a core needle diagnosis of a papillary lesion with atypia is associated with a 20–30% likelihood of coexisting DCIS or invasive cancer on complete excision. However, for benign papillary lesions without atypia, excisional biopsy will diagnose a cancer in less than 10% of cases and may not be necessary [9–11, 38].

Fibroadenomas

Fibroadenomas (FAs) are benign fibroepithelial masses (see pathology section) that usually present as smooth, lobulated mobile masses, most often in young women (teens and 20s). They may be asymptomatic or mildly painful. If asymptomatic and less than 2 cm in greatest diameter, they can be followed clinically. For FAs that have grown relatively rapidly, attained a size greater than 2 cm, or if they are painful, excision, usually under local anesthesia, is indicated. A wide margin is not required. If there is any doubt about the diagnosis, ultrasound and/or needle biopsy can be used to confirm the clinical impression. If the size of the mass increases over time, exceeds 2 cm, or becomes painful, excision should be considered. These tumors are sometimes found on routine screening, and if the imaging is typical for fibroadenoma, they can be followed, or if there is some concern that the lesion is atypical or enlarging, needle biopsy can be done for reassurance. Because fibroadenomas are usually very mobile, they can usually be reached through a circumareolar incision, resulting in minimal deformity. Even very large fibroadenomas (sometimes referred to as "giant") can be excised readily, and the breast size and shape will gradually return to normal. Occasional recommendations to undergo mastectomy for very large fibroadenomas are inappropriate, as these benign tumors compress the surrounding breast tissue, which then fills in the space left behind. An alternative to surgical excision is cryotherapy ablation, using US guidance [52–55]. This leaves minimal scar, but the tumor may take some time to regress after freezing.

One should be cautious about apparent FAs that are very large or have grown rapidly, as these may be phyllodes tumors. Needle biopsy will sometimes raise this issue but often is not definitive, with a diagnosis of "fibroepithelial lesion, cannot rule out phyllodes." These require excision to make a definitive diagnosis. Excision should include a margin of normal breast tissue if possible. If it turns out that the tumor is a benign phyllodes, then excision with a negative margin should be adequate treatment [56–59]. Most phyllodes tumors are benign but can recur locally; some (about 10–25%) are malignant [60, 61], and these can be locally aggressive and may even metastasize, usually hematogenously. Some have recommended excision with at least a 1 cm margin for phyllodes tumors, although the most important factor is achieving a histologically negative margin. For high-grade phyllodes tumors treated with breast-conserving surgery, radiation to the breast may improve local control [62–64]. If wide excision with a negative margin is not feasible, total mastectomy may be necessary. However, since phyllodes tumors rarely spread via lymphatics, surgical staging of regional nodes is unnecessary [61, 63].

Duct Ectasia

Dilated lactiferous ducts may be detected on mammogram or may present clinically as spontaneous or elicited nipple discharge. The nipple discharge may be clear or serous, yellow, brown, or green, among other colors. If the discharge only occurs with squeezing or manipulation of the breast, it is generally considered nonpathologic and should be ignored. If it is spontaneous, additional workup, such as galactography or, in some centers, mammary duct endoscopy, may be warranted [65]. Ectatic ducts may also be the underlying cause of breast abscesses, particularly retroareolar/central infections (see below). Dilated ducts appearing as a new finding on mammogram are considered by some to be a possible sign of a cancer and should be evaluated further, with US and/or galactograms.

Breast Infections

We will not consider postpartum mastitis here, since this is not usually a surgical disease and is generally treated conservatively with antibiotics [66, 67]. Diffuse mastitis otherwise is unusual but can be quite painful and may even be associated with systemic sepsis. This can occasionally occur as a complication of breast lymphedema associated with lymph node dissection and breast irradiation. This should be evaluated with breast imaging to rule out an underlying mass or abscess and needs to be distinguished from inflammatory breast cancer, which can have a similar appearance. If there is not a mass or abscess, treatment with antibiotics, usually to cover gram-positive bacteria, should be prescribed. If the process does not improve, a punch biopsy of the erythematous skin may be necessary to rule out inflammatory breast cancer, which can present without a mass.

Breast abscesses, which are usually evident clinically, present as painful fluctuant masses under or adjacent to the areola, with associated cellulitis surrounding the mass. The patient may also report purulent drainage from the nipple. Until recently, these were generally managed with surgical incision and drainage (I&D) under anesthesia, followed by wound care and gradual healing. At advanced stages, these are often fluctuant clinically, or they may show as fluid-filled spaces on ultrasound. The management of breast abscesses has changed in recent years, from routine I&D in the operating room to ultrasound-guided needle aspiration and antibiotics. The latter strategy is successful in most cases [68–70]. If the abscess recurs or has loculated or complex fluid that is too thick for aspiration, I&D may be necessary. Surgical drainage may also be preferred in patients with signs and symptoms of systemic sepsis, particularly in diabetic patients. In the past, it was routinely recommended that once the acute process had resolved, central duct excision should be performed to reduce the risk of subsequent recurrences [71, 72]. However, this has become more controversial, and some have suggested that duct excision should only be performed if multiple episodes occur. It should be pointed out that multiple other entities, such as infected sebaceous cysts, hidradenitis of the axilla, or inframammary fold area, are managed differently (managed in the same manner as in other parts of the body) as they are not the same as breast abscesses arising in milk ducts.

Idiopathic Granulomatous Mastitis

This may be one of the most mysterious diseases of the breast, with a myriad of presentations and no clear-cut etiology or best treatment. This may present as a discrete mass, which may be painful, a chronic abscess with or without spontaneous drainage to the skin, or a diffuse mass effect involving large areas of the breast. The cause is not clear, and recommended treatments range from antibiotics to steroids to methotrexate to I&D to excision of discrete masses to total mastectomy. The only clear recommendation is to start conservatively and reserve more radical treatments for diffuse disease that does not respond to other therapies [73–75].

Trauma/Hematoma

Blunt trauma to the breast, such as from a seatbelt or airbag in a motor vehicle accident, may result in a mass lesion in the breast, which may be a hematoma or an area of fat necrosis. This can cause considerable pain, with ecchymosis and a palpable mass. Although these may take a considerable time to resolve, surgery is rarely indicated unless a hematoma becomes secondarily infected, requiring drainage. If there is uncertainty about the diagnosis, breast imaging, with mammograms and ultrasound, can usually clarify the problem.

Radial Sclerosing Lesions (Radial Scar)

A diagnosis of radial scar usually results from image-guided needle biopsy of a clinically occult lesion seen on mammography. The common recommendation for this result has long been to surgically excise the area, because an underlying cancer can be missed [39–42]. However, this may only be the case if the mammographic finding was a spiculated density that looks very much like cancer. More recently, data have suggested that when radial scar is strictly a microscopic finding associated with a needle biopsy for other types of abnormalities, such as microcalcifications, the likelihood of missing a cancer is quite low and surgical excision may not be indicated [40–42, 76].

Atypical Hyperplasia

Atypical ductal or lobular hyperplasia has clearly been shown to be a risk factor for subsequent development of breast cancer long term [37, 77]. It may be appropriate, based on these diagnoses, especially if combined with other risk factors such as positive family history, to recommend chemoprevention with estrogen receptor modulators or aromatase inhibitors [78–81]. When these diagnoses, or lobular carcinoma in situ (which is NOT really cancer), are made with core needle biopsy, it is generally recommended that the lesion be entirely excised to rule out coexisting cancer, which may be found in up to 30% of cases [82, 83]. However, it has been suggested that if the biopsy is done with a large bore needle and vacuum-assisted equipment, especially if all of the calcifications on mammogram have been removed, that surgical excision may not be required.

Workup of a Patient with Breast Cancer

Imaging of the Breast

For patients with a biopsy-proven diagnosis of breast cancer, in addition to a complete history, review of systems, and physical examination, a complete set of current bilateral mammograms (within the last 3–6 months) should be available. Ultrasound of the breast may or may not be needed but sometimes can help delineate the extent of disease in the breast when breast density or other factors (such as invasive lobular cancer) make this difficult to determine on mammography. Routine breast MRI has been advocated by some for women with a new diagnosis of breast cancer, based on the likelihood of a change in management based on MRI findings [84–92]. A significant proportion of women (up to 25%) will have additional sites or extent of disease defined by MRI, and 3–5% of women will have otherwise undetected contralateral cancers found on MRI. However, other retrospective studies and at least two randomized trials have not shown that MRI decreases the need for re-excision or the rate of local recurrence after BCT [93–97]. It has been argued that although MRI does detect unsuspected additional lesions in the affected or the contralateral breast, the very low ipsilateral breast tumor recurrence (IBTR) and contralateral recurrence rates indicate that radiation to the affected breast, along with better systemic therapy, makes the discovery of these lesions irrelevant. Indeed, some have suggested that the routine use of MRI may unnecessarily delay the start of treatment and may increase the likelihood of total mastectomy. An intermediate stance holds that MRI should be used selectively for younger patients, patients with very dense breasts, patients with invasive lobular cancer (which can be very indistinct on other imaging), patients who will undergo primary or neoadjuvant systemic therapy, and in patients for whom accelerated partial breast irradiation is anticipated.

What NOT to do for Most Patients

One of the greatest drivers of excessive healthcare costs in the United States of America (USA) has been the profligate use of complex advanced imaging looking for systemic metastases in patients with early-stage cancers. For patients with breast cancer up to Stage II, and perhaps Stage IIIA, and with no symptoms to indicate the presence of metastases, the addition of studies such as CT scans, PET scans, or bone scans has clearly been shown to be of little or no benefit [98]. These expensive tests rarely turn up unsuspected metastatic cancer and often lead to additional unnecessary tests to clarify the results of the first unnecessary test. The recommendation NOT to perform these tests has been laid out clearly in guidelines from professional societies, such as the American Society of Clinical Oncology, and listed in the "Choosing Wisely" list maintained by the American Board of Internal Medicine Foundation at www.choosingwisely.org.

Staging for More Advanced Cancers

For women with locally or regionally advanced breast cancer (i.e., AJCC Stage III), CT scans of the chest, abdomen, and pelvis would be appropriate. PET-CT scans may be more convenient but are more expensive, are not always definitive for breast cancer metastases, and may not be covered by insurance. Alternative would be CT scans of the chest abdomen and pelvis, plus a nuclear medicine bone scan. For women with symptoms that suggest the presence of metastatic disease, regardless of stage, focused imaging may be justified (e.g., plain X-rays and bone scan for severe bone pain of recent onset, chest X-ray and chest CT for dyspnea or chronic cough of recent onset, head CT or MRI for neurologic symptoms or severe headache).

Treatment Options for Breast Cancer

Appropriate Sequence of Surgery and Other Treatments

In general, primary surgery has been the standard approach to breast cancer treatment, followed by adjuvant systemic therapy and radiation. However, in the past three decades or so, it has been demonstrated that neoadjuvant systemic therapy can be used to make locally advanced inoperable breast cancers more amenable to surgical resection and can convert patients from total mastectomy to breast conservation [99–107]. Depending on the phenotype of the cancer, and possibly the molecular profile, primary systemic therapy may be either cytotoxic chemotherapy or hormonal therapy. Neoadjuvant systemic therapy should be considered for any patient with a tumor ≥2 cm and/or with positive nodes, and the use of neoadjuvant chemotherapy (NCT) is particularly likely to be useful for tumors that are triple negative (TNBC, i.e., negative for estrogen and progesterone receptors and HER-2) and those that are HER-2 amplified. Potential advantages, in addition to reducing the scope of surgery for the breast primary, are (1) allowing time for genetic counseling and plastic surgery consultations without delaying treatment; (2) assessing the response to therapy, which may result in changes in treatment, either pre- or postoperatively; and (3) reducing the scope of surgery to axillary lymph nodes, avoiding the need for full axillary node dissection.

Surgical Options for the Breast Primary: Breast Conservation Versus Total Mastectomy

Surgical extirpation of the breast primary most simply comes down to breast conservation treatment (BCT—partial or segmental mastectomy, often called "lumpectomy") versus simple or total mastectomy. A number of factors have been suggested to be contraindications to BCT, but some of these have been disputed or even dispelled in the past two decades [108, 109]. Listed in Table 3.1 are factors that *no*

Table 3.1 Non-contraindications to breast conservation treatment for breast cancer

Extensive intraductal component
High grade
Positive nodes
Large breast
Small breast
Patient age (too young or too old)
Multifocal disease
Central location/nipple involvement
Second or third trimester of pregnancy

longer should be considered contraindications to BCT. Extensive intraductal component (EIC, defined as DCIS comprising more than 25% of the tumor area) was found to predict a higher likelihood of ipsilateral breast tumor recurrence, but only if negative margins were *not* routinely obtained [110–113]. More recent series have not found this to be an issue, if margins are negative and treatment includes irradiation to the breast [114–116]. Young age does indeed portend a higher risk of local recurrence, but total mastectomy and BCT still have equal outcomes [117–125]. Large tumor size has now been shown to be overcome by neoadjuvant systemic therapy, either chemotherapy or hormonal therapy, depending on the biologic features of the tumor [99–107, 126]. Even multicentric disease or large areas of DCIS have now given way to multiple lumpectomies in selected cases or to oncoplastic resections and rearrangement of breast tissue, which allow for removal of large segments of breast tissue and acceptable to excellent cosmetic outcomes [127–135]. Cancers presenting during pregnancy, while once considered indications for termination of the pregnancy and/or total mastectomy, can be safely treated with neoadjuvant chemotherapy, with minimal risk to the fetus, and breast-conserving surgery near or after delivery and radiation after delivery. The remaining relative and absolute or true indications for total mastectomy over BCT are listed in Tables 3.2 and 3.3. By far the most frequent of these should be patient choice, for reasons that are as varied as the patients themselves (e.g., fear of recurrence, not wanting to have further mammograms, strong family history [with or without a documented germline mutation]).

Staging of Regional Lymph Nodes with Clinically Negative Nodes

This aspect of breast cancer management has undergone major changes in the past two decades. For patients with clinically negative axillary lymph nodes, sentinel node biopsy has largely supplanted axillary lymph node dissection (ALND, usually removal of level I and II nodes) for providing staging information about the presence or absence of microscopic cancer in the nodes [136–139]. Sentinel lymph

Table 3.2 Relative contraindications to breast conservation treatment for breast cancer

Multicentric disease
Prior breast irradiation
Radiation therapy inaccessible
First trimester of pregnancy
Large tumor relative to breast size—can be overcome by neoadjuvant systemic therapy and/or oncoplastic methods
Connective tissue diseases (e.g., scleroderma or systemic lupus involving skin)

Table 3.3 Absolute contraindications to breast conservation treatment for breast cancer

Diffuse disease (e.g., malignant calcifications or biopsy-proven diffuse cancer found on MRI)
Inability to achieve negative margins
Patient choice

node (SLN) biopsy has been shown to result in equivalent outcomes to routine axillary node dissection in randomized trials. This has greatly decreased the morbidity of surgical management, particularly the incidence of lymphedema of the upper extremity [140]. This procedure is performed by injection into the breast of a radiotracer that can be taken up by the lymphatics and/or a colored dye that also helps to identify the sentinel nodes visually. We generally inject 1 microcurie of ^{99}Technetium sulfur colloid into the breast, while the patient is in the pre-op holding area, split between retroareolar injection and injection intradermally overlying the tumor site, in a total volume of 0.5 cc. Some have advocated and practiced injection after induction of anesthesia in the operating room [141, 142]. The advantage of this is that the patient does not experience the pain associated with the injection. However, those that favor the later injection have generally been using much larger volumes (4–5 cc), which is certainly more painful. We have found that with careful explanation and sometimes administration of mild sedation or after a regional block if being administered prior to mastectomy, the patients generally tolerate the injection well, and this allows more time for the tracer to reach the nodes. However, the later injection has been reported to work equally well. After induction of anesthesia and prepping, we then inject 3–5 cc of isosulfan blue, part retroareolar and part peri-tumoral, and massage the breast for 3–5 min before making an incision in the axilla and searching for the "hot" and blue nodes. Some centers use only one dye or tracer to identify the SLN, but dual dye techniques may improve the yield and accuracy, especially after neoadjuvant chemotherapy (see below). A variety of other radioactive, nonradioactive, and colored dyes have also been used to map the SLN for excision. It is also possible to find and remove the sentinel node through the mastectomy incision if a total mastectomy is being performed.

After the surgeon removes the nodes that are identified by a gamma probe and/or visual inspection, they are carefully examined by the pathologist, either immediately (intraoperative consultation) or by permanent section, depending on the situation. Randomized trials have demonstrated the accuracy of this approach, with false-negative rates in the range of 10% and no difference in patient outcomes compared to ALND [136–139]. If the sentinel nodes are negative, then no further surgery for regional nodes is needed. Initially, finding positive sentinel nodes would lead to a completion axillary node dissection. More recently, however, several studies have questioned whether the remaining lymph nodes need to be removed. For patients undergoing BCT followed by radiation and with one or two positive SLNs, the Z1011 trial found that completion ALND was not beneficial [143, 144]. The AMAROS trial in the United Kingdom found that for patients undergoing total mastectomy who had positive SLN, axillary radiation was as effective as ALND with less morbidity [145]. Some studies have now shown that if axillary US is negative for suspicious nodes in the axilla, then surgical staging is unlikely to find significant disease in axillary nodes that would lead to changes in patient treatment [146, 147]. In fact, decisions about systemic adjuvant therapy are now driven more by molecular characterization of breast cancers than by anatomic/pathologic staging.

Whether or not to perform SLN biopsy for patients with DCIS has been controversial [148]. Although positive SLN has been reported in about 5% of patients with "pure" DCIS, this does not appear to impact prognosis significantly and generally is not recommended. However, in certain circumstances, SLN may be appropriate for patients with a core biopsy diagnosis of DCIS. Patients undergoing total mastectomy because of the extent of disease or by patient choice should be considered for SLN biopsy because of the possibility of finding invasive cancer in the mastectomy specimen, which can occur in 20–25% of patients. If this occurs, one cannot go back to map the SLN after the breast has been removed. Similarly, imaging findings (e.g., a mass or extensive disease, especially if high grade) or pathology findings suspicious for invasion increase the likelihood of DCIS being upstaged to invasive cancer and should lead to consideration of a SLN biopsy.

Surgical Management of Regional Nodes for Patients with Clinically Positive Nodes

This is a particularly controversial area, particular in an era when MRI and US often detect abnormal nodes that may not be appreciated on physical exam. Regardless of the method of detection, abnormal nodes should generally be sampled by either FNA or core biopsy to document involvement prior to treatment. Whether the patient is considered to be a candidate for neoadjuvant therapy or primary surgery, pathologic confirmation of node involvement impacts the options for management. In the case of those who are not candidates for chemotherapy, then an axillary dissection will generally be appropriate for patients with clinically and pathologically positive nodes. On the other hand, neoadjuvant chemotherapy will often be chosen for women with positive nodes, and the management of the regional nodes for those patients is an evolving issue. With pathologic complete response rates for some subsets of patients (TNBC and HER-2 overexpressing cancers, in particular) ranging from 40 to 70%, the potential to avoid full axillary dissection even in patients presenting with positive nodes has become a reality. Although some still advocate SLN biopsy prior to receiving NCT, finding a positive SLN in this setting may obligate the surgeon to complete an ALND after treatment. Therefore, a number of studies have examined the accuracy of SLN biopsy in patients presenting with positive nodes after NCT. False-negative rates (FNR) of 10–15% have raised concerns that this could result in understaging and undertreatment, but these rates are little different from the FNR for primary SLN biopsy with no prior treatment. Furthermore, a number of maneuvers can reduce the rate of missing residual cancer in nodes, including the use of two dyes (radionuclide and colored dye), removing three or more nodes (if they exist), and marking the positive node with a clip and then confirming removal of the clipped node by specimen mammography [149–156]. In 80% of patients, the clipped node will be one of the nodes that maps with one of the dyes, but in the other 20%, the formerly positive clipped node will be different from the mapped nodes [157, 158]. Finding and removing the clipped node can be facilitated by also marking with India ink or a radioactive seed. With the combination of these techniques, the false-negative rate for post-NCT SLN biopsy for patients with initially positive nodes can be reduced to low single digits [157, 158]. Exceptions to this approach in our institution would be patients with multiple (three or more) nodes that are abnormal prior to therapy or those whose nodes remain abnormal clinically or on imaging at the end of treatment. These patients should generally have a standard axillary node dissection.

The subsequent management of the axilla in patients presenting with positive nodes and receiving NCT is also evolving. For patients whose SLN and clipped node are negative after NCT, most would agree that axillary dissection is unnecessary, but at this time addition of regional nodal irradiation would be considered standard for these patients. In the face of retrospective data suggesting that such patients are at low risk for regional recurrence [159], a clinical trial is currently underway which randomizes patients with documented pathologically positive nodes whose nodes are negative after NCT to regional nodal irradiation versus no irradiation after total mastectomy or breast-only irradiation for patients undergoing BCT [160–162]. Conversely, for patients with persistent cancer in the axilla, the current standard would be to complete an ALND and to add regional nodal irradiation. For these patients, a current clinical trial is randomizing patients with positive SLN after NCT to ALND + regional nodal irradiation versus omitting the ALND. Hopefully, these trials will be completed and provide answers to the questions that remain regarding the management of regional nodes in patients receiving NCT.

Breast Conservation Methods

Importance of Margins

The appropriate width of margins has been debated for decades. For invasive cancer, early studies of total mastectomy specimens found that "skip" areas of cancer separate from the primary site can be found frequently [163]. This has certainly been supported by the high incidence of IBTR in patients who underwent segmental mastectomy without radiation in the NSABP B-06 trial (40% at 10 years), despite negative margins [164, 165]. However, the addition of radiation and current systemic therapies has reduced the IBTR rate to the range of 5% or even less at 10 years [166]. Nevertheless, margins ranging from "no tumor on ink" to >5 mm have been advocated [163, 167–178]. The early NSABP B-06 trials defined negative margins as "no tumor on ink," referring to the pathologist's method of inking the surface of the submitted specimen prior to fixation. A recent meta-analysis and consensus statement, however, led to the recommendation that "no tumor on ink" is adequate for invasive breast cancer and that additional surgery to obtain a wider or "better" margin is not justified [179]. If a margin is truly positive, with tumor on ink, a second or even a third attempt to obtain negative margins by selective re-excision along the corresponding wall of the cavity can be successful. However, if multiple margins are very close (<1 mm) over an extensive area, rather than being "focal," we may still re-excise more tissue adjacent to the close margins.

For DCIS, the story on margins has been more difficult to settle. Again, a recent meta-analysis and consensus statement from multiple organizations support the recommendation that a minimal margin of 2 mm should ideally be achieved for DCIS [180]. However, this does not necessarily mean that a second operation should be performed to achieve a "better" margin if the initial excision margin is negative but less than 2 mm. However, a wider margin than "no tumor on ink" may be particularly advisable in patients for whom omission of breast irradiation is being considered [181–183].

Methods for Margin Marking and Assessment

There have been a number of methods used for orienting, marking, and/or analyzing the margins [184–193], but at the very least, the specimen should routinely be oriented for the pathologist. If the specimen is clearly oriented, then if any margin is positive, it may only be necessary to re-excise one margin in the excision cavity. Orientation methods include sutures of different lengths, clips that are labeled, and "painting" the six sides of the specimen with different colors, each specific to a designated margin. Assessment of margins using a variety of intraoperative imaging methods, including "three-dimensional" imaging, and a chemical probe that can detect cancer cells at the margins of the specimen have also been advocated. Intraoperative cytologic and histologic assessment of the resected specimen have both been used in some centers. Routine "shaving" of specimens from the margins of the resection cavity at the initial resection of cancers has been shown by some to reduce the incidence of re-excision, although the criteria for re-excision may not have been just "tumor on ink" in all cases, and it has not been shown that this procedure reduced the incidence of ipsilateral breast tumor recurrences [194].

Oncoplastic Resections

So-called oncoplastic techniques can be used to optimize the cosmetic result of breast conserving surgery (BCS) and extend BCS to patients who would otherwise need to have a total mastectomy. However, a detailed description of the many oncoplastic procedures that are used is beyond the scope of this chapter. Some surgeons use these approaches for nearly all of their BCS procedures, while others use these selectively. A number of these are based on plastic surgery methods used for reduction mammoplasty and the Wise pattern incisions often used for that procedure [127–135]. For women with sufficient breast tissue and small tumors, resections in the upper part of the breast usually have quite good results without these specialized techniques. But for larger tumors (including extensive DCIS), and especially for tumors in the lower half of the breast, oncoplastic methods can produce much better results than simple excision, allowing the breast to fill in the cavity naturally. In the lower half of the breast, excision without any reconstruction can lead to an unsatisfactory "bird beak" deformity. An example of oncoplastic resection and the outcome achievable is illustrated in Fig. 3.2. In some patients with very large or ptotic breasts, oncoplastic resection done as a reduction, with concomitant reduction of the contralateral breast, may be used with excellent outcomes and a high level of patient satisfaction (Fig. 3.3).

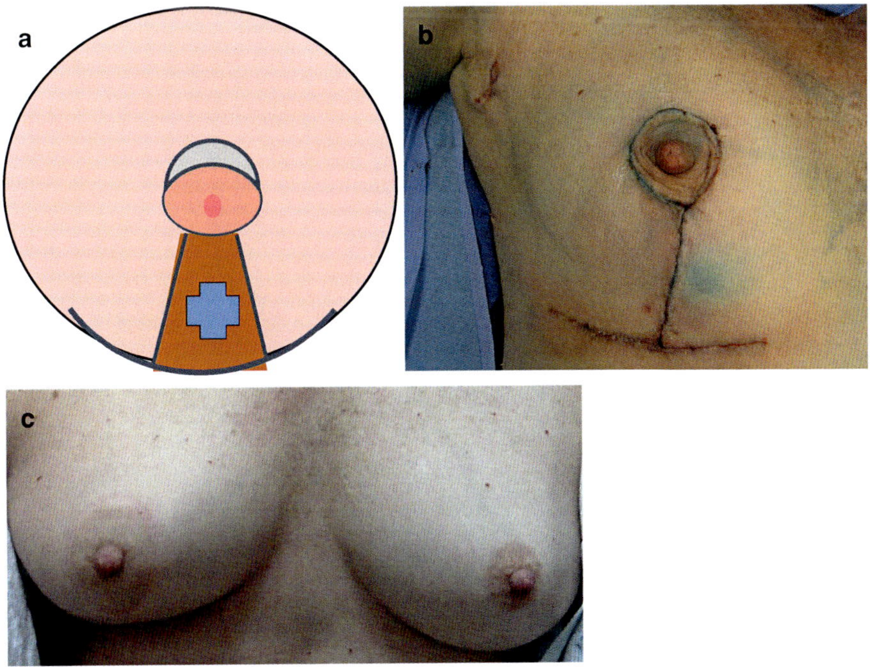

Fig. 3.2 Oncoplastic resection of cancer of lower central aspect of the breast. (**a**) Cartoon illustrating incisions (*dark blue*), tumor site (*blue cross*), resected tissue (*brown*), and de-epithelialized skin above areola (*gray crescent*). (**b**) Immediately after resection and reconstruction. (**c**) Appearance 1 year after surgery and irradiation

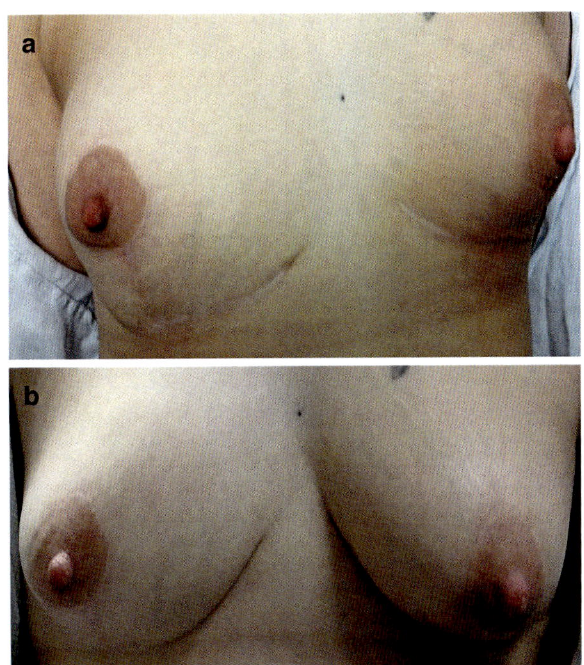

Fig. 3.3 (**a**) Result after bilateral reduction mammoplasties for ptotic breasts, including the cancer in the left breast, which is slightly hyperpigmented secondary to irradiation. Shown supine to illustrate scars. (**b**) Shown upright to illustrate cosmetic result

Total Mastectomy, with or Without Reconstruction

For patients who either choose or need to have a total or simple mastectomy, the standard incision has been to excise an ellipse of the skin centered on the nipple-areolar complex. If the patient is not undergoing immediate reconstruction, then enough skin is generally removed to allow a tension-free closure of the superior and inferior flaps, but without leaving excessive skin on the chest wall. Variations on V-Y plasties can be used to avoid excessive tissue or "dog ears" at the lateral corners [195]. However, for patients undergoing reconstruction, skin-sparing mastectomy, removing only the nipple and areola, or "total" skin-sparing or nipple-areola complex (NAC)-conserving mastectomies can be performed [196]. Preserving most or all of the skin of the breast has *not* been found to increase the risk of local recurrences significantly [196]. With appropriate patient selection, NAC-preserving mastectomies have also been found to be safe. The latter approach can be performed through a variety of incisions, including circumareolar, lateral radial, or inframammary crease, depending on the size and shape of the breast and surgeon preference. The last is perhaps the most challenging but offers excellent cosmetic outcomes. Aside from concern about recurrence, the other main concern with NAC-sparing mastectomy is the risk of nipple ischemia, which may occur in up to 5–10% of cases, depending on the approach and other factors. With careful technique and meticulous reconstruction, excellent cosmetic outcomes can be achieved (see Fig. 3.4). However, the preserved nipple will have minimal if any sensation.

Options for Reconstruction

Prosthetic Implants

For patients in whom total mastectomy is necessary or preferred by the patient, options for reconstruction may be either immediate or delayed and are performed with prosthetic implants or autologous tissue transfer [197]. The advantages of implants are that the surgery is less prolonged, as is the postoperative recovery. In most cases, this approach is started with a temporary tissue expander that has a port

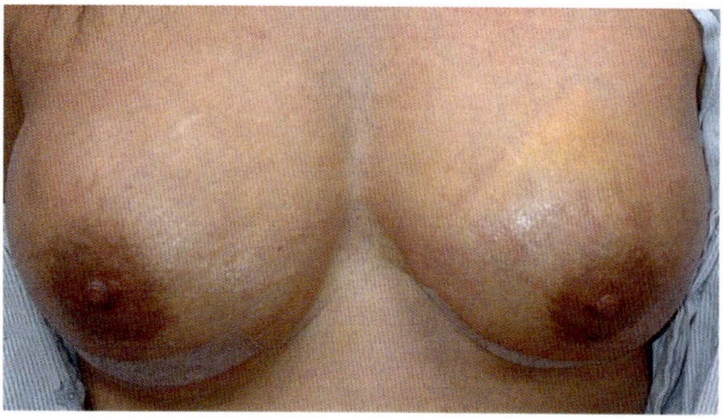

Fig. 3.4 Bilateral nipple-areolar mastectomies, performed through inframammary crease incisions, for germline genetic mutation. Photographed shortly after exchange of tissue expanders for permanent implants

and which is gradually inflated with saline over several months and then exchanged for a permanent implant. Recently, the FDA has approved a device that is inflated with CO_2 gas from a cylinder that is controlled by the patient. In some cases, immediate insertion of a permanent implant is possible. In general, these implants are placed behind the pectoralis major muscle, with or without a sling of collagen material to reinforce the inferior aspect. More recently, interest has grown in placing prosthetic implants superficial to the muscle and covered by a collagen sheet. This may give a more natural appearance and may be associated with less discomfort than stretching the pectoralis muscles with a submuscular implant. This has been made more feasible by the advent of newer devices that are semisolid rather than filled with fluid.

Autologous Tissue Reconstructions

An alternative approach to implant-based reconstruction is the transfer of the patient's own tissue from a remote site to replace the tissue lost with total mastectomy. For many years, the most common source of tissue was the lower abdominal fat and skin, rotated to the chest wall with its blood supply based on the superior epigastric vessels, along with the rectus abdominis muscle. This transverse rectus abdominis myocutaneous (TRAM) flap provided very good results, albeit at the expense of a more extensive surgical procedure and longer recovery time. The other major disadvantage was the functional deficit, making it difficult for women to sit up from a supine position, particularly with bilateral TRAMs. A number of alternatives, including myocutaneous latissimus dorsi flaps, have also been used. More recently, the trend has been to use so-called free flaps transferred with blood supply that is divided at the site of harvest and reanastomosed to vessels at the recipient site, using microvascular techniques. This requires special training and equipment, generally available only in larger hospitals. The surgery is of much longer duration, as is the recovery period; this is an obstacle to patients who have comorbidities or who want to return to full activities as quickly as possible. Nevertheless, the cosmetic results, barring significant complications, are excellent, and many patients prefer this approach, avoiding implanted artificial materials. For patients with limited skin or autologous tissue available or irradiated skin, a combination of implant and an autologous tissue flap to cover the implant with non-irradiated tissue may be used.

References

1. Moriarty AT, et al. Cytology of spontaneous nipple discharge—is it worth it? Performance of nipple discharge preparations in the College of American Pathologists Interlaboratory Comparison Program in Nongynecologic Cytopathology. Arch Pathol Lab Med. 2013;137:1039–42.
2. Kalu ON, Chow C, Wheeler A, Kong C, Wapnir I. The diagnostic value of nipple discharge cytology: breast imaging complements predictive value of nipple discharge cytology. J Surg Oncol. 2012;106:381–5.
3. Dawes LG, Bowen C, Venta LA, Morrow M. Ductography for nipple discharge: no replacement for ductal excision. Surgery. 1998;124:685–91.

4. King TA, Carter KM, Bolton JS, Fuhrman GM. A simple approach to nipple discharge. Am Surg. 2000;66:960–5.
5. Simmons R, et al. Nonsurgical evaluation of pathologic nipple discharge. Ann Surg Oncol. 2003;10:113–6.
6. Cabioglu N, et al. Surgical decision making and factors determining a diagnosis of breast carcinoma in women presenting with nipple discharge. J Am Coll Surg. 2003;196:354–64.
7. Liberman L, et al. Is surgical excision warranted after benign, concordant diagnosis of papilloma at percutaneous breast biopsy? AJR Am J Roentgenol. 2006;186:1328–34.
8. Tatarian T, et al. Intraductal papilloma with benign pathology on breast core biopsy: to excise or not? Ann Surg Oncol. 2016;23:2501–7.
9. Moon HJ, Jung I, Kim MJ, Kim EK. Breast papilloma without atypia and risk of breast carcinoma. Breast J. 2014;20:525–33.
10. Wyss P, Varga Z, Rossle M, Rageth CJ. Papillary lesions of the breast: outcomes of 156 patients managed without excisional biopsy. Breast J. 2014;20:394–401.
11. Menes TS, et al. Upgrade of high-risk breast lesions detected on mammography in the Breast Cancer Surveillance Consortium. Am J Surg. 2014;207:24–31.
12. Shamonki J, et al. Management of papillary lesions of the breast: can larger core needle biopsy samples identify patients who may avoid surgical excision? Ann Surg Oncol. 2013;20:4137–44.
13. Swapp RE, et al. Management of benign intraductal solitary papilloma diagnosed on core needle biopsy. Ann Surg Oncol. 2013;20:1900–5.
14. Wen X, Cheng W. Nonmalignant breast papillary lesions at core-needle biopsy: a meta-analysis of underestimation and influencing factors. Ann Surg Oncol. 2013;20:94–101.
15. Mansel RE, Dogliotti L. European multicentre trial of bromocriptine in cyclical mastalgia. Lancet. 1990;335:190–3.
16. Mansel RE, Wisbey JR, Hughes LE. Controlled trial of the antigonadotropin danazol in painful nodular benign breast disease. Lancet. 1982;1:928–30.
17. Pye JK, Mansel RE, Hughes LE. Clinical experience of drug treatments for mastalgia. Lancet. 1985;2:373–7.
18. Sandoval-Leon AC, Drews-Elger K, Gomez-Fernandez CR, Yepes MM, Lippman ME. Paget's disease of the nipple. Breast Cancer Res Treat. 2013;141:1–12.
19. Chen CY, Sun LM, Anderson BO. Paget disease of the breast: changing patterns of incidence, clinical presentation, and treatment in the U.S. Cancer. 2006;107:1448–58.
20. Yim JH, Wick MR, Philpott GW, Norton JA, Doherty GM. Underlying pathology in mammary Paget's disease. Ann Surg Oncol. 1997;4:287–92.
21. Helme S, Harvey K, Agrawal A. Breast-conserving surgery in patients with Paget's disease. Br J Surg. 2015;102:1167–74.
22. Siu AL, U.S. Preventive Services Task Force. Screening for breast cancer: U.S. Preventive Services Task Force recommendation statement. Ann Intern Med. 2016;164(4):279–96. Epub PMID 26757170
23. Oeffinger KC, et al. Breast cancer screening for women at average risk: 2015 guideline update from the American Cancer Society. JAMA. 2015;314:1599–614.
24. Burkett BJ, Hanemann CW. A review of supplemental screening ultrasound for breast cancer: certain populations of women with dense breast tissue may benefit. Acad Radiol. 2016;23:1604–9.
25. Melnikow J, et al. Supplemental screening for breast cancer in women with dense breasts: a systematic review for the U.S. Preventive Services Task Force. Ann Intern Med. 2016;164:268–78.
26. Hooley RJ, et al. Screening US in patients with mammographically dense breasts: initial experience with Connecticut Public Act 09-41. Radiology. 2012;265:59–69.
27. Hodgson R, et al. Systematic review of 3D mammography for breast cancer screening. Breast. 2016;27:52–61. doi:10.1016/j.breast.2016.01.002. Epub 2016 Mar 25.
28. Gilbert FJ, Tucker L, Young KC. Digital breast tomosynthesis (DBT): a review of the evidence for use as a screening tool. Clin Radiol. 2016;71:141–50.
29. Morrow M, Waters J, Morris E. MRI for breast cancer screening, diagnosis, and treatment. Lancet. 2011;378:1804–11.

30. Kuhl CK, et al. Abbreviated breast magnetic resonance imaging (MRI): first postcontrast subtracted images and maximum-intensity projection-a novel approach to breast cancer screening with MRI. J Clin Oncol. 2014;32:2304–10.
31. Mango VL, et al. Abbreviated protocol for breast MRI: are multiple sequences needed for cancer detection? Eur J Radiol. 2015;84:65–70.
32. Friese CR, Neville BA, Edge SB, Hassett MJ, Earle CC. Breast biopsy patterns and outcomes in Surveillance, Epidemiology, and End Results-Medicare data. Cancer. 2009;115:716–24.
33. Williams RT, et al. Needle versus excisional biopsy for noninvasive and invasive breast cancer: report from the National Cancer Data Base, 2003–2008. Ann Surg Oncol. 2011;18:3802–10.
34. James TA, Mace JL, Virnig BA, Geller BM. Preoperative needle biopsy improves the quality of breast cancer surgery. J Am Coll Surg. 2012;215:562–8.
35. Burkhardt JH, Sunshine JH. Core-needle and surgical breast biopsy: comparison of three methods of assessing cost. Radiology. 1999;212:181–8.
36. VandenBussche CJ, et al. Reflex estrogen receptor (ER) and progesterone receptor (PR) analysis of ductal carcinoma in situ (DCIS) in breast needle core biopsy specimens: an unnecessary exercise that costs the United States $35 million/y. Am J Surg Pathol. 2016;40:1090–9.
37. Hartmann LC, Degnim AC, Santen RJ, Dupont WD, Ghosh K. Atypical hyperplasia of the breast—risk assessment and management options. N Engl J Med. 2015;372:78–89.
38. Khan S, et al. Papillary lesions of the breast: to excise or observe? Breast J. 2017.
39. Donaldson AR, Sieck L, Booth CN, Calhoun BC. Radial scars diagnosed on breast core biopsy: frequency of atypia and carcinoma on excision and implications for management. Breast. 2016;30:201–7. doi:10.1016/j.breast.2016.06.007. Epub 2016 Jun 29.
40. Kalife ET, Lourenco AP, Baird GL, Wang Y. Clinical and radiologic follow-up study for biopsy diagnosis of radial scar/radial sclerosing lesion without other atypia. Breast J. 2016;22:637–44.
41. Leong RY, Kohli MK, Zeizafoun N, Liang A, Tartter PI. Radial scar at percutaneous breast biopsy that does not require surgery. J Am Coll Surg. 2016;223:712–6.
42. Kim EM, et al. Isolated radial scar diagnosis by core-needle biopsy: is surgical excision necessary? Springerplus. 2016;5:398. doi:10.1186/s40064-016-1993-z. eCollection 2016.
43. Bloomquist EV, et al. A randomized prospective comparison of patient-assessed satisfaction and clinical outcomes with radioactive seed localization versus wire localization. Breast J. 2016;22:151–7.
44. Langhans L, et al. Radioguided surgery for localization of nonpalpable breast lesions a mini-review. Curr Radiopharm. 2016;9:114–20.
45. Chan BK, Wiseberg-Firtell JA, Jois RH, Jensen K, Audisio RA. Localization techniques for guided surgical excision of non-palpable breast lesions. Cochrane Database Syst Rev. 2015;12:CD009206.
46. Diego EJ, et al. Localizing high-risk lesions for excisional breast biopsy: a comparison between radioactive seed localization and wire localization. Ann Surg Oncol. 2014;21:3268–72.
47. Cox CE, et al. Pilot study of a new nonradioactive surgical guidance technology for locating nonpalpable breast lesions. Ann Surg Oncol. 2016;23:1824–30.
48. Allen SS, Froberg DG. The effect of decreased caffeine consumption on benign proliferative breast disease: a randomized clinical trial. Surgery. 1987;101:720–30.
49. Gumm R, Cunnick GH, Mokbel K. Evidence for the management of mastalgia. Curr Med Res Opin. 2004;20:681–4.
50. Chase C, Wells J, Eley S. Caffeine and breast pain: revisiting the connection. Nurs Womens Health. 2011;15:286–94.
51. Horner NK, Lampe JW. Potential mechanisms of diet therapy for fibrocystic breast conditions show inadequate evidence of effectiveness. J Am Diet Assoc. 2000;100:1368–80.
52. Kaufman CS, et al. Office-based ultrasound-guided cryoablation of breast fibroadenomas. Am J Surg. 2002;184:394–400.
53. Zhao Z, Wu F. Minimally-invasive thermal ablation of early-stage breast cancer: a systemic review. Eur J Surg Oncol. 2010;36:1149–55.

54. Manenti G, et al. Percutaneous local ablation of unifocal subclinical breast cancer: clinical experience and preliminary results of cryotherapy. Eur Radiol. 2011;21:2344–53.
55. Tafra L, et al. Pilot trial of cryoprobe-assisted breast-conserving surgery for small ultrasound-visible cancers. Ann Surg Oncol. 2003;10:1018–24.
56. Khosravi-Shahi P. Management of non metastatic phyllodes tumors of the breast: review of the literature. Surg Oncol. 2011;20:e143–8.
57. Tan BY, et al. Phyllodes tumours of the breast: a consensus review. Histopathology. 2016;68:5–21.
58. Spitaleri G, et al. Breast phyllodes tumor: a review of literature and a single center retrospective series analysis. Crit Rev Oncol Hematol. 2013;88:427–36.
59. Shaaban M, Barthelmes L. Benign phyllodes tumours of the breast: (over) treatment of margins—a literature review. Eur J Surg Oncol. 2016;10. Epub PMID 27939569
60. Guillot E, et al. Management of phyllodes breast tumors. Breast J. 2011;17:129–37.
61. Chen WH, et al. Surgical treatment of phyllodes tumors of the breast: retrospective review of 172 cases. J Surg Oncol. 2005;91:185–94.
62. Kim YJ, Kim K. Radiation therapy for malignant phyllodes tumor of the breast: an analysis of SEER data. Breast. 2016;32:26–32. doi:10.1016/j.breast.2016.12.006.
63. Adesoye T, et al. Current trends in the management of phyllodes tumors of the breast. Ann Surg Oncol. 2016;23:3199–205.
64. Barth RJ Jr, Wells WA, Mitchell SE, Cole BF. A prospective, multi-institutional study of adjuvant radiotherapy after resection of malignant phyllodes tumors. Ann Surg Oncol. 2009;16:2288–94.
65. Van Zee KJ, Pérez GO, Minnard E, Cohen MA. Preoperative galactography increases the diagnostic yield of major duct excision for nipple discharge. Cancer. 1998;82:1874–80.
66. Irusen H, Rohwer AC, Steyn DW, Young T. Treatments for breast abscesses in breastfeeding women. Cochrane Database Syst Rev. 2015; doi:10.1002/14651858.CD010490.pub2.
67. Marchant DJ. Inflammation of the breast. Obstet Gynecol Clin North Am. 2002;29:89–102.
68. Giess CS, Golshan M, Flaherty K, Birdwell RL. Clinical experience with aspiration of breast abscesses based on size and etiology at an academic medical center. J Clin Ultrasound. 2014;42:513–21.
69. Lam E, Chan T, Wiseman SM. Breast abscess: evidence based management recommendations. Expert Rev Anti Infect Ther. 2014;12:753–62.
70. Wang K, Ye Y, Sun G, Xu Z. The Mammotome biopsy system is an effective treatment strategy for breast abscess. Am J Surg. 2013;205:35–8.
71. Taffurelli M, et al. Recurrent periductal mastitis: surgical treatment. Surgery. 2016;160:1689–92.
72. Lannin DR. Twenty-two year experience with recurring subareolar abscess and lactiferous duct fistula treated by a single breast surgeon. Am J Surg. 2004;188:407–10.
73. Sheybani F, Sarvghad M, Naderi HR, Gharib M. Treatment for and clinical characteristics of granulomatous mastitis. Obstet Gynecol. 2015;125:801–7.
74. Fazzio RT, Shah SS, Sandhu NP, Glazebrook KN. Idiopathic granulomatous mastitis: imaging update and review. Insights Imaging. 2016;7:531–9.
75. Benson JR, Dumitru D. Idiopathic granulomatous mastitis: presentation, investigation and management. Future Oncol. 2016;12:1381–94.
76. Gautam S, Tebo JM, Hamilton TA. IL-4 suppresses cytokine gene expression induced by IFN- gamma and/or IL-2 in murine peritoneal macrophages. J Immunol. 1992;148:1725–30.
77. Mooney KL, Bassett LW, Apple SK. Upgrade rates of high-risk breast lesions diagnosed on core needle biopsy: a single-institution experience and literature review. Mod Pathol. 2016;29:1471–84.
78. Russo IH, Russo J. Hormonal approach to breast cancer prevention. J Cell Biochem. 2000;34:1–6.
79. Chlebowski RT, Collyar DE, Somerfield MR, Pfister DG, American Society of Clinical Oncology Breast Cancer Technology Assessment Working Group. American Society of Clinical Oncology technology assessment on breast cancer risk reduction strategies: tamoxifen and raloxifene. J Clin Oncol. 1999;17:1939–55.

80. Fisher B, et al. Tamoxifen for prevention of breast cancer: report of the National Surgical Adjuvant Breast and Bowel Project P-1 Study. J Natl Cancer Inst. 1998;90:1371–88.
81. Mocellin S, Pilati P, Briarava M, Nitti D. Breast cancer chemoprevention: a network meta-analysis of randomized controlled trials. J Natl Cancer Inst. 2015;108. djv318.
82. Brem RF, et al. Lobular neoplasia at percutaneous breast biopsy: variables associated with carcinoma at surgical excision. AJR Am J Roentgenol. 2008;190:637–41.
83. Liberman L, et al. Lobular carcinoma in situ at percutaneous breast biopsy: surgical biopsy findings. AJR Am J Roentgenol. 1999;173:291–9.
84. Lehman CD, et al. MRI evaluation of the contralateral breast in women with recently diagnosed breast cancer. N Engl J Med. 2007;356:1295–303.
85. Liberman L, et al. MR imaging findings in the contralateral breast of women with recently diagnosed breast cancer. AJR Am J Roentgenol. 2003;180:333–41.
86. Esserman L, et al. Utility of magnetic resonance imaging in the management of breast cancer: evidence for improved preoperative staging. J Clin Oncol. 1999;17:110–9.
87. Mameri CS, Kemp C, Goldman SM, Sobral LA, Ajzen S. Impact of breast MRI on surgical treatment, axillary approach, and systemic therapy for breast cancer. Breast J. 2008;14:236–44.
88. Hlawatsch A, Teifke A, Schmidt M, Thelen M. Preoperative assessment of breast cancer: sonography versus MR imaging. AJR Am J Roentgenol. 2002;179:1493–501.
89. Hollingsworth AB, Stough RG, O'Dell CA, Brekke CE. Breast magnetic resonance imaging for preoperative locoregional staging. Am J Surg. 2008;196:389–97.
90. Grady I, Gorsuch-Rafferty H, Hadley P. Preoperative staging with magnetic resonance imaging, with confirmatory biopsy, improves surgical outcomes in women with breast cancer without increasing rates of mastectomy. Breast J. 2012;18:214–8.
91. Quan ML, et al. Magnetic resonance imaging detects unsuspected disease in patients with invasive lobular cancer. Ann Surg Oncol. 2003;10:1048–53.
92. Bedrosian I, et al. Changes in the surgical management of patients with breast carcinoma based on preoperative magnetic resonance imaging. Cancer. 2003;98:468–73.
93. Solin LJ, Orel SG, Hwang WT, Harris EE, Schnall MD. Relationship of breast magnetic resonance imaging to outcome after breast-conservation treatment with radiation for women with early-stage invasive breast carcinoma or ductal carcinoma in situ. J Clin Oncol. 2008;26(3):386–91.
94. Turnbull L, et al. Comparative effectiveness of MRI in breast cancer (COMICE) trial: a randomised controlled trial. Lancet. 2010;375:563–71.
95. Turnbull LW, et al. Multicentre randomised controlled trial examining the cost-effectiveness of contrast-enhanced high field magnetic resonance imaging in women with primary breast cancer scheduled for wide local excision (COMICE). Health Technol Assess. 2010;14:1–182.
96. Peters NH, et al. Preoperative MRI and surgical management in patients with nonpalpable breast cancer: the MONET—randomised controlled trial. Eur J Cancer. 2011;47:879–86.
97. Pilewskie M, et al. Effect of MRI on the management of ductal carcinoma in situ of the breast. Ann Surg Oncol. 2013;20:1522–9.
98. Carlson RW, et al. Invasive breast cancer. J Natl Compr Cancer Netw. 2011;9:136–222.
99. Gianni L, et al. Phase III trial evaluating the addition of paclitaxel to doxorubicin followed by cyclophosphamide, methotrexate, and fluorouracil, as adjuvant or primary systemic therapy: European Cooperative Trial in Operable Breast Cancer. J Clin Oncol. 2009;27:2474–81.
100. Fisher B, et al. Effect of preoperative chemotherapy on local-regional disease in women with operable breast cancer: findings from National Surgical Adjuvant Breast and Bowel Project B-18. J Clin Oncol. 1997;15:2483–93.
101. Chen AM, et al. Breast conservation after neoadjuvant chemotherapy: the MD Anderson Cancer Center experience. J Clin Oncol. 2004;22:2303–12.
102. Peintinger F, et al. The safety of breast-conserving surgery in patients who achieve a complete pathologic response after neoadjuvant chemotherapy. Cancer. 2006;107:1248–54.
103. Shen J, et al. Effective local control and long-term survival in patients with T4 locally advanced breast cancer treated with breast conservation therapy. Ann Surg Oncol. 2004;11:854–60.

104. Shin HC, et al. Breast-conserving surgery after tumor downstaging by neoadjuvant chemotherapy is oncologically safe for stage III breast cancer patients. Ann Surg Oncol. 2013;20:2582–9.
105. Wolmark N, Wang J, Mamounas E, Bryant J, Fisher B. Preoperative chemotherapy in patients with operable breast cancer: nine-year results from National Surgical Adjuvant Breast and Bowel Project B-18. J Natl Cancer Inst Monogr. 2001;30:96–102.
106. Mittendorf EA, et al. Impact of chemotherapy sequencing on local-regional failure risk in breast cancer patients undergoing breast-conserving therapy. Ann Surg. 2013;257:173–9.
107. Mauri D, Pavlidis N, Ioannidis JP. Neoadjuvant versus adjuvant systemic treatment in breast cancer: a meta-analysis. J Natl Cancer Inst. 2005;97:188–94.
108. Kaviani A, et al. From radical mastectomy to breast-conserving therapy and oncoplastic breast surgery: a narrative review comparing oncological result, cosmetic outcome, quality of life, and health economy. ISRN Oncol 2013;742462:1–6.
109. Nijenhuis MV, Rutgers EJ. Who should not undergo breast conservation? Breast. 2013;22(Suppl 2):S110–4. doi:10.1016/j.breast.2013.07.021.
110. Holland R, et al. The presence of an extensive intraductal component following limited excision correlates with prominent residual disease in the remainder of the breast. J Clin Oncol. 1990;8:113–8.
111. Schnitt SJ, Connolly JL, Harris JR, Cohen RB. Pathologic predictors of early local recurrence in stage I and II breast cancer treated by primary radiation therapy. Cancer. 1984;53:1049–57.
112. Osteen RT, Steele GD Jr, Menck HR, Winchester DP. Regional differences in surgical management of breast cancer. CA Cancer J Clin. 1992;42:39–43.
113. Osteen RT, et al. Identification of patients at high risk for local recurrence after conservative surgery and radiation therapy for stage I and II breast cancer. Arch Surg. 1987;122:1248–53.
114. Gage I, et al. Long-term outcome following breast-conserving surgery and radiation therapy. Int J Radiat Oncol Biol Phys. 1995;33:245–51.
115. Gage I, et al. Pathologic margin involvement and the risk of recurrence in patients treated with breast-conserving therapy. Cancer. 1996;78:1921–8.
116. Houssami N, et al. Meta-analysis of the impact of surgical margins on local recurrence in women with early-stage invasive breast cancer treated with breast-conserving therapy. Eur J Cancer. 2010;46:3219–32.
117. Fowble BL, et al. The influence of young age on outcome in early stage breast cancer. Int J Radiat Oncol Biol Phys. 1994;30:23–33.
118. Recht A, et al. The effect of young age on tumor recurrence in the treated breast after conservative surgery and radiotherapy. Int J Radiat Oncol Biol Phys. 1988;14:3–10.
119. Bartelink H, et al. Recurrence rates after treatment of breast cancer with standard radiotherapy with or without additional radiation. N Engl J Med. 2001;345:1378–87.
120. Bonnier P, et al. Age as a prognostic factor in breast cancer: relationship to pathologic and biologic features. Int J Cancer. 1995;62:138–44.
121. Borger J, et al. Risk factors in breast-conservation therapy. J Clin Oncol. 1994;12:653–60.
122. Mamounas EP, et al. Association between the 21-gene recurrence score assay and risk of locoregional recurrence in node-negative, estrogen receptor-positive breast cancer: results from NSABP B-14 and NSABP B-20. J Clin Oncol. 2010;28:1677–83.
123. Litiere S, et al. Breast conserving therapy versus mastectomy for stage I-II breast cancer: 20 year follow-up of the EORTC 10801 phase 3 randomised trial. Lancet Oncol. 2012;13:412–9.
124. Miles RC, et al. Local recurrence after breast-conserving surgery: multivariable analysis of risk factors and the impact of young age. Ann Surg Oncol. 2012;19:1153–9.
125. Bartelink H, et al. Impact of a higher radiation dose on local control and survival in breast-conserving therapy of early breast cancer: 10-year results of the randomized boost versus no boost EORTC 22881-10882 trial. J Clin Oncol. 2007;25:3259–65.
126. Chiba A, et al. Trends in neoadjuvant endocrine therapy use and impact on rates of breast conservation in hormone receptor-positive breast cancer: a national cancer data base study. Ann Surg Oncol. 2016;24(2):418–24. doi:10.1245/s10434-016-5733-y. Epub ahead of print.

127. Grisotti A, Calabrese C. Conservative treatment of breast cancer: reconstructive problems. In: Spear SL, Willey SC, Robb GL, Hammond DC, Nahabedian MY, editors. Surgery of the breast: principles and art. Philadelphia, PA: Lippincott, Williams & WIlkins; 2006. p. 147–78.
128. Audretsch WP. Reconstruction of the partial mastectomy defect: classification and method. In: Spear SL, Willey SC, Robb GL, Hammond DC, Nahabedian MY, editors. Surgery of the breast: principles and art. Philadelphia, PA: Lippincott, Williams & WIlkins; 2006. p. 179–216.
129. Brunnert KE. The Osnabrueck experience with reconstruction of the partial mastectomy defect. In: Spear SL, Willey SC, Robb GL, Hammond DC, Nahabedian MY, editors. Surgery of the breast: principles and art. Philadelphia, PA: Lippincott, Williams & WIlkins; 2006. p. 217–43.
130. Clough KB, et al. Oncoplastic techniques allow extensive resections for breast-conserving therapy of breast carcinomas. Ann Surg. 2003;237:26–34.
131. Clough KB, Kaufman GJ, Nos C, Buccimazza I, Sarfati IM. Improving breast cancer surgery: a classification and quadrant per quadrant atlas for oncoplastic surgery. Ann Surg Oncol. 2010;17:1375–91.
132. Down SK, Jha PK, Burger A, Hussien MI. Oncological advantages of oncoplastic breast-conserving surgery in treatment of early breast cancer. Breast J. 2013;19:56–63.
133. Fitzal F, et al. Breast-conserving therapy for centrally located breast cancer. Ann Surg. 2008;247:470–6.
134. Kronowitz SJ, et al. Practical guidelines for repair of partial mastectomy defects using the breast reduction technique in patients undergoing breast conservation therapy. Plast Reconstr Surg. 2007;120:1755–68.
135. Haloua MH, et al. A systematic review of oncoplastic breast-conserving surgery: current weaknesses and future prospects. Ann Surg. 2013;257:609–20.
136. Galimberti V, et al. Long-term follow-up of 5262 breast cancer patients with negative sentinel node and no axillary dissection confirms low rate of axillary disease. Eur J Surg Oncol. 2014;40:1203–8.
137. Krag DN, et al. Sentinel-lymph-node resection compared with conventional axillary-lymph-node dissection in clinically node-negative patients with breast cancer: overall survival findings from the NSABP B-32 randomised phase 3 trial. Lancet Oncol. 2010;11:927–33.
138. Veronesi U, et al. Sentinel lymph node biopsy in breast cancer: ten-year results of a randomized controlled study. Ann Surg. 2010;251:595–600.
139. Krag DN, et al. Technical outcomes of sentinel-lymph-node resection and conventional axillary-lymph-node dissection in patients with clinically node-negative breast cancer: results from the NSABP B-32 randomised phase III trial. Lancet Oncol. 2007;8:881–8.
140. Ashikaga T, et al. Morbidity results from the NSABP B-32 trial comparing sentinel lymph node dissection versus axillary dissection. J Surg Oncol. 2010;102:111–8.
141. Johnson CB, Boneti C, Korourian S, Adkins L, Klimberg VS. Intraoperative injection of subareolar or dermal radioisotope results in predictable identification of sentinel lymph nodes in breast cancer. Ann Surg. 2011;254:612–8.
142. Vu HN, et al. Intraoperative injection of radiocolloid for sentinel node biopsy in breast cancer. J Nucl Med Technol. 2013;41:263–7.
143. Li Q, Carr A, Ito F, Teitz-Tennenbaum S, Chang AE. Polarization effects of 4-1BB during CD28 costimulation in generating tumor-reactive T cells for cancer immunotherapy. Cancer Res. 2003;63:2546–52.
144. Giuliano AE, et al. Axillary dissection vs no axillary dissection in women with invasive breast cancer and sentinel node metastasis: a randomized clinical trial. JAMA. 2011;305:569–75.
145. Donker M, et al. Radiotherapy or surgery of the axilla after a positive sentinel node in breast cancer (EORTC 10981-22023 AMAROS): a randomised, multicentre, open-label, phase 3 non-inferiority trial. Lancet Oncol. 2014;15:1303–10.
146. Choi HY, et al. Preoperative axillary lymph node evaluation in breast cancer: current issues and literature review. Ultrasound Q. 2017;33(1):6–14.

147. Barco I, et al. Role of axillary ultrasound, magnetic resonance imaging, and ultrasound-guided fine-needle aspiration biopsy in the preoperative triage of breast cancer patients. Clin Transl Oncol. 2016;19:704–710
148. Tunon-de-Lara C, et al. The role of sentinel lymph node biopsy and factors associated with invasion in extensive dcis of the breast treated by mastectomy: the Cinnamome prospective multicenter study. Ann Surg Oncol. 2015;22:3853–60.
149. Boughey JC, et al. Sentinel lymph node surgery after neoadjuvant chemotherapy in patients with node-positive breast cancer: the ACOSOG Z1071 (Alliance) clinical trial. JAMA. 2013;310:1455–61.
150. Mamounas E, et al. Sentinel node biopsy (SNB) following neoadjuvant chemotherapy in breast cancer (BC): results from NSABP B-27. Abstracts from the Society of Surgical Oncology 54th Annual Cancer Symposium, 21; 2001. [Ref type: Abstract].
151. Kuehn T, et al. Sentinel-lymph-node biopsy in patients with breast cancer before and after neoadjuvant chemotherapy (SENTINA): a prospective, multicentre cohort study. Lancet Oncol. 2013;14:609–18.
152. Xing Y, et al. Meta-analysis of sentinel lymph node biopsy after preoperative chemotherapy in patients with breast cancer. Br J Surg. 2006;93:539–46.
153. Kelly AM, Dwamena B, Cronin P, Carlos RC. Breast cancer sentinel node identification and classification after neoadjuvant chemotherapy-systematic review and meta analysis. Acad Radiol. 2009;16:551–63.
154. van Deurzen CH, et al. Accuracy of sentinel node biopsy after neoadjuvant chemotherapy in breast cancer patients: a systematic review. Eur J Cancer. 2009;45:3124–30.
155. Hunt KK, et al. Sentinel lymph node surgery after neoadjuvant chemotherapy is accurate and reduces the need for axillary dissection in breast cancer patients. Ann Surg. 2009;250:558–66.
156. Hieken TJ, Boughey JC, Jones KN, Shah SS, Glazebrook KN. Imaging response and residual metastatic axillary lymph node disease after neoadjuvant chemotherapy for primary breast cancer. Ann Surg Oncol. 2013;20:3199–204.
157. Diego EJ, et al. Axillary staging after neoadjuvant chemotherapy for breast cancer: a pilot study combining sentinel lymph node biopsy with radioactive seed localization of pre-treatment positive axillary lymph nodes. Ann Surg Oncol. 2016;23:1549–53.
158. Caudle AS, et al. Improved axillary evaluation following neoadjuvant therapy for patients with node-positive breast cancer using selective evaluation of clipped nodes: implementation of targeted axillary dissection. J Clin Oncol. 2016;34:1072–8.
159. Mamounas EP, et al. Predictors of locoregional recurrence after neoadjuvant chemotherapy: results from combined analysis of National Surgical Adjuvant Breast and Bowel Project B-18 and B-27. J Clin Oncol. 2012;30:3960–6.
160. Liu J, et al. The role of postmastectomy radiotherapy in clinically node-positive, stage II-III breast cancer patients with pathological negative nodes after neoadjuvant chemotherapy: an analysis from the NCDB. Oncotarget. 2016;7:24848–59.
161. Chapman CH, Jagsi R. Postmastectomy radiotherapy after neoadjuvant chemotherapy: a review of the evidence. Oncology (Williston Park). 2015;29:657–66.
162. Garg AK, Buchholz TA. Influence of neoadjuvant chemotherapy on radiotherapy for breast cancer. Ann Surg Oncol. 2015;22:1434–40.
163. Holland R, Veling SH, Mravunac M, Hendriks JH. Histologic multifocality of Tis, T1-2 breast carcinomas. Implications for clinical trials of breast-conserving surgery. Cancer. 1985;56:979–90.
164. Fisher B, et al. Reanalysis and results after 12 years of follow-up in a randomized clinical trial comparing total mastectomy with lumpectomy with or without irradiation in the treatment of breast cancer. New Engl J Med. 1995;333:1456–61.
165. Fisher B, et al. Twenty-year follow-up of a randomized trial comparing total mastectomy, lumpectomy, and lumpectomy plus irradiation for the treatment of invasive breast cancer. N Engl J Med. 2002;347:1233–41.
166. Morrow M. Rethinking the local therapy of breast cancer: integration of biology and anatomy. Ann Surg Oncol. 2015;22:3168–73.

167. McKenzie-Johnson T, Grover A, Bear HD. Appropriate margin width in breast-conserving surgery. Curr Breast Cancer Rep. 2010;2:67–74.
168. Cellini C, et al. Factors associated with residual breast cancer after re-excision for close or positive margins. Ann Surg Oncol. 2004;11:915–20.
169. Zavagno G, et al. Role of resection margins in patients treated with breast conservation surgery. Cancer. 2008;112:1923–31.
170. Dillon MF, et al. Identifying patients at risk of compromised margins following breast conservation for lobular carcinoma. Am J Surg. 2006;191:201–5.
171. Smitt MC, Nowels K, Carlson RW, Jeffrey SS. Predictors of reexcision findings and recurrence after breast conservation. Int J Radiat Oncol Biol Phys. 2003;57:979–85.
172. Swanson GP, Rynearson K, Symmonds R. Significance of margins of excision on breast cancer recurrence. Am J Clin Oncol. 2002;25:438–41.
173. McCahill LE, et al. Variability in reexcision following breast conservation surgery. JAMA. 2012;307:467–75.
174. Morrow M, et al. Surgeon recommendations and receipt of mastectomy for treatment of breast cancer. JAMA. 2009;302:1551–6.
175. O'Sullivan MJ, Li T, Freedman G, Morrow M. The effect of multiple reexcisions on the risk of local recurrence after breast conserving surgery. Ann Surg Oncol. 2007;14:3133–40.
176. Moran MS, et al. Society of Surgical Oncology-American Society for Radiation Oncology consensus guideline on margins for breast-conserving surgery with whole-breast irradiation in stage I and II invasive breast cancer. Ann Surg Oncol. 2014;21:704–16.
177. Jaffre I, et al. Margin width should not still enforce a systematic surgical re-excision in the conservative treatment of early breast infiltrative ductal carcinoma. Ann Surg Oncol. 2013;20:3831–8.
178. Adams BJ, et al. The role of margin status and reexcision in local recurrence following breast conservation surgery. Ann Surg Oncol. 2013;20:2250–5.
179. Moran MS, Schnitt SJ, Giuliano AE, Harris JR, Khan SA, Horton J, et al. Society of Surgical Oncology-American Society for Radiation Oncology consensus guideline on margins for breast-conserving surgery with whole-breast irradiation in stages I and II invasive breast cancer. J Clin Oncol. 2014;32(14):1507–15.
180. Morrow M, et al. Society of Surgical Oncology-American Society for Radiation Oncology-American Society of Clinical Oncology consensus guideline on margins for breast-conserving surgery with whole-breast irradiation in ductal carcinoma in situ. Ann Surg Oncol. 2016;23:3801–10.
181. Silverstein MJ. An argument against routine use of radiotherapy for ductal carcinoma in situ. Oncology (Williston Park). 2003;17:1511–33.
182. MacDonald HR, et al. Margin width as the sole determinant of local recurrence after breast conservation in patients with ductal carcinoma in situ of the breast. Am J Surg. 2006;192:420–2.
183. Silverstein MJ, Lagios MD. Treatment selection for patients with ductal carcinoma in situ (DCIS) of the breast using the University of Southern California/Van Nuys (USC/VNPI) prognostic index. Breast J. 2015;21:127–32.
184. Henry-Tillman R, Johnson AT, Smith LF, Klimberg VS. Intraoperative ultrasound and other techniques to achieve negative margins. Semin Surg Oncol. 2001;20:206–13.
185. Cox CE, et al. Touch preparation cytology of breast lumpectomy margins with histologic correlation. Arch Surg. 1991;126:490–3.
186. Moore MM, et al. Intraoperative ultrasound is associated with clear lumpectomy margins for palpable infiltrating ductal breast cancer. Ann Surg. 2001;233:761–8.
187. Sauter ER, et al. Is frozen section analysis of reexcision lumpectomy margins worthwhile? Margin analysis in breast reexcisions. Cancer. 1994;73:2607–12.
188. Allweis TM, et al. A prospective, randomized, controlled, multicenter study of a real-time, intraoperative probe for positive margin detection in breast-conserving surgery. Am J Surg. 2008;196:483–9.
189. Nguyen FT, et al. Intraoperative evaluation of breast tumor margins with optical coherence tomography. Cancer Res. 2009;69:8790–6.

190. Rizzo M, et al. The effects of additional tumor cavity sampling at the time of breast-conserving surgery on final margin status, volume of resection, and pathologist workload. Ann Surg Oncol. 2010;17:228–34.
191. Esbona K, Li Z, Wilke LG. Intraoperative imprint cytology and frozen section pathology for margin assessment in breast conservation surgery: a systematic review. Ann Surg Oncol. 2012;19:3236–45.
192. Hequet D, Bricou A, Delpech Y, Barranger E. Surgical management modifications following systematic additional shaving of cavity margins in breast-conservation treatment. Ann Surg Oncol. 2011;18:114–8.
193. Cabioglu N, et al. Role for intraoperative margin assessment in patients undergoing breast-conserving surgery. Ann Surg Oncol. 2007;14:1458–71.
194. Chagpar AB, et al. A randomized, controlled trial of cavity shave margins in breast cancer. N Engl J Med. 2015;373:503–10.
195. Gibbs ER, Kent RB III. Modified V-Y advancement technique for mastectomy closure. J Am Coll Surg. 1998;187:632–3.
196. Hieken TJ, Boolbol SK, Dietz JR. Nipple-sparing mastectomy: indications, contraindications, risks, benefits, and techniques. Ann Surg Oncol. 2016;23:3138–44.
197. Yu P. Breast reconstruction at the MD Anderson Cancer Center. Gland Surg. 2016;5:416–21.

Breast Cancer: Overview of Decision Making by the Medical Oncologist

4

Mary Helen Hackney

Optimal management of breast cancer patients requires collaboration with surgical and radiation oncologists. Treatment planning depends on an accurate diagnosis and characterization of the cancer phenotype. Sources of information for proper treatment planning include breast imaging (bilateral mammograms supplemented by ultrasound and sometimes MRI) and careful pathologic review supported by assessment for estrogen receptor, progesterone receptor, and HER2 status. The increasing use of systemic therapy prior to definitive surgery requires medical oncology involvement in development of the initial treatment plan. Medical oncologists are responsible for chemotherapy, endocrine therapy, HER2-directed therapy, long-term care, and when necessary end-of-life care.

Breast cancer care can be broadly divided into two groups, early-stage disease and distant disease (stage 4 disease at presentation or recurrence after treatment for early-stage disease). Approximately 10% of new cases in the United States present as stage 4 disease.

There are several broad principles that should be considered in patients presenting with early breast cancer.

1. Estrogen receptor-positive cancers should always be considered for endocrine therapy.
2. Estrogen receptor-negative cancers should be considered for chemotherapy.
3. HER2-expressing cancers should be considered for trastuzumab and/or other HER2-targeted agents along with chemotherapy.
4. All patients should be evaluated for clinical research trials, if available, at each phase of their treatment [16].

These rules are just guidelines as other factors such as TNM stage impact the final treatment plans.

M.H. Hackney, MD, MS, FACP
Division of Hematology Oncology and Palliative Care, Department of Internal Medicine, Virginia Commonwealth University Health System (VCU HEALTH), Richmond, VA, USA
e-mail: mhhackne@vcu.edu

M.O. Idowu et al. (eds.), *Diagnosis and Management of Breast Tumors*,
DOI 10.1007/978-3-319-57726-5_4

Early-Stage Disease

The increased use of breast cancer screening has led to increased detection of smaller cancers. Many of the original adjuvant studies did not include patients with tumors under 1.0 cm. The use of central venous access devices and the improvement in antiemetics have made it easier to give chemotherapy. New chemotherapy and endocrine and targeted therapies are increasingly available. The challenge becomes determining who needs which treatment, how much and for how long.

Treatment planning depends on the tumor type and grade, the size of the cancer, and the extent of metastatic tumor (if any) in lymph nodes. For some patients, newer genomic-based studies may contribute information that impacts decision making, particularly the use of chemotherapy. Estrogen receptor status remains a key factor for decision making. All patients with positive estrogen receptors should be considered for endocrine therapy as a component of their systemic therapy. Generally, estrogen receptor-positive patients have a better prognosis. The higher levels of estrogen receptor expression (over 10%) probably respond better to endocrine therapy, but patients with any level of estrogen receptor staining should be considered for a trial of endocrine therapy. Estrogen receptor-negative cancers should be considered for chemotherapy.

Progesterone receptor levels are also routinely measured. A patient with an estrogen-negative/progesterone-positive tumor should be considered for endocrine therapy though these patients have a poorer prognosis than patients with estrogen- and progesterone-positive tumor [19].

HER2 expression was once considered a poor prognostic feature. However, the remarkable efficacy of trastuzumab added to systemic therapy has resulted in significant improvement in prognosis [19]. Newer studies support the addition of pertuzumab to trastuzumab for neoadjuvant and metastatic therapy regimens.

Ki-67 provides information on the proliferation status of the cancer, but the utility of the assay remains limited due to challenges in standardization of the assay. In general, lower scores, less than 15%, suggest that the patient has a less aggressive cancer. Higher scores suggest faster growth and potentially more aggressive cancers. Ongoing clinical trials are evaluating the change in Ki-67 levels during neoadjuvant endocrine treatment and attempting to standardize the assay. Sustained reduction in the Ki-67 to <10% appears to predict excellent outcomes with endocrine therapy alone.

Several genomic-based tests are available to help in decision making for stage 1 and 2 breast cancers. All breast cancer patients may derive benefit from chemotherapy to reduce the chance of recurrence. Genomic-based assays have been developed to identify those patients most likely to benefit from chemotherapy. They are most useful for the estrogen receptor-positive cancers, particularly those with minimal or no nodal involvement. They are generally not useful for patients with HER2 overexpression. Oncotype DX, MammaPrint, and Prosigna (formerly called PAM50) are three of the better known gene expression assays that provide prognostic information [13, 18, 22]. Though the three tests provide slightly different information, they all stratify patients into higher risk versus lower risk for recurrence. Oncotype DX stratifies patients into low risk, moderate risk, and high risk of recurrence [18]. Patients at low risk for recurrence should only be treated with endocrine therapy since chemotherapy does not provide significant improvement to their excellent prognosis with endocrine therapy alone. High-risk patients should be offered chemotherapy followed by endocrine therapy to give them the best opportunity for long-term survival without recurrence. The results from the TAILORx clinical trial evaluating the best treatment for moderate-risk patients should be reported in the near future. Mammaprint provides a high risk/low risk stratification.

The tumor size and the extent of lymph node involvement remain important in the treatment decision making process. Neoadjuvant endocrine and systemic therapies had previously been reserved for locally advanced and inflammatory breast cancer [11]. Based on data from several clinical trials, neoadjuvant chemotherapy can now be considered for any patient with a tumor larger than 2 cm or with biopsy-documented lymph node involvement [14]. Neoadjuvant therapy may allow the patient to have lesser surgery and have fewer nodes removed. It also demonstrates the responsiveness of the cancer to treatment. Pathologic response to treatment may be useful in determining need for additional therapy and the risk of recurrence.

Patient Discussions

Education and collaboration are keys to identifying optimal therapy for a breast cancer patient. Once a diagnosis has been established with characterization of the phenotype and the proper imaging has been completed, the medical oncologist and the patient are ready to begin the interactive process that will determine the systemic treatment plan. Sometimes this will begin after a patient has surgery and the pathologic stage is known. A critical aspect of these discussions is helping patients understand their risk of disease recurrence balanced against the potential side effects of the therapies. Patients with comorbid conditions including complications of advanced age, renal failure, or liver failure may not be able to tolerate some therapies. A clear discussion of side effects and providing the patient with information that can be reviewed again at home help with patient and caregiver understanding. Online models such as Adjuvant! Online can be useful to visually demonstrate the risks of recurrence and the benefits of treatment. However, a challenge to use of these tools is the need for updating as new information becomes available. Adjuvant! Online also does not incorporate data on HER2 status in its current model.

Professional societies and organizations have increasingly provided guidelines for treatment. One of the more important organizations is the NCCN which has established programs for developing and updating treatment algorithms for most cancers. Information is available both for clinicians and patients [16]. The breast cancer algorithms are comprehensive and are frequently updated. ASCO guidelines are not as comprehensive but also include many guides for supportive care such as antiemetic use and growth factor use.

Women of childbearing potential who wish to optimize the possibility of pregnancy following systemic cancer therapies need referral to a fertility specialist for discussion about treatment options. Chemotherapy may cause early menopause with permanent ovarian failure. Long-term endocrine therapy may impact decision making about pregnancy following the treatment for cancers.

During treatment it is important to emphasize global patient health and wellness particularly for those women who have an excellent prognosis. Patients should be encouraged to exercise and stay active. Although tobacco is not directly linked to breast cancer, counseling for tobacco cessation should be offered as part of good global health practice. It is often difficult to lose weight during treatment for breast cancer. Women should be encouraged to seek a healthy weight as part of their long-term survival plan. Comprehensive care requires programs to provide support for patients during and after cancer treatment. Nutrition classes should be available on a regular basis with individual counseling if possible. Lymphedema management should be available to all patients who have had nodal surgery or irradiation. Counseling and guidance for navigating the financial challenges of cancer management are essential. A process for directing patients to legal support is important particularly for help with medical directives, wills, guardianship, and job discrimination during and after the treatment. Medical patient education is a very important piece of comprehensive patient care. An educated patient and caregiver team will be better equipped to face the rigors of treatment with greater confidence and assurance.

Endocrine Therapy

Endocrine therapy is the oldest systemic therapy for breast cancer. The original treatments with bilateral oophorectomies and adrenalectomies have been replaced by medications that interfere with the estrogen receptor function or block postmenopausal estrogen production. Tamoxifen, a selective estrogen receptor modulator, is approved for use at any age and at any stage and can be used for both male and female breast cancers. The side effects include hot flashes, a risk of deep vein thrombosis, and a rare risk of uterine cancer. The third-generation aromatase inhibitors (anastrozole, letrozole, exemestane) are also approved for any stage of estrogen-positive breast cancer [5, 6]. These medications are only effective if the ovaries are nonfunctioning either in natural menopause or in women with premature ovarian failure due to chemotherapy or oophorectomies. There is a slight benefit to using aromatase inhibitors rather than tamoxifen in postmenopausal women. Side effects can include diffuse arthralgia, hair thinning, and bone loss. Compliance can be an issue if the side effects of hormonal therapy are intolerable. Clinicians need to monitor compliance and work with patients to find suitable interventions or change the medication to support compliance with treatment.

Ovarian ablation either by use of LHRH (luteinizing hormone-releasing hormone) analogs or surgery can improve outcomes in premenopausal women with high-risk, estrogen-positive, early-stage disease when administered with an aromatase inhibitor or tamoxifen. Ovarian ablation is also indicated for premenopausal women with estrogen receptor-positive, recurrent breast cancer. Oophorectomies also reduce the risk of ovarian cancer in women who have tested positive for deleterious BRCA gene mutations.

Other hormonal therapies with specific breast cancer indications are fulvestrant and toremifene. Historically, megestrol acetate, estrogen, and halotestin were used for metastatic disease. They are no longer available or have been surpassed by the newer agents such as fulvestrant.

The standard duration for endocrine therapy in early-stage disease is 5 years. Several studies now support the use of hormonal therapy for 10 years. Ten-year data is available for tamoxifen and anastrozole and the combination of 5 years of tamoxifen and letrozole [10]. Long-term risks and side effects must be weighed against benefits.

Chemotherapy

The first successful chemotherapy regimen to gain widespread use was CMF (cyclophosphamide, methotrexate, and 5-fluorouracil). This regimen is still in use but has been supplanted by the combinations of anthracyclines and taxanes. Cyclophosphamide remains the backbone of many regimens. Platinums, particularly carboplatin, have a role in triple-negative breast cancer and HER2-positive treatment regimens.

Several guidelines are available to use for decision making and to provide information regarding the different regimens. Chemotherapy can be given after definitive surgery or as neoadjuvant therapy prior to surgery. Patients with locally advanced or inflammatory breast cancer should always have chemotherapy prior to surgery. Increasingly chemotherapy is used in the neoadjuvant setting for patients with biopsy-proven positive lymph nodes or larger, palpable tumors [11].

Patients with HER2-positive cancers should have trastuzumab added to the chemotherapy regimen [21]. Pertuzumab is approved for administration with trastuzumab and chemotherapy in the neoadjuvant setting. The dual HER2 blockade with both trastuzumab and pertuzumab in the neoadjuvant setting provides an increased response to treatment [9]. The most common chemotherapy combinations with HER2-targeted therapy are carboplatin and docetaxel or anthracycline, cyclophosphamide, and weekly paclitaxel.

The use of antiemetic medications and white cell growth factors has made the administration of chemotherapy safer and easier for patients. Breast cancer chemotherapy is administered in an outpatient setting. Rarely are patients admitted. The most common reason for admission is fever with neutropenia.

Side effects of treatment can be challenging. Hair loss is common and may be emotionally troubling. There are several methods using cold that might reduce hair loss but these can be costly and burdensome. Hair usually returns, but in some women it may be thinner or minimal. Neuropathy is common with the use of taxanes. Dose adjustment may be necessary. The neuropathy usually presents as a "pins and needles" feeling in the fingertips and toes. Recovery may take months with the toes often the slowest to fully recover. The neuropathy may cause pain as well as numbness which can compromise the ability to work or do some tasks. Medications to relieve neuropathic discomfort may be required. One of the most challenging side effects is cognitive dysfunction associated with chemotherapy, also known as "chemo brain" or "chemo fog". High-functioning patients are most likely to notice the challenge to short-term memory, name recall, and slowness of learning new material. Generally, this improves over time. Good sleep and limits to multitasking may help. Sometimes it is useful to refer patients for neurocognitive testing. Cardiomyopathy and heart failure can develop after anthracycline chemotherapy or trastuzumab. Left chest radiation therapy may also be an additive factor. There are guidelines regarding cardiac function monitoring before, during and after treatment. This may help detect early dysfunction prior to symptoms. Referral to a cardiologist, particularly one familiar with chemotherapy agents, may be helpful. Bone marrow failure or acute leukemia is very rare but can be seen as a consequence of chemotherapy particularly the anthracyclines and to a lesser extent cyclophosphamide. Acute leukemias following chemotherapy have poorer outcomes as compared to de novo acute leukemia.

Breast Cancer Risk Reduction: Atypical Ductal Hyperplasia and Ductal Carcinoma In Situ

The increased use of routine mammography screening has led to the discovery of many breast lesions that are not invasive cancer. The question is whether there are interventions that can reduce or prevent women from getting breast cancer especially if there are non-cancerous changes found in the breasts. Approximately one in eight women will develop breast cancer over their lifetime. Lifestyle risk reduction strategies include limitation of alcohol consumption, maintenance of appropriate body weight, and no use or very limited use of hormone replacement therapy. Although there is a big market for special diets and supplements to reduce cancer risks, the data to support these is weak. Two large national trials demonstrated the efficacy of tamoxifen and raloxifene as risk reduction agents (chemoprevention) in women who meet a certain level of risk as determined by the Gail Model [7, 26]. The Gail Model is a breast cancer risk calculator utilizing current age, age of menarche, number of prior breast biopsies, and the presence of atypical ductal hyperplasia in prior breast biopsies to determine a woman's lifetime risk for breast cancer. Women who have a 5-year risk level of 1.66% or higher can be considered for tamoxifen or raloxifene. Both are selective estrogen receptor modulators with slightly different side effect profiles. Although the data has been available for years, fewer women than expected have chosen to start one of these medications. The side effect risks as compared to the relatively low risk of breast cancer have discouraged many women from taking these medications. Even so, women with a new diagnosis of atypical ductal hyperplasia should have a discussion with a medical oncologist or other clinician who can review the risk calculator and discuss the pros and cons of risk reduction therapy [24].

Ductal carcinoma in situ is currently treated with segmental mastectomy and radiation therapy or if extensive with a mastectomy. There may be a subsegment of patients who can just have local excision without radiation therapy. Since DCIS is considered a high risk for the development of additional DCIS lesions or invasive cancer in the ipsilateral and contralateral breast, these patients should be considered for discussions about chemoprevention to reduce the risk of developing breast cancer. Trials have shown risk reduction with endocrine therapies in DCIS is limited to women with estrogen receptor-positive DCIS [8]. Only patients with estrogen-positive disease should be considered for endocrine-based chemoprevention. Patients who opt for bilateral mastectomies have no significant residual breast tissue, so they are not candidates for chemoprevention. Patients who have had a segmental mastectomy or have an intact contralateral breast after unilateral mastectomy can be considered for either tamoxifen or anastrozole. Tamoxifen has been the longest used drug for risk reduction. Two studies have demonstrated that aromatase inhibitors are slightly more effective than tamoxifen as a breast cancer risk reduction agent. The decision to use one or the other is based on menopausal state and a discussion about side effects and tolerability.

Special Populations

Age

There are no upper age limits for administration of chemotherapy in early breast cancer. Consideration for chemotherapy in the elderly requires careful discussion regarding the risk of distant recurrence weighed against the benefit of locoregional therapy only and the impact on the quality of life, the comorbidities and the performance status. The patient who is more likely to die of comorbid conditions within a few years should be spared the side effects of chemotherapy. Unfortunately elderly patients have been underrepresented in clinical trials due to limitations on age and comorbidities.

The aromatase inhibitors have a significant risk of arthralgias that in conjunction with arthritis pain may compromise a patient's quality of life and functional status. Aromatase inhibitors also impact bone health, and a patient with significant osteoporosis may need to be evaluated for alternative endocrine therapy. Risk of serious bone fractures in the elderly can be more important than a low risk of cancer recurrence [1].

Pregnancy

Breast cancer occurs in about 1 out of 3000 pregnancies. Women are usually in their early 30s. Diagnosis may be delayed or complicated by the pregnancy-induced breast changes. Mastitis and inflammatory breast cancer can look very similar until the inflammatory changes do not respond to antibiotics.

Radiology imaging is limited particularly in the first trimester. Ultrasound is the preferred imaging modality and biopsies can be performed under ultrasound guidance. Clinical exam is important, but it may be difficult in the pregnant breast. When the diagnosis is made, the medical oncologist and the support team need to have an informed discussion with the patient about the treatment choices. As with all patients, the choices will be based in part on the breast cancer characteristics. It is important to have an obstetrician with high-risk pregnancy training involved to help with decision making and support. Beyond the first trimester, women can receive chemotherapy and maintain their pregnancy. Pregnant women should be referred for genetic counseling since the results may impact future surgical and long-term decisions.

Neoadjuvant chemotherapy can be safely given starting in the second trimester. Anthracyclines and cyclophosphamide are the backbones of neoadjuvant therapy and have not been shown to affect fetal development. Cardiac assessment is required due to the risk of cardiomyopathy with both pregnancy and anthracyclines. There is less data on the safety of taxanes and carboplatin on fetal development, but both have been used. Methotrexate and endocrine therapy are absolutely contraindicated. White cell growth factors have limited safety data. Of note, most pregnancy-associated breast cancers are estrogen receptor negative. Limited data is available about the safety of trastuzumab although at least one case report raises concerns about safety of the fetus (changes reported in the amniotic fluid). The goal of any pregnancy is the delivery of a healthy baby as close to term as possible. The obstetrician should monitor fetal growth at regular intervals during the treatment. If changes occur, then discussions timing of delivery will need to occur. Generally, the chemotherapy agents used during pregnancy do not cause significant thrombocytopenia or anemia. The counts recover quickly with the cessation of chemotherapy to make delivery safer.

With the use of neoadjuvant chemotherapy, women can continue a pregnancy to term prior to surgery. Her surgical options will be the same as a nonpregnant patient with the same stage. Since the baby will be delivered before surgery, she is able to receive radiation therapy if required as part of her treatment. Hormonal-based therapy, if appropriate, can be delayed until after delivery.

Pregnancy After Breast Cancer Treatment

Breast cancer is relatively uncommon in women of childbearing age, but women who develop breast cancer prior to childbearing may desire pregnancy after treatment for early breast cancer. Retrospective studies have not demonstrated an increased risk of recurrent breast cancer if a woman chooses to become pregnant after completing her cancer treatment. Women should not be on tamoxifen if they wish to attempt pregnancy. There are no clear guidelines, but some physicians suggest that patients wait a minimum of 2 years after treatment before attempting pregnancy. The remaining degree of risk for recurrence will vary widely based on the phenotype and stage of the initial cancer, in conjunction with the time since initial treatment. It is important for medical oncologists to help the patient understand the degree of residual risk, but ultimately the decision to have another child must be made by the individual woman.

Stage 4 or Metastatic Disease

Approximately 10% of US patients present with metastatic disease at the time of diagnosis. A number of women will develop their metastatic disease following initial treatment for early-stage disease. Breast cancers recur over a wide range of time, in some case up to 20 years after the initial diagnosis. A biopsy should be done for any suspected recurrence. It is important to confirm if it is really a breast cancer recurrence or a different cancer. Repeat biomarker studies should be performed to include the estrogen receptor, progesterone receptor and the Her2 expression. Recurrent breast cancers may have changes in these profile markers that could impact treatment decisions [20].

Treatment for recurrent cancer generally is more individualized than early-stage disease. Clinical trials, if available, should be considered throughout the treatment process. Endocrine therapies are generally the initial therapy for estrogen receptor-positive patients. However, if there is significant visceral disease, then chemotherapy may be considered first for a more rapid response to then be followed by endocrine therapy. Endocrine therapies are now often combined with newer agents that target specific growth pathways. Palbociclib, an inhibitor of cell proliferation, and everolimus [25], an mTor inhibitor that works at the master switch of cell growth, are two examples of newer agents that substantially improve disease-free progression when combined with endocrine therapy. Multiple lines of these therapies can be employed until the cancer becomes refractory to endocrine therapies which require switching to chemotherapy.

Patients with estrogen-negative recurrent cancers are ideal candidates for clinical trials evaluating newer agents. If trials are not available, then single agent chemotherapy is preferred. Although doublets may have some limited use, they generally have more toxicity. There are multiple drugs that may have some activity in recurrent breast cancer. The number of lines is dependent on performance status, prior response to treatment, and patient desires. Generally as the line of chemotherapies increases, the likelihood of a significant effect diminishes steadily.

Recurrent breast cancer is not generally considered curable. One exception is a local recurrence in a previously treated breast or chest wall following mastectomy. There may be some other situations of isolated metastasis that can be focally treated. It is important for the clinician to discuss the goals of care and end-of-life decisions with all patients but particularly those with metastatic disease. The discussions may evolve as the disease evolves. Since recurrence is generally not curable, the patient and their support system need to be involved in decisions regarding the balance of treatment and its side effects versus quality of life versus chance to prolong life. It is important for the patient not to feel abandoned when the decisions to stop anticancer therapies are made. Supportive care and palliative care services can provide symptom management and help with the transition to hospice care.

References

1. ASCO Guidelines—Geriatric Oncology. n.d.
2. ASCO Guidelines on Survivorship Care. n.d.
3. ASCO Guidelines: Hormone Use. n.d.
4. Baum M. Adju vant endocrine therapy in postmenopausal women with early breast cancer: where are we now. Lancet. 2002;359:2131–9.
5. Coates A. Letrozole compared with tamoxifen as initial adjuvant therapy for breast cancer. J Clin Oncol. 2007;25(15):2148.
6. Cuzick J, Sestak I. Effect of anastrozole and tamoxifen as adjuvant treatment for early-stage breast cancer: 10 year analysis of the ATAC trial. Lancet Oncol. 2010;11(12):1135–41.

7. Fisher B, Costantino JP, Wickerham DL, Redmond CK, Kavanah M, Cronin WM, et al. Tamoxifen for prevention of breast cancer: report of the National Surgical Adjuvant Breast and Bowel Project P-1 Study. J Natl Cancer Inst. 1998;90(18):1371–88.
8. Forbes JF, Sestak I, Howell A, Bonanni B, Bundred N, Levy C, et al. Anastrozole versus tamoxifen for the prevention of locoregional and contralateral breast cancer in postmenopausal women with locally excised ductal carcinoma in situ (IBIS-II DCIS): a double-blind, randomised controlled trial. Lancet. 2016;387:866–73.
9. Gianni L, Pienkowski T, Im YH, Roman L, Tseng LM, Liu MC, et al. Efficacy and safety of neoadjuvant pertuzumab and trastuzumab in women with locally advanced, inflammatory, or early HER2-positive breast cancer (NeoSphere): a randomized multicentre, open-label, phase 2 trial. Lancet Oncol. 2012;13:25–32.
10. Goss P. Preventing relapse beyond 5 years: the MA, 17 extended adjuvant trial. Semin Oncol. 2006;33(2 Suppl 7):S8–12.
11. Gralow J. Preoperative therapy in invasive breast cancer: pathologic assessment and systemic therapy issues in operable disease. J Clin Oncol. 2008;26(5):814–9.
12. Khatcheressian J. Breast cancer follow-up and management after primary treatment: American Society of Clinical Oncology clinical practice guideline update. J Clin Oncol. 2013;31(7):961–5.
13. Knauer M. The predictive value of the 70-gene signature for adjuvant chemotherapy in early breast cancer. Breast Cancer Res Treat. 2010;120(3):655–61.
14. Mauri D. Neoadjuvant versus adjuvant systemic treatment in breast cancer: a meta-analysis. J Natl Cancer Inst. 2005;97(3):188–94.
15. Monnier AM. The Breast International Group 1-98 trial: big results for women with hormone-sensitive early breast cancer. Expert Rev Anticancer Ther. 2007;7(5):627–34.
16. Gradishar W, Salerno KE. NCCN Guidelines Update: Breast cancer. J Natl Compr Cancer Netw. 2016;14(5 Suppl):641–4.
17. National Cancer Institute: Breast Cancer. https://www.cancer.gov/types/breast/hp/breast-treatment-pdq. (Accessed on June 12, 2017).
18. Paik S, Shak S, Tang G, Kim C, Baker J, Cronin M, et al. A multigene assay to predict recurrence of tamoxifen-treated, node-negative breast cancer. N Engl J Med. 2004;351(27):2817–26.
19. Purdie C, Quinlan P, Jordan L, Ashfield A, Ogston S, Dward J, et al. Progesterone receptor expression is an independent prognostic variable in early breast cancer: a population-based study. Br J Cancer. 2014;110(3):565–72.
20. Simmons C, Miller N, Geddie W, Gianfelice D, Oldfield M, Dranistsaris G, et al. Does confirmatory tumor biopsy alter the management of breast cancer patients with distant metases? Ann Oncol. 2009;20(9):1499–504.
21. Slamon D, Eiermann W, Robert N, Pienkowski T, Martin M, Press M, et al. Adjuvant trastuzumab in HER2—positive breast cancer. N Engl J Med. 2011;365(14):1273–83.
22. Sparano JA, Gray RJ, Makower DF, Pritchard KI, Albain KS, Hayes DF, et al. Prospective validation of a 21-gene expression assay in breast cancer. N Engl J Med. 2015;373(21):2005–14.
23. Virnig B, Tuttle T, Shamliyan T, Kane R. Ductal carcinoma in situ of the breast: a systematic review of incidence, treatment, and outcomes. J Natl Cancer Inst. 2010;102(3):170–8.
24. Visvanathan K, Hurley P, Bantug E, Brown P, Col NF, Cuzick J, et al. Use of Pharmacologic Interventions for Breast Cancer Risk Reduction: American Society of Clinical Oncology Clinical Practice Guideline. J Clin Oncol. 2013;31(23):2942–62.
25. Yardley DA, Noguchi S, Pritchard KI, Burris HA 3rd, Baselga J, Gnant M, et al. Everolimus plus exemestane in postmenopausal patients with HR+ breast cancer: BOLERO-2 final progression-free survival analysis. Adv Ther. 2013;30:870–84.
26. Wickerman DL, Costantino JP, Vogel V, Cronin R, Cecchini J. The study of tamoxifen and raloxifene (STAR): Initial findings from the NSABP P-2 breast cancer prevention study. J Clin Oncol 24, no. 18 suppl.

5 Overview of Radiation Oncology Evaluation and Management of Breast Tumors

Todd C. Adams, Nicholas Serrano, Christopher Chipko, and Douglas W. Arthur

Radiation therapy is indicated as part of the standard of care treatment for the majority of patients with breast cancer. Large clinical trials evaluating the efficacy of radiation treatment for breast cancer date back more than a half century. This chapter discusses the indications for adjuvant radiation therapy for ductal carcinoma in situ and invasive breast cancer. It explores the data supporting the indications for radiation therapy and the benefit of radiation therapy in various clinical settings. Also discussed are the role of regional nodal irradiation, the indications for shorter radiation treatment schedules, and the benefit of a radiation boost. This chapter further addresses the role of partial breast irradiation, and lastly, it discusses the clinical scenarios where omission of radiation may be considered. The role of radiation in treating breast angiosarcomas and malignant phyllodes tumors is not addressed here because these topics are more appropriately discussed in the context of the management of sarcomas.

Ductal Carcinoma In Situ (DCIS)

Local Management Options

Breast-conserving surgery alone, breast-conserving surgery followed by partial-breast irradiation, breast-conserving surgery followed by whole-breast radiotherapy, and mastectomy

T.C. Adams, MD (✉) • N. Serrano, MD • C. Chipko, MD • D.W. Arthur, MD
Department of Radiation Oncology, Virginia Commonwealth University Health (VCU HEALTH), Richmond, VA, USA
e-mail: todd.adams@vcuhealth.org; serranona@vcu.edu; chipkocr@vcu.edu; douglas.arthur@vcuhealth.org

M.O. Idowu et al. (eds.), *Diagnosis and Management of Breast Tumors*,
DOI 10.1007/978-3-319-57726-5_5

Ideal Candidate for Breast-Conserving Treatment

The ideal candidate for breast-conserving treatment is a patient with a unifocal, less than 5 cm breast tumor resected with negative margins at least 2 mm margins for DCIS. The tumor size should be relatively small in comparison to the breast size such that a good postsurgical cosmetic outcome can be achieved. The ideal candidate would be nonpregnant and absent of a history of scleroderma or lupus skin involvement.

Indications for Radiation

Local management decisions for DCIS are influenced by patient preference, patient age, tumor size, tumor grade, and the ability of the resection to achieve both a negative surgical margin and acceptable cosmetic result. Pure DCIS is an in-breast control issue as it lacks the ability to metastasize and therefore has no bearing on overall survival if properly managed. The addition of adjuvant radiation improves local control for all subsets of DCIS patients treated with breast-conserving surgery with no impact on overall survival. The decision to add postoperative radiotherapy is principally a relative risk reduction of in-breast failure (recurrence in the treated breast). Therefore, as the age of the presenting patient becomes younger and the tumor features become more threatening, the risk of in-breast failure following lumpectomy increases and the recommendation for postoperative radiotherapy becomes stronger. General guidelines governing recommendations are as follows: Omission of radiation should be considered as an appropriate option for those women aged 60 and older who receive endocrine therapy; have a small (<2 cm), low- or intermediate-grade, estrogen receptor-positive tumor resected with wide (>2 mm) surgical margins; and have a sufficiently small in-breast recurrence rate without adjuvant radiotherapy, assuming the patient has been informed and accepts the relatively small increase in disease recurrence. For those women presenting with more significant features (who have estrogen-negative disease, who have estrogen-positive disease but are not undergoing endocrine therapy, who are less than 60 years old and have tumors larger than 2 cm, grade 3 tumors, and/or tumors resected with <2 mm margins), the risk of in-breast failure is sufficiently higher that postoperative radiotherapy is considered the standard of care and should be strongly considered. Postmastectomy radiation for DCIS is generally not indicated.

Benefit of Radiation

Adjuvant radiation significantly improves local control but does not affect breast cancer-specific survival or overall survival.

Absolute Radiation Contraindications

Radiation therapy during pregnancy

Relative Contraindications

Active scleroderma or lupus involving the skin, focally positive surgical margin, close surgical margin (1 mm or less), known BRCA1/BRCA2 mutation, and previous radiation therapy to the breast or chest wall

Radiation Technique

Radiation may be given to the *whole breast with standard fractionation* (50 Gy in 25 fractions) or *hypofractionation* (42.56 Gy in 16 fractions). A boost is typically recommended, but omission can be considered for patients aged 60 or older with low volume disease resected with acceptable surgical margins. In appropriately selected patients, radiation may be given to a partial-breast target with *accelerated partial-breast irradiation* (APBI). Patient selection guidelines for APBI use with DCIS are available from several societies [1–3]. APBI can be delivered with *brachytherapy*, 34 Gy in ten fractions given twice daily, or *highly conformal external beam irradiation*, 38.5 Gy in ten fractions given twice daily.

Factors for Consideration

Patient age, patient life expectancy, comorbidities which may increase the risk of complications, tumor size, margin width, tumor grade, tumor histology (i.e., comedonecrosis), hormone receptor status, cosmetic result, and patient expectations

Selected Studies

Mastectomy vs. Breast-Conserving Therapy

There are no DCIS randomized trials comparing mastectomy and breast-conserving therapy (local resection plus radiation). The equivalency of mastectomy and breast-conserving therapy in DCIS can be extrapolated from the rich invasive breast cancer literature comparing these two modalities. Postmastectomy radiation for DCIS is generally not indicated. Breast-conserving surgery followed by adjuvant radiation is a standard-of-care option for the treatment for DCIS. Data supporting the recommendation for postoperative radiation therapy comes from four randomized trials. In sum, these trials showed that adjuvant whole-breast irradiation reduced ipsilateral breast tumor recurrence by approximately 50% compared to observation; overall survival was not improved with radiation.

The National Surgical Adjuvant Breast and Bowel Project (NSABP) B-17 trial randomized 818 patients with DCIS to lumpectomy plus adjuvant radiation or lumpectomy alone [4, 5]. Patients were required to have negative surgical margins, and radiation was delivered to the whole breast to a dose of 50 Gy in 25 fractions without a boost. At a 15-year follow-up, radiation significantly reduced the rate of ipsilateral breast tumor recurrence from 35.0% in the lumpectomy alone group to 19.8% in the lumpectomy plus adjuvant radiation group (HR 0.48; $P < 0.001$). The decrease in local recurrence was for both invasive and noninvasive recurrences.

The European Organization for Research and Treatment of Cancer (EORTC) produced similar results in their EORTC 10853 trial where they randomized 1010 patients with DCIS to lumpectomy or lumpectomy plus radiation [6]. As in NSABP-B17, patients were required to have clear surgical margins and a radiation dose of 50 Gy in 25 fractions was delivered to the whole breast. While a boost was not recommended, 5% of patients received a tumor bed boost. At 15 years, there was a significant reduction in local recurrences with the addition of radiation therapy, from 31% with lumpectomy alone to 18% with lumpectomy plus radiation (HR 0.52; $P < 0.001$). Subgroup analysis showed there was a benefit of radiation in all subgroups.

The SweDCIS Trial randomized 1067 patients with DCIS to lumpectomy or lumpectomy plus radiation [7]. In this study, patients underwent sector resection which required 1 cm gross surgical margins; microscopically clear margins were not required. Although most patients received conventional radiation of 50 Gy in 25 fractions to the whole breast, a split course of 54 Gy in 28 fractions with a mid-treatment 2-week break was allowed. No boost was allowed. At 20-year follow-up, the ipsilateral breast event cumulative risk was 20.0% in the radiation arm and 32.0% in the lumpectomy alone arm ($P < 0.001$). Subgroup analysis showed that for patients with tumors 14 mm or smaller with negative surgical margins, there was no statistical difference in breast events between lumpectomy plus radiation and lumpectomy alone.

The UK Coordinating Committee on Cancer Research collaborated with Australia and New Zealand to conduct the UK/ANZ DCIS trial which incorporated a 2 × 2 factorial design to evaluate the benefit of the adjuvant radiation, tamoxifen, or both to breast-conserving surgery [8]. After undergoing lumpectomy with negative margins, patients were randomized to observation, radiation alone, tamoxifen alone, or radiation plus tamoxifen. Randomization was independently performed for radiation and tamoxifen, or the surgeon selected one treatment modality with randomization to the other modality. Radiation was given to the whole breast to a dose of 50 Gy in 25 fractions without a boost. Tamoxifen was given 20 mg daily. After 12.7-year median follow-up of 1071 patients, post-lumpectomy radiation reduced all ipsilateral breast events from 19.4% in patients treated without radiation to 7.1% in patients treated with radiation (HR 0.32; $P < 0.0001$). Radiation reduced ipsilateral invasive disease and ipsilateral DCIS but had no effect on contralateral breast events. The benefit of radiation was irrespective of tamoxifen use. Tamoxifen reduced the incidence of recurrent ipsilateral DCIS and contralateral breast cancer but did not have a significant effect on ipsilateral invasive disease.

At least two meta-analyses have established the role of adjuvant radiation in the treatment of DCIS. In 2010, an Early Breast Cancer Trialists' Collaborative Group (EBCTCG) meta-analysis of 3729 DCIS patients treated with breast-conserving surgery showed that adjuvant radiation compared to observation provided a significant reduction in 10-year ipsilateral breast events from 28.1% without radiation to 12.9% with radiation ($p < 0.00001$) [9]. The benefit was significant regardless of age of the patient, extent of breast-conserving surgery, tamoxifen use, negative versus positive margins, unifocal versus multifocal disease, nuclear grade, presence of comedonecrosis, tumor architecture, or tumor size. The proportional benefit was greater in women aged 50 or older compared to women younger than age 50, but otherwise did not differ with any other evaluable factors. Even for women with small, low-grade tumors resected to negative margins, adjuvant radiation reduced the 10-year risk of ipsilateral breast tumor recurrence from 30.1 to 12.1%.

A Cochrane Database review of the four randomized trials mentioned above confirmed a statistically significant benefit of the addition of adjuvant radiation therapy on ipsilateral recurrent DCIS (HR 0.61; $P = 0.03$), ipsilateral recurrent invasive cancer (HR 0.50; $P = 0.001$), and all ipsilateral breast events (HR 0.49; $P < 0.00001$) [10]. On multivariate analysis, there were no subgroups which did not benefit from the addition of radiation, regardless of completeness of excision, patient age, size of the primary lesion, or the presence or absence of comedonecrosis.

Omission of Adjuvant Radiation in DCIS

Multiple studies have examined the safety of omission of radiation in subsets of DCIS patients. Collectively, these studies show that adjuvant radiation significantly reduces the risk of in-breast failure for all subsets of patients. However, for patients aged 60 and older who receive endocrine therapy and have a small (<2 cm), low- or intermediate-grade, estrogen receptor-positive tumor resected with wide (>2 mm) surgical margins, the risk of in-breast recurrence may be sufficiently low that adjuvant radiation may be avoided if the patient accepts the increased risk of recurrence.

The Van Nuys Prognostic Index uses tumor size, margin width, and pathologic classification as predictors of local recurrence of DCIS to create a score which predicts the risk of local recurrence and the benefit of adjuvant radiation [11, 12]. The scores are used to make treatment recommendations regarding surgery and radiation. The predictors of local recurrence and index scores are based on regression analysis of nonrandomized patient data contained in a prospective database from two institutions.

A single arm prospective trial by Harvard/Dana-Farber Institute evaluated 158 patients with predominantly low- or intermediate-grade DCIS mammographically measuring ≤2.5 cm with surgical margins ≥1 cm [13]. Patients were treated with wide local excision alone without adjuvant radiation or tamoxifen. The 10-year cumulative local recurrence rate was 15.6%. Sixty-nine percent of local recurrences were DCIS and 31% were invasive. The annual rate of local recurrence was 1.9% per patient year.

The Radiation Therapy Oncology Group (RTOG) 9804 study was a randomized trial for patients with good-risk DCIS which compared postoperative radiation therapy with observation alone [14]. Patients had low- or intermediate-grade DCIS measuring less than 2.5 cm resected with margins ≥3 mm. The expected enrollment on the trial was 1790 patients, but the trial closed early due to poor accrual after 636 patients. Tamoxifen, which was optional, was used by 62% of patients. The median pathologic tumor size was 0.5 cm with the pathological margin being between 3–9 mm in 36% of patients and 10 mm or more in 16% of patients. Almost half (48%) of patients underwent re-excision. The 7-year local failure rate was 0.9% in the radiation arm versus 6.7% in the observation arm (HR 0.11; $P < 0.001$). There was no difference in grade 3 or 4 toxicities between the two treatment arms.

Similarly, the Eastern Cooperative Oncology Group (ECOG) E-5194 trial prospectively evaluated two cohorts of low-risk DCIS patients treated with wide local excision alone [15]. Cohort 1 included patients with low- or intermediate-grade DCIS measuring ≤2.5 cm; cohort 2 included patients with high-grade DCIS measuring ≤1 cm. A minimum 3 mm margin was required. At 12-year follow-up, the ipsilateral breast event rate was 14.4% for cohort 1 and 24.6% for cohort 2. Approximately half (52%) of recurrences were invasive. Although tumor size up to 2.5 cm and margin width as close as 3 mm were allowed, the median tumor size was 5 mm and the median margin width was 1 cm. Even in this favorable-risk population, recurrence rates were significant without radiation.

Radiation Boost and Hypofractionation in DCIS

There are no randomized trials looking specifically at the role of a radiation boost in DCIS patients treated with radiation. The recommendation for a radiation boost is based on extrapolation from randomized trials of patients with low-risk early-stage invasive breast cancer. Similarly, the recommendation for hypofractionation for DCIS patients aged 50 or older is based on prospective randomized trials of patients with early-stage invasive disease.

Invasive Breast Cancer: The Role of Adjuvant Radiation in Breast-Conserving Therapy

Local Management Options

Breast-conserving surgery alone, breast-conserving surgery followed by partial-breast irradiation, and breast-conserving surgery followed by whole-breast radiotherapy (Figs. 5.1 and 5.2).

Ideal Candidate for Breast-Conserving Treatment

The ideal candidate for breast-conserving treatment is a patient with a unifocal, less than 5 cm breast tumor resected with negative margins for invasive disease. The tumor size should be relatively small in comparison to the breast size such that a good postsurgical cosmetic outcome can be achieved. The ideal candidate would be nonpregnant and absent a history of scleroderma or lupus skin involvement.

Indications for Radiation

Adjuvant radiation following breast-conserving surgery for invasive breast cancer improves local control, breast cancer-specific survival, and overall survival. Adjuvant radiation is indicated for patients under the age of 70 who undergo lumpectomy and for patients aged 70 or older who wish to maximize local control. Adjuvant radiation provides a local control benefit for all subgroups of patients, including those aged 70 or older. The absolute local control benefit, however, is less for patients aged 70 or older than for younger patients. Omission of adjuvant radiation is an appropriate option in patients aged 70 or older who will receive 5 years of endocrine therapy and who have small (T1), low- or intermediate-grade, estrogen receptor-positive tumors resected with good margins assuming the patient has been informed and accepts the relatively small increase in disease recurrence.

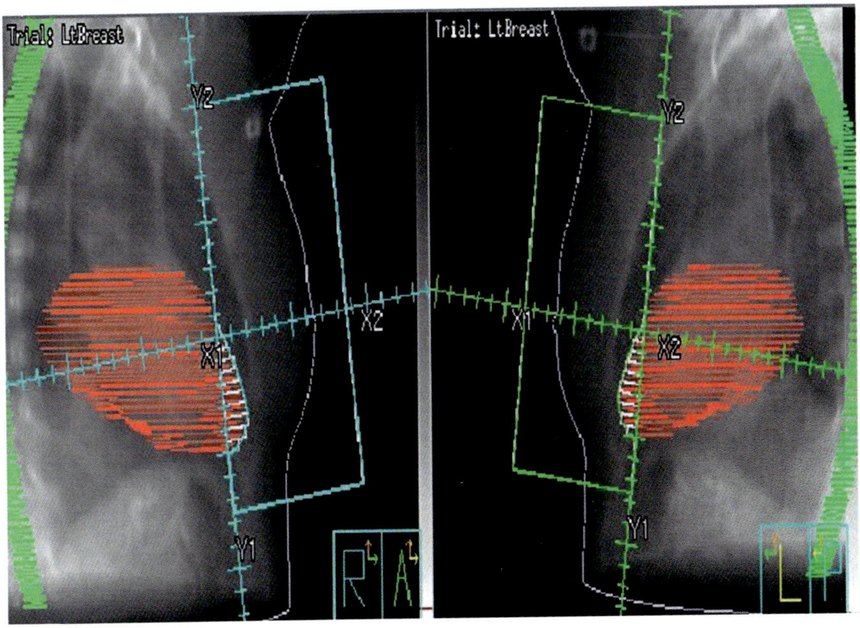

Fig. 5.1 Beam's eye view of tangential whole-breast radiation treatment fields

Fig. 5.2 Skin rendering view of a medial tangential whole-breast radiation treatment field

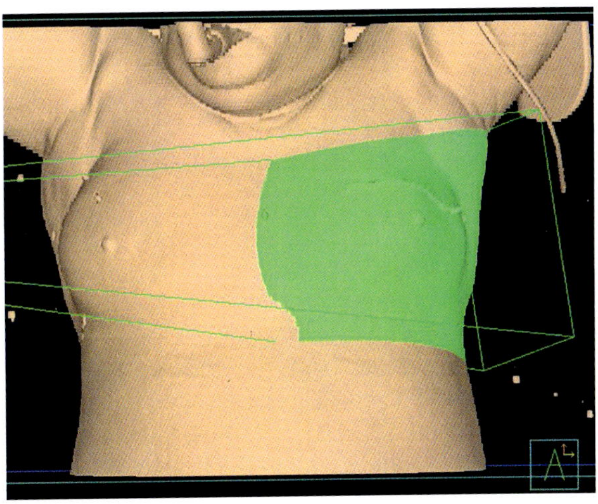

Benefit of Radiation

Adjuvant radiation following breast-conserving surgery for invasive breast cancer improves local control, breast cancer-specific survival, and overall survival.

Absolute Contraindications

Radiation therapy during pregnancy

Relative Contraindications

Active scleroderma or lupus involving the skin, positive surgical margin, known BRCA1/BRCA2 mutation, and previous radiation therapy to the breast

Radiation Technique

Radiation may be given to the whole breast with standard fractionation (50 Gy in 25 fractions) or hypofractionation (42.56 Gy in 16 fractions). A boost is typically recommended, but omission can be considered for patients aged 60 or older with low volume disease resected with acceptable surgical margins. In appropriately selected patients, radiation may be given to the partial-breast target with accelerated partial-breast irradiation (APBI). Patient selection guidelines for APBI use for invasive disease are available from several societies [1–3]. APBI can be delivered with brachytherapy, 34 Gy in ten fractions given twice daily, or highly conformal external beam irradiation, 38.5 Gy in ten fractions given twice daily.

The addition of regional nodal irradiation is recommended for patients with one or more pathologically positive lymph nodes evaluated at surgery or prior to neoadjuvant chemotherapy. Regional nodal irradiation includes the undissected axilla, supraclavicular-axillary apical nodes, and internal mammary nodes.

Factors for Consideration

Patient age, patient life expectancy, comorbidities which may increase the risk of complications, tumor size, margin width, lymphovascular space invasion, number of lymph nodes involved, volume of lymph node involvement, extranodal extension, number of lymph nodes removed, tumor grade, tumor histology, hormone receptor status, HER2/neu status, response to neoadjuvant chemotherapy, cosmetic result, and patient expectations

Selected Studies

Mastectomy vs. Breast-Conserving Therapy for Invasive Breast Cancer

Randomized trials have established that breast-conserving surgery followed by radiation therapy is equivalent to mastectomy for appropriately selected patients with early-stage breast cancer. In all of these trials, segmental mastectomy combined with breast irradiation resulted in survival and local control rates similar to those achieved by modified radical or radical mastectomy.

In 1973 Veronesi et al. began a prospective trial in Milan comparing radical mastectomy to breast-conserving surgery followed by radiation [16]. The study enrolled 701 patients with no palpable axillary lymph nodes and tumors up to 2 cm in diameter. Patients were randomly assigned to receive Halsted radical mastectomy, or quadrantectomy, axillary dissection, and radiation. A radiation dose of 50 Gy given over 5 weeks was delivered to the breast followed by a boost dose of 10 Gy. Patients found to have positive axillary lymph nodes at surgery received 12 cycles of adjuvant cyclophosphamide, methotrexate, and fluorouracil. The 20-year mortality rate from all causes was 41.2% in the radical-mastectomy arm and 41.7% in the breast-conserving surgery plus radiation arm ($P = 1.0$). Mortality from breast cancer was not significantly different, at 24.3 and 26.1%, respectively ($P = 0.8$). The cumulative incidence of local failure was 2.3% in the mastectomy group and 8.8% in the breast-conserving surgery and radiation group ($P < 0.001$). There was no difference between the groups in the incidence of contralateral breast cancer, distant metastases, or second primary cancers.

The National Surgical Adjuvant Breast and Bowel Project (NSABP) initiated the NSABP B-06 trial in the United States in 1976 which enrolled 1843 women with clinical stage I or II breast cancer [17]. Patients were randomly assigned to treatment with total mastectomy, lumpectomy, or lumpectomy with radiation. The prescribed radiation dose was 50 Gy to the breast without a lumpectomy cavity boost. At 20-year follow-up, there was no significant difference in overall survival, disease-free survival, or distant disease-free survival among any of the groups. However, the addition of radiation to lumpectomy significantly decreased the local recurrence rate by half compared to lumpectomy alone with the cumulative ipsilateral breast recurrence being 14.3% in the lumpectomy and radiation group and 39.2% in the lumpectomy alone group ($P < 0.001$).

EORTC 10801 was a randomized trial which compared mastectomy to breast-conserving therapy in 868 women with stage I and II breast cancer [18]. The European Organization for Research and Treatment of Cancer (EORTC) conducted the trial in the United Kingdom, the Netherlands, Belgium, and South Africa and initiated enrollment in 1980. Patients were randomized to modified radical mastectomy or breast-conserving therapy. Breast-conserving therapy consisted of lumpectomy with a 1 cm margin, axillary dissection, and whole-breast irradiation prescribed to 50 Gy with a 25 Gy lumpectomy site boost. At 20-year follow-up, the mortality rate was 55% in the modified radical mastectomy group and 61% in the breast-conserving therapy group, with no significant difference in time to death (HR 1.11; $p = 0.23$). There was also no significant difference in time to distant metastases (HR 1.13; $P = 0.23$) with a distant metastasis rate of 42% in the modified radical mastectomy group and 46% in the breast-conserving therapy group. Time to distant metastases and overall survival were stratified by age less than 50 versus age greater than or equal to 50, and there was no difference between treatment groups. The 15-year overall survival rate was 53.6% in the mastectomy group and 51.6% in the breast-conserving therapy group.

The Institut Gustave Roussy conducted a prospective trial in which 179 patients under age 70 with T1 N0-N1 M0 invasive breast cancer were randomized to modified radical mastectomy or wide lumpectomy, axillary surgery, and adjuvant radiation [19, 20]. Eligible patients had tumors macroscopically measuring 2 cm or less on frozen section at the time of surgery. Lymph node-negative patients received a whole-breast irradiation dose of 45 Gy given in 18 fractions with a 15 Gy tumor bed boost. Patients with positive lymph nodes received whole-breast irradiation and were randomized to radiation treatment of the regional lymph nodes. The 15-year rates of local recurrence, locoregional recurrence, contralateral breast cancer, distant metastases, and overall survival were not statistically different between surgical treatment arms and radiation treatment arms. The 15-year cumulative local recurrence rate was 13% in the lumpectomy and radiation group and 18% in the mastectomy group ($P = 0.48$). The 15-year rate of any first event was 45% with lumpectomy and radiation and 56% with mastectomy ($P = 0.23$) with 15-year overall death rates of 27 and 35%, respectively ($P = 0.19$).

Radiation vs. Hormonal Therapy

There have been at least nine clinical trials evaluating endocrine therapy as a substitute for radiation. All trials have shown that radiation therapy alone provides improved local control compared to endocrine therapy alone.

Radiation vs. Observation

There have been a number of randomized trials investigating the local control benefit of the addition of postoperative radiation to breast-conserving surgery. In these studies, the addition of postoperative radiation reduced the risk of local recurrence by 50% or more compared to breast-conserving surgery alone. These studies support the role of adjuvant radiation as part of standard-of-care treatment for younger women who select breast-conserving treatment.

Beginning in 1981, the Uppsala-Orebro Breast Cancer Study conducted a randomized trial of breast-conserving surgery with or without radiation in 381 Swedish women with stage I breast cancer [21]. Patients were treated with sector resection and axillary dissection and then randomized adjuvant breast irradiation to 54 Gy or observation. At 5 years, the local recurrence rate was 2.3% in the group that received adjuvant radiation versus 18.4% in the group in which radiation was omitted. Overall survival, regional recurrence-free survival, and distant recurrence-free survival were not different between groups.

As discussed above, NSABP B-06 compared total mastectomy, lumpectomy alone, and lumpectomy plus radiation in 1851 women with clinical stage I and II breast cancer. In 1137 women with negative surgical margins, the 20-year cumulative incidence of ipsilateral breast tumor recurrence was 39.2% in the lumpectomy alone group compared to 14.3% in the lumpectomy plus radiation group ($p < 0.0001$) [17]. For women with negative lymph nodes, the 20-year ipsilateral breast tumor recurrence rates were 36.2% with lumpectomy alone and 17.0% with lumpectomy plus radiation; for women with positive lymph nodes, the ipsilateral breast tumor recurrence rates were 44.2% without radiation versus 8.8% with radiation. Disease-free survival, distant disease-free survival, and overall survival did not differ between any of the groups. Breast cancer-specific mortality was decreased in patients treated with lumpectomy plus radiation compared to lumpectomy alone (HR 0.82, $P = 0.04$). This marginally significant decrease in breast cancer mortality may have been partially offset by deaths from other causes (HR 1.23; $P = 0.23$).

Because of the uncertainty regarding the need for radiation in women with favorable risk factors, the NSABP initiated NSAPB B-21 which enrolled 1009 women with tumors clinically or pathologically <1 cm in size who were treated with lumpectomy and axillary dissection [22]. Patients were required to have negative lymph nodes and negative margins on pathology review. Patients were randomized to tamoxifen only, radiation and placebo, or radiation and tamoxifen. At 8 years, the cumulative incidence of local relapse was 16.5% in the tamoxifen alone group, 9.3% in the radiation and placebo group, and 2.8% in the radiation and tamoxifen group. The respective hazard ratios for ipsilateral breast tumor recurrence were HR 0.51 ($P = 0.008$) for radiation plus placebo versus tamoxifen alone, HR 0.37 ($P = 0.01$) for radiation plus tamoxifen versus radiation plus placebo, and HR 0.19 ($P < 0.0001$) for radiation plus tamoxifen versus tamoxifen alone. Tamoxifen decreased the occurrence of contralateral breast cancer compared to radiation plus placebo (HR 0.45; $P = 0.039$). There was no difference in overall survival or distant metastases between groups.

Veronesi et al. at the Milan National Cancer Institute also investigated the efficacy of breast-conserving surgery without radiation in a study where 579 women under the age of 70 with breast cancer less than 2.5 cm in size were randomized to quadrantectomy, axillary dissection, and radiation, or the same surgery without radiation [23]. The 10-year crude ipsilateral breast tumor recurrence rate was 23.5% for patients treated without radiation and 5.8% for patients who received radiation. The cumulative hazard rate for ipsilateral recurrence was significant ($P < 0.001$). Overall survival was not statistically different between the treatment arms; however, on subset analysis, patients with node-positive disease had improved survival with radiation ($P = 0.038$) with a crude mortality rate of 34.1% in the radiation omission group versus 19.1% for group who received radiation. Subset analysis also showed that the group which radiation provided the greatest decrease in ipsilateral recurrence was patients aged 45 and younger. In older age groups, the difference in ipsilateral recurrence tended decrease until no difference was seen after age 65.

Meta-analyses of Radiation in Breast-Conserving Therapy

Two comprehensive meta-analyses of the benefit of postoperative radiation added to breast-conserving surgery suggest that adjuvant radiation significantly decreases local recurrence, breast cancer mortality, and overall mortality.

In 2005, the Early Breast Cancer Trialists' Collaborative Group (EBCTCG) published a meta-analysis of individual patient data from 7311 patients with invasive breast cancer treated on clinical trials comparing breast-conserving surgery with radiation to breast-conserving surgery without radiation [24]. The meta-analysis showed that radiation significantly improved 15-year local recurrence and 15-year breast cancer-specific survival compared to no radiation and radiation significantly improved 15-year overall mortality by 5.3% (35.2 versus 40.5%). The analysis also showed three-fourths of breast recurrences occurred in the first 5 years following treatment.

The Early Breast Cancer Trialists' Collaborative Group updated the meta-analysis in 2011 to include individual data on 10,801 patients treated on 17 randomized trials comparing adjuvant radiation versus observation after breast-conserving surgery [25]. The update showed that compared to observation, adjuvant radiation significantly decreased the 10-year risk of any first recurrence from 35.0 to 19.3% (RR 0.52). Radiation also significantly reduced the 10-year risk of breast cancer mortality from 25.2 to 21.4% (RR 0.82) and significantly decreased the 15-year risk of overall mortality from 37.6 versus 34.6% (RR 0.92). For women with node-positive disease, the benefits of radiation were even greater with radiation reducing the 10-year risk of any first recurrence from 63.7 to 42.5% and improving the 15-year risk of breast cancer mortality from 51.3 to 42.8%.

Omission of Radiation in Older Patients

Lumpectomy followed by radiation is a standard of care option for the majority of women with early-stage invasive breast cancer. As observed in randomized trials, lumpectomy without radiation results in increased local relapse. However, trials examining the omission of radiation found that in elderly women, local relapse rates were lower and radiation provided a lower absolute local control benefit without improving overall survival. The question of whether radiation can be safely eliminated following breast-conserving therapy for elderly patients has been studied with retrospective and prospective studies which are reviewed below. In sum, these studies show adjuvant radiation improves local control for older women with favorable-risk disease without improving overall survival. For patients aged 70 or older who will receive 5 years of endocrine therapy and who have small (T1), low- or intermediate-grade, estrogen receptor-positive tumors resected with good margins, the risk of disease recurrence may be acceptably low such that adjuvant radiation may be omitted if the patient accepts the increased risk of recurrence associated with radiation omission.

CALGB (Cancer and Leukemia Group B) 9343 was a trial which evaluated the effect of radiation omission in older patients with favorable-risk breast cancer [26]. The trial evaluated 636 women aged 70 or older with clinically node-negative, estrogen receptor-positive breast cancer measuring 2 cm or less who were treated with lumpectomy with negative pathological margins. Axillary dissection was permissible but not required. Patients were randomized to receive tamoxifen 20 mg for 5 years plus whole-breast irradiation with a boost or tamoxifen alone for 5 years. With a median follow-up of 12.6 years, the 10-year rate of locoregional recurrence was 10% in the tamoxifen alone arm versus 2% in the tamoxifen plus radiation arm (HR 0.18; $p < 0.001$). The published study did not analyze pathologic tumor size or margin width. Overall survival at 10 years was 67% in the tamoxifen plus radiation group and 66% in the tamoxifen alone group. Overall survival, breast cancer-specific survival, time to mastectomy, and time to distant metastasis were not statistically different between groups.

Fyles et al. performed a trial in Canada which enrolled 769 women aged 50 or older with node-negative invasive breast cancer and tumor size of 5 cm or less on pathologic review [27]. Patients were treated with breast-conserving surgery with negative pathologic margins and then randomized to whole-breast irradiation plus tamoxifen 20 mg for 5 years or tamoxifen alone. Most patients were aged 60 or older, most tumors were less than 2 cm, and more than 80% of tumors were hormone receptor positive. The 5-year rate of local recurrence was 0.6% for patients receiving radiation plus tamoxifen and 7.7% for patients receiving tamoxifen alone (HR 8.3; $P < 0.001$). The 5-year disease-free survival rates were 91% for patients receiving radiation and tamoxifen versus 84% for patients receiving tamoxifen alone ($P = 0.004$). In a planned subset analysis of women with the most favorable-risk disease, the 5-year rate of local recurrence of women with estrogen receptor-positive tumors measuring 2 cm or less was 0.5% for patients receiving radiation and tamoxifen and 5.9% for patients receiving tamoxifen alone ($P < 0.001$). The 5-year rate of axillary recurrence was also less with radiation versus no radiation (0.5 versus 2.5% ($P = 0.049$), respectively). Overall survival and distant recurrence rates were not statistically different between groups.

The most recent study evaluating the role of radiation omission in patients with low-risk invasive breast cancer is the PRIME II which enrolled 1326 women in the United Kingdom, Greece, Australia, and Serbia from 2003 to 2009 [28]. All women were 65 years or older and had low-risk disease defined as node-negative, hormone receptor-positive breast cancer measuring 3 cm or less. The study allowed for tumors with lymphovascular invasion or nuclear grade 3 histology, but not both. Following surgical axillary staging and breast-conserving surgery with pathologic margins of 1 mm or more, patients were randomized to receive endocrine therapy and whole-breast irradiation with a boost or endocrine therapy alone. The 5-year rate of ipsilateral breast tumor recurrence was 4.1% in the endocrine therapy alone arm and 1.3% in the endocrine therapy plus radiation arm. The hazard ratio for ipsilateral breast tumor recurrence for the endocrine therapy alone arm was 5.19 ($P = 0.0007$). Five-year overall survival was 93.9% in both treatment arms. Regional recurrence, distant metastases, contralateral breast cancers, and new breast cancers were not significantly different between groups. Analysis of patient characteristics showed 88% of patients had tumors 2 cm or smaller with roughly 40% of tumors measuring 1 cm or less. In more than half of patients, the surgical margin was either greater than 5 mm or re-excision was performed. Ninety percent of patients had estrogen receptor-rich tumors, and more than 95% of patients had tumors of low or intermediate grade.

Collectively these studies suggest the local control benefit of adjuvant radiation for elderly patients with low-risk features is statistically significant, but the absolute value may be relatively small. Adjuvant radiation for this subgroup of patients has not been shown to improve overall survival or distant metastasis-free survival. The decision to give radiation to these patients must weigh improvement in local recurrence against the overall risk of disease recurrence and the risk of radiation treatment side effects. Patient longevity must also be considered because the cumulative risk of disease recurrence increases over time so patients with a long life expectancy will experience a higher risk of disease recurrence than patients with a shorter life expectancy.

Regional Nodal Irradiation in Breast-Conserving Therapy

Whole-breast irradiation often includes treatment of level 1 and part of level 2 axillary lymph nodes. The addition of regional nodal irradiation expands the treated nodal basins to include level 3 axillary nodes, supraclavicular nodes, and internal mammary nodes. The addition of regional nodal radiation to whole-breast radiation typically occurs when encountering positive axillary lymph nodes and its role in breast-conserving treatment has historically been extrapolated from trials evaluating locoregional radiotherapy in the postmastectomy setting. Two recently published randomized trials have explored the benefit of regional nodal radiotherapy in the setting of breast conservation and whole-breast radiotherapy. Although the results are supportive of a benefit of regional nodal irradiation in high-risk or node-positive patients, the relative benefit is small and the trials have generated discussion regarding how to best identify those patients who will receive a meaningful benefit from added therapy in both the breast conservation and postmastectomy scenarios. The NCIC (National Cancer Institute of Canada) Clinical Trials Group MA.20 trial evaluated the benefit of regional nodal irradiation in node-positive or high-risk early-stage invasive breast cancer patients treated with breast-conserving surgery and adjuvant chemotherapy [29]. Eligible patients underwent breast-conserving surgery and axillary staging with sentinel lymph node biopsy or axillary dissection. Patients were required to have positive axillary nodes on pathologic review or have a pathologically negative axilla, but have high-risk features. High-risk features included a primary breast tumor measuring at least 5 cm, or a breast tumor measuring at least 2 cm with fewer than ten axillary nodes removed and at least one of the following: estrogen receptor negativity, grade 3 histology, or lymphovascular invasion. Following surgery, patients received adjuvant chemotherapy, endocrine therapy, or both. The study enrolled 1832 eligible patients who were randomized to adjuvant whole-breast irradiation (control arm) or adjuvant whole-breast and regional nodal irradiation which included treatment of the internal mammary, supraclavicular, and axillary lymph nodes. The radiation dose was 50 Gy given over 25 fractions. Ninety-nine percent of patients had T1 or T2 disease and 75% of patients had estrogen receptor-positive tumors. Two-thirds of patients had ten or more axillary lymph nodes removed. Half of patients had one pathologically positive node, and three-fourths of patients had one or two positive nodes. At 10 years of follow-up, the primary outcome of overall survival was not statistically different between groups, 81.8% in the whole-breast irradiation group and 82.8% in the whole-breast and regional nodal irradiation group (HR 0.91; $P = 0.38$). Disease-free survival was improved with regional nodal irradiation compared to whole-breast irradiation (82 versus 77%; HR 0.76; $P = 0.01$). Regional nodal irradiation also improved 10-year isolated locoregional disease-free survival compared to whole-breast-only irradiation (95.2 versus 92.2%; HR 0.59; $P = 0.009$) and 10-year distant disease-free survival (86.3 versus 82.4%; HR 0.76; $P = 0.03$). Breast cancer-specific mortality did not differ statistically between groups. On preplanned subgroup analysis of patients with estrogen receptor-negative disease, regional nodal irradiation improved 10-year overall survival compared to whole-breast-only irradiation (81.3 versus 73.9%; HR 0.69; $P = 0.05$).

The European Organization for Research and Treatment of Cancer (EORTC) 22922/10925 trial enrolled 4004 women in 13 countries to evaluate the survival benefit of elective internal mammary and medial supraclavicular irradiation in patients with stage I, II, or III invasive breast cancer [30]. Patients were eligible if their primary breast tumor was centrally or medially located, with or without axillary nodal involvement, or if the primary breast tumor was externally located with axillary nodal involvement. Following mastectomy or breast-conserving surgery, patients were randomized to elective radiation to the internal mammary and medial supraclavicular nodal basins or no radiation treatment to these nodal basins. Most patients (76%) underwent breast-conserving surgery followed by whole-breast irradiation, and 85% received a tumor bed boost. A minority of patients (24%) underwent mastectomy of which approximately three-fourths received chest wall irradiation. Systemic therapy was given to almost all node-positive patients (99%) and to two-thirds of node-negative patients. The axillary disease burden was low in most patients with 44.5% of patients having no pathologically involved lymph nodes and 43% of patients having 1–3 pathologically involved nodes. Sixty percent of patients had a primary breast tumor 2 cm or smaller, and 36% of patients had a primary breast tumor measuring 2–5 cm. The median patient age was 54. Ten-year overall survival was borderline statistically different between groups, with an 82.3% overall survival rate in the elective nodal irradiation group and 80.7% in the group without elective nodal irradiation (HR 0.87; $P = 0.06$). Elective nodal radiation improved 10-year breast cancer mortality from 14.4 to 12.5% (HR 0.082; $P = 0.02$) and improved 10-year disease-free survival from 69.1 to 72.1% (HR 0.89; $P = 0.04$). Distant disease-free survival was also higher in the elective nodal irradiation group compared to no elective irradiation, 78 versus 75%, respectively (HR 0.86; $P = 0.02$).

Radiation Boost

A radiation boost is a short course of focused tumor bed irradiation additional to whole-breast irradiation. Studies have shown that a tumor bed boost improves local control, especially in younger patients.

The EORTC boost trial was a multicenter trial which examined the benefit of a lumpectomy cavity boost in 2657 patients with early-stage breast cancer [31]. Patients were eligible if they were age 70 or younger and had T1-T2 N0-1 M0 invasive breast cancer. Patients underwent axillary dissection and local excision of the primary breast tumor with a 1–2 cm margin. Patients with microscopically negative margins underwent whole-breast irradiation of 50 Gy over 5 weeks and were then randomized to a 16 Gy boost to the tumor bed or no boost. Overall survival at 20 years was not statistically different between groups with survival at 59.7% in the boost group compared to 61.1% in the no boost group (HR 1.05; $P = 0.323$). The boost group had decreased local recurrence as the first treatment failure compared to the no boost group (9 versus 13%) (HR 0.65; $P < 0.001$). Twenty-year ipsilateral breast tumor recurrence was 12.0% in the boost group compared to 16.4% in the no boost group. At 20 years, a higher rate of severe fibrosis was seen in the boost group compared to the no boost group, 5.2 versus 1.8% ($P < 0.0001$). The absolute reduction in local recurrence provided by a boost was greatest in younger patients and progressively decreased in older subgroups of patients. For example, the boost decreased 20-year local recurrence in patients younger than age 40 from 36.0 to 24.4%, while in patients older than age 60, local recurrence decreased from 12.7 to 9.7%.

The Lyon Breast Cancer Trial also investigated the role of a tumor bed boost. The study enrolled 1024 patients less than 70 years of age with invasive ductal carcinoma measuring up to 3 cm [32]. All patients underwent breast-conserving surgery with negative pathologic margins followed by whole-breast irradiation of 50 Gy in 20 fractions. Patients were randomized to a 10 Gy boost to the tumor bed or no further treatment. With a median follow-up of 3.3 years, the 5-year rate of local recurrence was 3.6% in the patients who received a boost versus 4.5% in the patients who received no boost ($P = 0.044$). Although the rate of grade 1 or 2 telangiectasia was higher in the boost group (12.4 versus 5.9%), patient-reported assessment of cosmetic result was not different between treatment groups.

Hypofractionation

Traditionally, patients treated with whole-breast irradiation received 25–28 daily fractions (treatments) given at a dose of 1.8–2 Gy per day, potentially followed by a boost. Hypofractionation is treating patients with a fewer number of fractions than would traditionally take place usually with goal of reducing overall treatment duration. Hypofractionation typically involves giving patients a higher daily dose of radiation than one would receive with traditionally fractionated treatment. Hypofractionated treatment in breast cancer has reduced the number of whole-breast treatments from 25 to 28 fractions potentially followed by a boost to 15 or 16 fractions +/- a boost. This reduces treatment duration from 5–7 to 3–4 weeks.

The validity of hypofractionated whole-breast radiation treatment was established by three large randomized trials comparing hypofractionated to conventionally fractionated treatment. These trials suggest hypofractionated treatment provides equivalent local control and toxicity compared to traditionally fractioned treatment in appropriately selected patients.

The Ontario Clinical Oncology Group's hypofractionation trial was a multicenter trial in Canada which enrolled patients from April 1993 to September 1996 [29]. The trial included 1230 women with pathologically node-negative invasive breast cancer treated with lumpectomy. Patients were excluded if they had a tumor larger than 5 cm, clinical T4 disease, or breast width greater than 25 cm. Patients were randomized to whole-breast irradiation of 42.5 Gy in 16 fractions over 22 days or 50 Gy in 25 fractions over 35 days. Ten-year local recurrence was not significantly different between groups (6.2% in the 42.6 Gy group and 6.7% in the 50 Gy group). Ten-year overall survival was the same between groups (84%).

The START-A and START-B trials were multicenter hypofractionation trials which ran concurrently in the United Kingdom between 1999 and 2002 [33]. Eligible patients had pT1-T3a pN0-N1 M0 invasive breast cancer treated with breast-conserving surgery or mastectomy. The majority of patients received tamoxifen and/or chemotherapy.

The START-A trial randomized 2236 patients to three different radiation treatment schedules, all given over 5 weeks: 39 Gy in 13 fractions, 41.6 Gy in 13 fractions, or 50 Gy in 25 fractions (control group) [33]. A sequential tumor bed boost was allowed as was treatment of the regional lymph nodes if lymph nodes were positive. Eighty-five percent of patients received breast-conserving surgery and 61% received a tumor bed boost; 29% of patients had positive lymph nodes and 14% received locoregional irradiation. At a median follow-up of 9.3 years, the 10-year rate of locoregional relapse did not differ statistically between the 41.6 and 50 Gy groups (6.3 versus 7.4%, respectively; HR 0.91; $P = 0.65$) or between the 39 and 50 Gy groups (8.8 versus 7.4%, respectively; HR 1.18; $P = 0.41$).

The START-B hypofractionation trial enrolled patients concurrently with the START-A trial. Similar to the START-A trial, eligible patients on START-B were women who had pT1-T3a pN0-N1 M0 invasive breast cancer treated with breast-conserving surgery or mastectomy [33]. A majority of patients received tamoxifen and/or chemotherapy. The START-B trial randomized 2215 patients to two different radiation treatment schedules with differing durations of treatment: 40 Gy in 15 fractions over 3 weeks (experimental group) or 50 Gy in 25 fractions over 5 weeks (control group). A sequential tumor bed boost was allowed. Ninety-two percent of patients received breast-conserving surgery and 43% received a tumor bed boost; 23% of patients had positive lymph nodes but only 7% underwent locoregional irradiation. At a median follow-up of 9.9 years, the 10-year rate of locoregional relapse was not significantly different between the 40 Gy group and the 50 Gy group (4.3 versus 5.5%; HR 0.65; $P = 0.21$).

In START-A trial, there was significantly less breast edema, telangiectasias, and moderate or marked breast induration in the 39 Gy group compared to the 50 Gy group; there was no significant difference in toxicity between the 41.6 and 50 Gy groups. In START-B, there was significantly less breast edema, breast shrinkage, and telangiectasia development in the 40 Gy group compared to the 50 Gy group.

In 2011, the American Society for Radiation Oncology issued an evidence-based guideline for fractionation for whole-breast irradiation [34]. The guideline stated that for patients aged 50 or older with pT1-T2 pN0 breast cancer treated with breast-conserving surgery without adjuvant chemotherapy, hypofractionated whole-breast irradiation provides equivalent local control and toxicity compared to conventional fractionated whole-breast irradiation. When using hypofractionation, they recommended the radiation dose along the central axis of the breast deviate no more or less than 7% from the prescription dose. The task force behind the guideline favored giving hypofractionated radiotherapy using a dose schedule of 42.5 Gy in 16 fractions when a boost is not used. There was no consensus regarding the use of a tumor bed boost with hypofractionation. Additionally, the task force recommended the heart should be excluded from the primary treatment fields when hypofractionated whole-breast radiation is used due to the uncertainty regarding late effects of hypofractionation on cardiac function.

In 2014, the American Society for Radiation Oncology, as part of its Choosing Wisely campaign, recommended that in women who are aged 50 years or older with early-stage invasive breast cancer, whole-breast irradiation following breast-conserving surgery should not be given without consideration of shorter treatment schedules [35].

Accelerated Partial-Breast Irradiation

The previous sections have covered the literature supporting adjuvant whole-breast irradiation therapy as part of standard of care treatment after breast-conserving surgery, with hypofractionation shown to be a reasonable alternative to conventional fractionation in appropriately selected patients. However, whole-breast radiation therapy may be overtreating a significant volume of uninvolved breast tissue, and many hypothesize that this treatment of uninvolved tissue may be responsible for some of the acute and chronic toxicity associated with breast-conserving therapy. Accelerated partial-breast irradiation (APBI) has been investigated as a possible alternative to whole-breast radiation therapy for select patients with DCIS or low-risk invasive breast cancer [36]. The rationale behind APBI is that the majority of breast relapses occur within or near the tumor bed. Pathological studies from mastectomy specimens have demonstrated a lower probability of subclinical microscopic disease with increasing distance from the primary tumor [16, 36–40]. APBI targets only the surgical bed and a limited volume of normal tissue surrounding the surgical bed (Figs. 5.3 and 5.4). The accelerated treatment schedule reduces the overall radiation treatment duration to 1 week or less, which is more feasible for women with difficulty traveling to a radiation treatment center or women may not want to commit to the longer treatment duration associated with conventional or

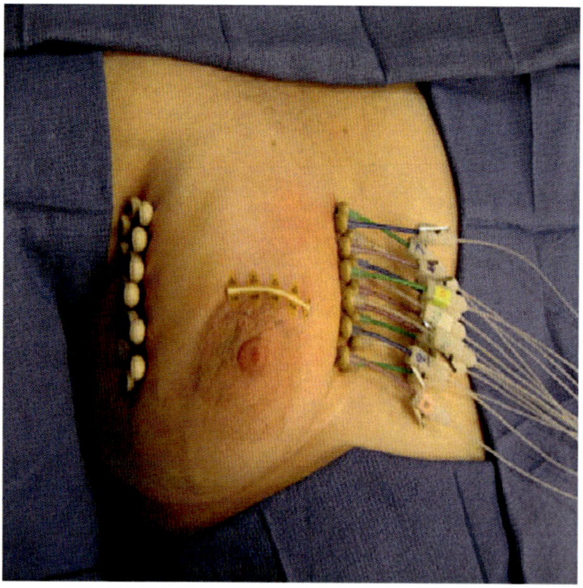

Fig. 5.3 External view of a multicatheter interstitial brachytherapy accelerated partial-breast irradiation treatment

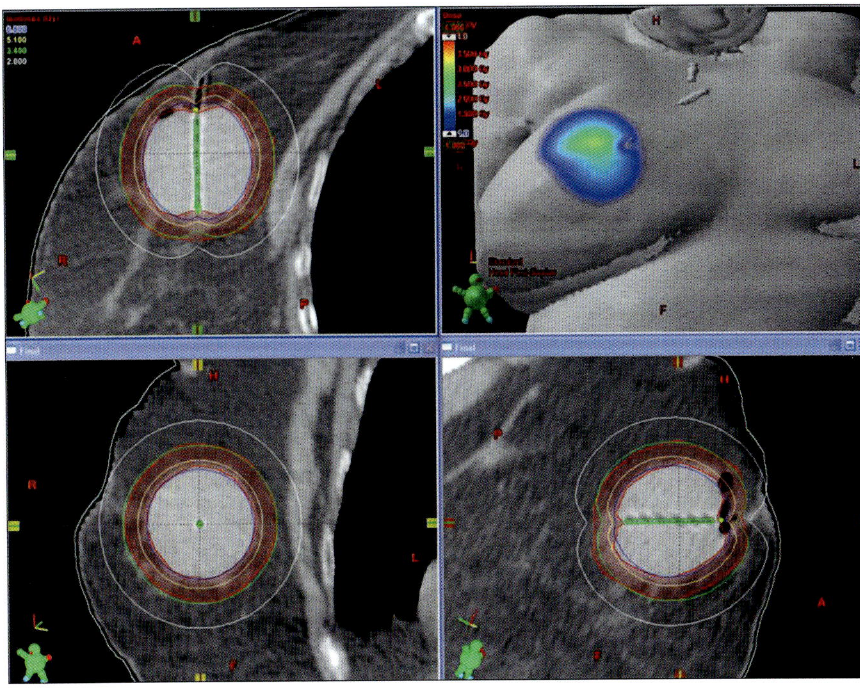

Fig. 5.4 Axial view, skin-rendering view, coronal view, and sagittal view of an intracavitary brachytherapy accelerated partial-breast irradiation treatment

hypofractionated whole-breast radiation. The advantages of APBI extend beyond convenience. APBI limits radiation exposure to only the part of the breast surrounding the tumor bed and can effectively minimize dose to the lungs, heart, chest wall, ribs, and normal breast or nodal tissue. APBI may also reduce certain radiation treatment-related toxicities, which may improve overall quality of life [41].

Historically, the first utilized APBI technique was multicatheter interstitial brachytherapy, which was primarily used as a boost technique after whole-breast irradiation [42, 43]. This technique involves the use of multiple catheters that are generally positioned at 1.0–1.5 cm intervals. The total number of catheters and planes employed is dependent on the size, extent, and shape of the tumor cavity. Multiple studies utilizing this technique have established multicatheter interstitial brachytherapy as an acceptable treatment option for appropriately selected patients [44–46]. Among partial-breast irradiation techniques, this technique has the longest patient follow-up, allowing for more accurate outcome analyses. However, it is both complex and technically challenging, limiting its widespread use.

Starting in 1998, the Hungarian National Institute of Oncology performed a prospective trial which enrolled 258 women with pT1 pN0-1mic, grade 1–2, non-lobular breast cancer resected with negative margins and randomized participants to conventionally fractionated whole-breast irradiation to 50 Gy in 2 Gy fractions (n = 130) or partial-breast irradiation. Partial-breast irradiation was delivered with HDR interstitial brachytherapy to a dose of 36.4 Gy given over seven twice-daily fractions of 5.2 Gy ($n = 88$) or electrons to a dose of 50 Gy in 2 Gy fractions ($n = 40$) [1]. With 10 years of follow-up, there was no statistical difference in local recurrence between whole-breast irradiation group and the partial-breast irradiation groups (5.9 vs. 5.1%, respectively; $p = 0.77$). Overall survival, disease-free survival, and cause-specific survival did differ between treatment arms. However, there was an improved good-excellent cosmetic outcome with partial-breast irradiation techniques.

From 2004 to 2009, the Groupe European de Curietherapie—European Society of Therapeutic Radiology and Oncology (GEC-ESTRO) conducted a multi-institutional, multinational, phase III, non-inferiority trial which randomized 1184 early-stage breast cancer patients to whole-breast irradiation or accelerated partial-breast irradiation using multicatheter interstitial brachytherapy [47]. Eligible patients had unifocal and unicentric stage 0, I, or IIa breast cancer (lesions ≤3 cm, pN0 or N1mi) treated with breast-conserving surgery with at least 2 mm margins. Whole-breast irradiation ($n = 551$) was prescribed to a dose of 50–50.4 Gy given in 1.8–2 Gy fractions followed by a 10 Gy boost. Accelerated partial-breast irradiation using a multicatheter interstitial technique was delivered using twice-daily high-dose rate brachytherapy to a dose of 32.0 Gy given in 8 fractions (8 × 4.0 Gy) or 30.3 Gy in 7 fractions (7 × 4.3 Gy), or pulsed-dose rate brachytherapy to a dose of 50 Gy with pulses of 0.60–0.80 Gy/h (1 pulse per hour, 24 h/day). The 5-year rate of local recurrence was 0.9% for the whole-breast irradiation group and 1.4% for the accelerated partial-breast irradiation group ($p = 0.42$) with the accelerated partial-breast technique being statistically non-inferior to whole-breast irradiation at 5 years. There was also no difference in the 5-year rates of grade 2–3 late skin side effects, grade 2–3 subcutaneous tissue late side effects, or grade 3 fibrosis. No patients experienced grade 4 toxicity.

Intracavitary brachytherapy is a less complex partial-breast technique with increased reproducibility. It has become the most widely used brachytherapy technique for APBI. The technique employs a single-balloon catheter introduced into the lumpectomy site either at the time of lumpectomy or percutaneously after surgery (Fig. 5.5). The catheter is located centrally within a distal balloon which is inflated after the catheter is placed in the lumpectomy cavity. Correct placement requires symmetry of the balloon, conformance of the balloon surface to the lumpectomy cavity, and a minimum distance between the surface of the balloon and skin of >5 mm (ideally >7 mm). Like the multicatheter technique, treatment is frequently delivered via an HDR remote afterloading system to a circumferential 1 cm distance from the balloon surface.

External beam APBI represents a noninvasive alternative with multiple techniques available. Three-dimensional conformal radiotherapy (3D-CRT) was the initial technique. Challenges with this technique include daily positioning of the target, movement with breathing, and delivery of higher doses to the surrounding normal breast tissue than with brachytherapy. Nonetheless, this approach has been widely embraced and has been shown to be reproducible [48, 49]. However, concerns regarding cosmesis and toxicity have emerged in more recent trials [50, 51]. The RAPID trial enrolled 2135 women (age > 40 years, tumor <3 cm) who underwent 3D-CRT APBI or hypofractionated whole-breast irradiation. Interim analysis demonstrated increased adverse cosmesis and grade

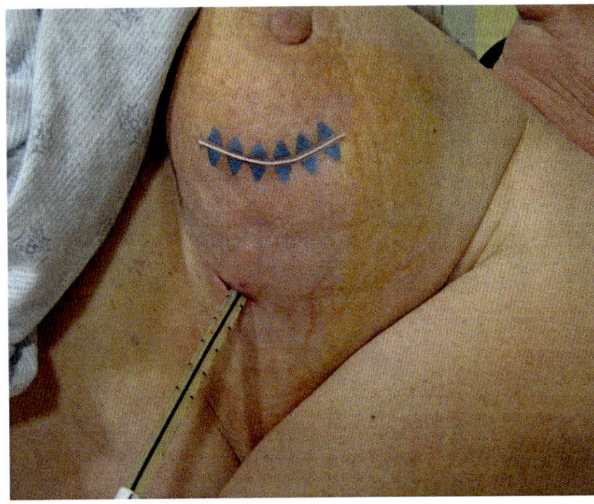

Fig. 5.5 External view of an intracavitary brachytherapy accelerated partial-breast irradiation treatment. A balloon attached to the end of the catheter is located within the lumpectomy cavity

1 and 2 toxicities with 3D-CRT APBI at 3 years [52]. Recent data supports the use of IMRT (intensity modulated radiation therapy) rather than 3D-CRT to deliver external beam APBI [53]. A University of Florence trial included 520 patients (age > 40 years, tumor size ≤2.5 cm) who received APBI via IMRT (30 Gy given over 5 fractions delivered every other day) or conventionally fractionated whole-breast irradiation. With 5-year follow-up, IMRT APBI showed reduced toxicity and improved cosmetic outcome compared to whole-breast treatment, with no difference in local control [54].

Intraoperative ABPI is a technique that has been studied primarily outside of the United States. Radiation is delivered in a single intraoperative dose to the lumpectomy site at the time of surgery using intraoperative electrons or intraoperative photons. TARGIT-A was a phase III, non-inferiority study which randomized over 3451 women to either targeted intraoperative radiation (TARGIT) or conventional whole-breast irradiation from 2000 to 2012 [55]. Per protocol, approximately 15% of patients receiving TARGIT also received whole-breast radiation because of unexpected adverse features seen on final pathology. Targeted intraoperative radiation was given to a dose of approximately 20 Gy at the tumor bed surface with the radiation dose decreasing to approximately 5–7 Gy at 1 cm from the tumor bed surface. At last reporting, 1222 patients had a median follow-up of 5 years. The 5-year risk of local recurrence was 3.3% for TARGIT and 1.3% for whole-breast irradiation (p = 0.042) [55]. There was no difference in complications between the two groups.

Postmastectomy Radiation

Indications for Postmastectomy Radiation for Invasive Breast Cancer

1. Patients with one or more pathologically positive lymph nodes evaluated at surgery or prior to neoadjuvant chemotherapy
2. Positive mastectomy surgical margin or mastectomy surgical margin of <1 mm
3. Tumor size >5 cm
4. Inflammatory breast cancer

Benefit of Postmastectomy Radiation

For patients with node-positive disease, postmastectomy radiation improves locoregional recurrence-free survival, recurrence-free survival, breast cancer-specific survival, and overall survival.

Patients Who May Avoid Postmastectomy Radiation

Patients with negative axillary lymph nodes and primary breast tumor 5 cm less with mastectomy margin 1 mm or greater

Absolute Contraindication

Pregnancy

Relative Contraindications

Active scleroderma or lupus involving the skin, previous radiation

Factors for Consideration

Patient age, patient life expectancy, comorbidities which may increase the risk of complications, tumor size, margin width, lymphovascular space invasion, number of lymph nodes involved, volume of lymph node involvement, extranodal extension, number of lymph nodes removed, tumor grade, tumor histology, hormone receptor status, HER2/neu status, response to neoadjuvant chemotherapy, cosmetic result, and patient expectations

Radiation Technique

Most patients receiving postmastectomy radiation should receive treatment to the chest wall and comprehensive regional nodes which includes the undissected axilla, supraclavicular-axillary apical nodes, and internal mammary nodes. Less extensive fields may be indicated for a subset of patients with a lower risk of recurrence at the discretion of the treating radiation oncologist. Postmastectomy radiation is given with external beam irradiation. The dose for postmastectomy radiation is 50 Gy in 25–28 fractions. A boost of 10–16 Gy may be added at the discretion of the treating radiation oncologist.

Selected Studies

Survival Improvement of Patients with Positive Lymph Nodes

The survival advantage of postmastectomy radiation for node-positive breast cancer patients was established by three modern postmastectomy radiation trials and a large meta-analysis.

The earliest of the modern postmastectomy radiation trials was performed by the British Columbia Cancer Agency in Vancouver and Victoria, British Columbia. From January 1979 to December 1986, the trial enrolled 318 premenopausal women with pathologically involved axillary lymph nodes [56]. The patients were treated with modified radical mastectomy followed by adjuvant cyclophosphamide, methotrexate, and 5-fluorouracil (CMF) chemotherapy. Patients were randomized to adjuvant locoregional radiation or no additional treatment. Radiation was targeted to the postmastectomy chest wall, supraclavicular lymph nodes, axillary lymph nodes, and bilateral internal mammary lymph nodes. Radiation treatment took place between the fourth and fifth cycles of chemotherapy. A dose of 37.5 Gy in 16 fractions was given to the chest wall, 35 Gy in 16 fractions to the supraclavicular and axillary lymph nodes, and 37.5 Gy in 16 fractions to the bilateral internal mammary lymph nodes. At 20-year follow-up (median follow-up of 249 months), the radiation group had significantly better isolated locoregional recurrence-free survival compared to the no additional treatment group (90 versus 74%; RR 0.36; $P = 0.002$) and better systemic relapse-free survival (48 versus 31%; RR 0.66; $P = 0.004$). The radiation group showed higher rates of breast cancer-free survival (48 versus 30%; RR 0.63; $P = 0.001$), event-free survival (35 versus 25%; RR 0.70; $P = 0.009$), and breast cancer-specific survival (53 versus 38%; RR 0.67; $P = 0.008$). Overall survival increased by 10% with radiation (47% with radiation versus 37% without radiation) (RR 0.73; $P = 0.03$).

The Danish Breast Cancer Cooperative Group protocol 82b enrolled 1708 high-risk premenopausal women from November 1982 to December 1989 [57]. High risk was defined as axillary lymph node involvement, tumor size greater than 5 cm, or breast cancer invasion into the skin or pectoral fascia. Patients were in pathologic stage II or III. All patients were treated with total mastectomy and axillary nodal dissection, with a median of seven lymph nodes removed. Following surgery, patients were randomized to receive 9 weeks of CMF chemotherapy alone or an 8-week split course of CMF chemotherapy with locoregional radiation occurring during the split. A third group received CMF plus tamoxifen, but enrollment was discontinued in June 1986 because of greater than expected mortality in this group. Radiation consisted of treatment to the chest wall, surgical scar, and regional lymph nodes (supraclavicular, infraclavicular, axillary, and internal mammary lymph nodes). The radiation dose was 50 Gy in 25 fractions given over 5 weeks or 48 Gy in 22 fractions given over 5½ weeks. At 10-year follow-up (median 114 months), there was improved locoregional recurrence in the group receiving CMF plus radiation compared to the group receiving CMF alone (9 versus 32%, $P < 0.001$). Disease-free survival was increased in the chemotherapy plus radiation group compared to the chemotherapy alone group (40 versus 34%, $P < 0.001$). Overall survival was higher with CMF plus radiation compared to CMF alone (54 versus 45%, $P < 0.001$). On multivariate analysis, postmastectomy radiation increased disease-free survival and overall survival regardless of tumor size, number of positive of nodes, or tumor grade.

The Danish Breast Cancer Cooperative Group protocol 82c included 1460 postmenopausal high-risk breast cancer patients with high-risk indicating axillary lymph node involvement, tumor size great than 5 cm, or cancer invasion into the skin or pectoral fascia [58]. Trial enrollment occurred between October 1982 and March 1990. Like Danish 82b, patients were treated with mastectomy and axillary lymph node dissection with a median of seven lymph nodes removed. Danish 82c randomized patients to adjuvant radiation plus 1 year of tamoxifen or 1 year of tamoxifen alone. A third group received adjuvant CMF plus tamoxifen and was reported separately. Radiation was targeted to the chest wall, surgical scar, and regional lymph nodes (supraclavicular, infraclavicular, axillary, and internal mammary lymph nodes). The radiation dose was 50 Gy in 25 fractions over 35 days or 48 Gy in 22 fractions over 38 days. At 10 years of follow-up (median 119 months), the trial results showed improved locoregional recurrence in the radiation plus tamoxifen group compared to the tamoxifen alone group (8 versus 35%, $P < 0.001$). Total recurrences were fewer in the radiation plus tamoxifen group compared to tamoxifen alone (47 versus 60%), and disease-free survival was better with radiation plus tamoxifen compared to tamoxifen alone (36 versus 24%, $P < 0.001$). Overall survival was increased with radiation plus tamoxifen compared to tamoxifen alone (45 versus 36%, $P = 0.03$).

In 2006, the Danish Breast Cancer Cooperative Group published a study of the long-term patterns of disease recurrence for 3083 patients enrolled in protocols 82b and 82c [59]. The 18-year probability of any first breast recurrence was 73% for patients who did not receive adjuvant radiation versus 59% for patients who received adjuvant radiation ($P < 0.001$). The probability of locoregional recurrence at 18 years was 49% for patients who did not receive adjuvant radiation versus 14% for patients who received adjuvant radiation ($P < 0.001$). The 18-year probability of distant metastases after locoregional recurrence was 35% for patients who did not receive adjuvant radiation versus 6% for patients who received adjuvant radiation ($P < 0.001$), and the probability of distant metastases was 64% for the no radiation group versus 53% for the radiation group.

In 2014 the Early Breast Cancer Trialists' Collaborative Group (EBCTCG) published a meta-analysis of individual patient data of 8135 women treated with mastectomy and axillary surgery in 22 clinical trials which took place from 1964 to 1986 [60]. It compared the outcomes of patients treated without radiation to patients treated with postmastectomy radiation to the chest wall and regional lymph nodes. Axillary surgery consisted of axillary dissection or axillary sampling. Axillary dissection was defined as dissection of levels I and II or a median of ten or more lymph nodes removed, and axillary sampling was defined as removal of less than levels I and II or less than a median of ten lymph nodes removed. The primary outcomes were 10-year locoregional recurrence, 10-year any first recurrence, 20-year breast cancer mortality, and 20-year overall mortality. Recurrence was analyzed at 10 years because many trials did not follow patients for recurrence beyond year 10.

The meta-analysis showed that for the 700 women who had pathologically negative lymph nodes after mastectomy and axillary dissection, postmastectomy radiation did not improve rates of locoregional recurrence, any first recurrence, or breast cancer mortality [60].

For the 3131 women with pathologically positive lymph nodes after mastectomy and axillary dissection, postmastectomy radiation improved locoregional recurrence from 26.0 to 8.1%, any first recurrence from 62.5 to 51.9%, and breast cancer mortality from 66.4 to 58.3%. Radiation decreased overall mortality from 70.4 to 65.4% [60].

For the 1314 women with 1–3 pathologically positive lymph nodes who were treated with mastectomy and axillary dissection, postmastectomy radiation decreased locoregional recurrence from 20.3 to 3.8%, any first recurrence from 45.7 to 34.2%, and breast cancer mortality from 50.2 to 42.3% [60]. For the 1772 women with four or more positive lymph nodes treated with mastectomy and axillary dissection, postmastectomy radiation improved locoregional recurrence from 32.1 to 13%, any first recurrence from 75.1 to 66.3%, and breast cancer mortality from 80.0 to 70.7% [60].

The benefit of postmastectomy radiation was sustained even if women received systemic therapy. For the 1133 women with 1–3 pathologically involve lymph nodes who were treated with mastectomy, axillary dissection, and systemic therapy, radiation decreased locoregional recurrence from 21.0 to 4.3%, any first recurrence from 45.5 to 33.8%, and breast cancer mortality from 49.4 to 41.5% [60]. For the 1677 women with four or more positive lymph nodes who were treated with mastectomy, axillary dissection, and systemic therapy, postmastectomy radiation improved locoregional recurrence from 31.5to 13.6%, any first recurrence from 74.0 to 65.8%, and breast cancer mortality from 78.0 to 70.0% [60].

There has been controversy whether radiation is needed if axillary dissection is performed and only one lymph node is pathologically involved. For the 318 women who had one pathologically positive lymph node and who were treated with mastectomy, axillary dissection, and systemic therapy, postmastectomy radiation improved locoregional recurrence from 20.2 to 3.0%, any first recurrence from 36.3 to 25.3%, and 15-year breast cancer mortality from 35.2 to 30.5% [60]. For the 365 women with 2–3 pathologically positive nodes who were treated with mastectomy, axillary dissection, and systemic therapy, postmastectomy radiation decreased locoregional recurrence from 19.3 to 4.7%, any first recurrence from 47.8 to 40.4%, and 15-year breast cancer mortality from 50.5 to 42.5%.

Overall the study showed that for women with node-positive disease who received postmastectomy radiation, one breast cancer death was prevented at 20 years for every 1.5 recurrences prevented at 10 years [60].

The American Society of Clinical Oncology, American Society for Radiation Oncology, and Society of Surgical Oncology issued a focused guideline update on postmastectomy radiation in 2016 [61]. There was unanimous agreement on the panel that for patients with T1-T2 tumors and 1–3 positive axillary lymph nodes who undergo axillary nodal dissection, postmastectomy radiation reduces the risk of locoregional failure, any recurrence, and breast cancer mortality. They indicated that for subsets of patients with a very low risk of locoregional failure, the absolute benefit of postmastectomy radiation may be outweighed by the potential toxicity; however, the panel could not clearly define those subsets. The panel recommended consideration of the following factors in deciding whether or not a patient will benefit from postmastectomy radiation: patient age, limited life expectancy, comorbidities which may increase the risk of complications, tumor size, lymphovascular invasion, number of lymph nodes involved, size of lymph node involvement, response to neoadjuvant systemic therapy, tumor grade, and strong hormonal sensitivity. The panel recommended that postmastectomy radiation be given to patients with axillary nodal involvement who receive neoadjuvant systemic therapy and have less than a pathological complete response. For clinically node-negative patients who receive neoadjuvant systemic therapy or those with a pathological complete response in the lymph nodes after neoadjuvant systemic therapy, the panel felt there was insufficient evidence to either recommend postmastectomy radiation or recommend omission of postmastectomy radiation. They recommended these patients be enrolled in clinical trials.

Neoadjuvant Chemotherapy

Traditional predictive factors such as tumor size, tumor grade, number of lymph nodes involved, volume of lymph node involvement, and extracapsular extension have been used by radiation oncologists to estimate the benefit of postmastectomy radiation and determine the appropriateness of postmastectomy radiation treatment. Because neoadjuvant chemotherapy can dramatically change one or all of these factors and introduce new predictive factors (such as pathological complete response), estimating the benefit of postmastectomy radiation after neoadjuvant chemotherapy is more difficult. There are no published randomized trials evaluating the role of postmastectomy radiation following neoadjuvant chemotherapy. However, there is retrospective analysis of patients treated prospectively on chemotherapy clinical trials. Presently there is insufficient evidence to suggest traditional predictive factors used to make postmastectomy radiation decisions are no longer beneficial or new predictive factors, such as pathological complete response, are equally or more predictive than traditional factors in making postmastectomy radiation treatment decisions. This is being evaluated on clinical trials such as NSABP B-51. Until the results of NSAB B-51and similar trials are published, postmastectomy radiation treatment decisions off clinical trial should be made using traditional predictive factors. Since these predictive factors may be altered by neoadjuvant chemotherapy, they should be determined using pretreatment workup and staging.

Huang et al. conducted a retrospective analysis of 744 patients enrolled on 6 consecutive prospective clinical trials at MD Anderson Cancer Center between 1974 and 2000 [62]. Patients had nonmetastatic, noninflammatory breast cancer and received doxorubicin-based chemotherapy and mastectomy. Outcomes from 542 patients who received postmastectomy radiation were compared to 134 patients who did not receive postmastectomy radiation. The study demonstrated that postmastectomy radiation reduced the rate of 10-year locoregional recurrence from 22 to 11%. On subset analysis, postmastectomy radiation significantly reduced the rate of locoregional recurrence for subsets of patients with clinical T3 or T4 tumors, stage IIB or greater disease, pathologic tumor size greater than 2 cm, and four or more positive lymph nodes. For patients with stage III or IV disease who achieved a pathological complete response after neoadjuvant chemotherapy, postmastectomy radiation reduced the rate of 10-year locoregional recurrence from 33 to 3%.

Postmastectomy radiation also improved 10-year cause-specific survival in patients with stage IIIB or greater disease (44 vs. 22%), clinical T4 tumors (45 vs. 24%), or four or more positive lymph nodes (44 vs. 18%). Overall survival was higher with postmastectomy radiation in patients with stage IIIB or greater disease (42 vs. 20%), clinical T4 tumors (42 vs. 20%), or four or more positive lymph nodes (38 vs. 15%).

Mamounas et al. performed a combined analysis of National Surgical Adjuvant Breast and Bowel Project (NSABP) trials B-18 and B-27 to determine the patterns and predictors of locoregional recurrence for patients treated with neoadjuvant chemotherapy [63]. In the two NSABP trials, patients who underwent lumpectomy after neoadjuvant chemotherapy received radiation to the breast alone, and patients who underwent mastectomy after neoadjuvant chemotherapy received no adjuvant radiation. In NSABP B-18, patients were randomized to receive neoadjuvant or adjuvant doxorubicin and cyclophosphamide (AC) given every 21 days for a total of four cycles. Patients aged 50 or older received tamoxifen for 5 years regardless of hormone receptor status. In NSABP B-27, patients were randomized to one of three treatment arms. Patients in group 1 received four cycles of neoadjuvant AC, patients in group 2 received four cycles of neoadjuvant AC followed by four cycles of neoadjuvant docetaxel given every 21 days, and patients in group 3 received four cycles of neoadjuvant AC followed by four cycles of adjuvant docetaxel. All patients received 5 years of tamoxifen regardless of hormone receptor status. In NSABP B-18, a total of 763 patients received adjuvant chemotherapy and 760 patients received neoadjuvant chemotherapy. All 2411 patients on NSABP B-27 received neoadjuvant chemotherapy. Mamounas performed a combined analysis of the 3171 patients who received neoadjuvant chemotherapy on the two trials. With 83 patients lost to follow-up, a total of 3088 patients were analyzed. Most patients in the trial had early-stage disease. In B-18, 65% of patients had clinical T1-2 N0 disease and 22% of patients had clinical T1-2 N1 disease. In B-27, 51% of patients had clinical T1-2 N0 disease and 20% of patients had clinical T1-2 N1 disease. Most patients were clinically node-negative; in B-18, 73% of patients were clinically node-negative; and in B-27, 70% of patients were clinically node-negative. On multivariate analysis of 1071 patients who were treated with mastectomy, independent predictors of 10-year locoregional recurrence were clinical tumor size greater than 5 cm versus less than 5 cm (HR 1.58), clinically node-positive versus node-negative (HR 1.53), pathological complete response in the breast versus no breast pathological complete response in node-negative patients (HR 2.21), and pathologically node-positive versus pathologically node-negative plus breast pathological complete response (HR 4.48).

In the 1890 patients who underwent lumpectomy, independent predictors of 10-year local regional recurrence on multivariate analysis included age 50 or older versus less than age 50 (HR 0.71), clinically node-positive versus node-negative (HR 1.70), pathological complete response in the breast versus no breast pathological complete response in node-negative patients (HR 1.44), and pathologically node-positive versus pathologically node-negative with breast pathological complete response (HR 2.25).

Table 5.1 Ten-year locoregional recurrence for patients treated with neoadjuvant chemotherapy followed by mastectomy without postmastectomy radiation [63]

	Clinically node negative		Clinically node positive	
	Tumor ≤5 cm	Tumor >5 cm	Tumor ≤5 cm	Tumor >5 cm
ypN(−)/breast pCR	6.6% ($n = 46$)	6.2% ($n = 16$)	0% ($n = 21$)	0% ($n = 11$)
ypN(−)/no breast pCR	6.3% ($n = 178$)	11.8% ($n = 95$)	10.8% ($n = 37$)	9.2% ($n = 84$)
ypN(+)	11.2% ($n = 184$)	14.6% ($n = 179$)	17.0% ($n = 143$)	22.4% ($n = 128$)

In general, the analysis showed a relatively low probability of locoregional recurrence for mastectomy patients who were clinically node-negative prior to neoadjuvant chemotherapy and pathologically node-negative after neoadjuvant chemotherapy. Locoregional recurrence was also low for patients who were clinically node-positive prior to neoadjuvant chemotherapy but had a pathological complete response in the breast and lymph nodes after neoadjuvant chemotherapy. Other subsets of patients had higher probabilities of locoregional recurrence. The incidence of locoregional recurrence at 10 years is summarized in Table 5.1 for mastectomy patients.

It is important to note that this analysis is a subset analysis of patients treated on two large chemotherapy clinical trials. Interpretation of the data is limited by many factors including the retrospective nature of the analysis, lack of a radiation treatment arm, small number of patients with a pathological complete response in the breast and lymph nodes, and most patients having early-stage, clinically node-negative disease. Patients with T4 or N2 disease at presentation were not eligible for treatment on either of the trials so this data does not apply to patients with more advanced disease. Furthermore, estrogen receptor, progesterone receptor, and HER2/neu status were not evaluated prior to chemotherapy, so these are not known for patients who had a pathological complete response in the breast and lymph nodes. Also, two different chemotherapy regimens were used, tamoxifen was given concurrently with chemotherapy rather sequentially, tamoxifen was given on the basis of age rather than ER status, and no patients received Herceptin. The greatest benefit of this analysis is hypothesis generation. This study and others led to the initiation of NSABP B-51. Table 5.2 highlights summary of radiation treatment recommendations at our institution.

Recurrent Disease

Patients with disease recurrence who did not previously receive radiation treatment are recommended to receive adjuvant radiation. Patients who previously received external beam irradiation may be eligible for re-irradiation with partial-breast radiation or external beam irradiation. Patients who previously received partial-breast irradiation may be eligible for re-irradiation with external beam irradiation.

Table 5.2 Summary of radiation treatment recommendations at VCU based on the above literature and acknowledging areas of controversy—this is how we do it.

Stage	Treatment recommendation
Mastectomy without neoadjuvant chemotherapy	
pT1/T2 N0 (positive or negative for ITC)	Observation is recommended if the surgical margins are negative. If the margins are positive, radiation to the chest wall and lower axilla is recommended.
pT1/T2 N1mic	If SLN biopsy only, radiation to the chest wall and lower axilla is recommended. If ALND (six nodes or more), observation is recommended if the surgical margins are negative. If the margins are positive, radiation to the chest wall and lower axilla is recommended.
pT1/T2 N1 with one node positive (macroscopic)	If SNL biopsy only, chest wall and regional nodal irradiation is recommended. If ALND (six nodes or more), observation may be considered if the patient has a less aggressive overall picture—e.g., older patients with small, low-grade, hormone receptor-positive, HER2-negative tumors resected with margins 2 mm or greater; otherwise chest wall and regional nodal irradiation is recommended.
pT1/T2 N1 with two nodes positive	Chest wall and regional nodal irradiation is recommended.
pT1/T2 N1 with three or more nodes positive	Chest wall and regional nodal irradiation is recommended.
pT3 N0	Chest wall and regional nodal irradiation is generally recommended. Observation may be considered for older patients with hormone receptor-positive, HER2-negative tumors measuring 5–6 cm and resected with good surgical margins.
pT4 N0 or inflammatory breast cancer	Chest wall and regional nodal irradiation is recommended.
Neoadjuvant chemotherapy followed by mastectomy	
Local regional irradiation is recommended for patients with evidence of preoperative nodal involvement until further evidence suggests otherwise. *Preoperative nodal evaluation includes imaging studies and/or biopsy	
cT1/T2 N1 with pCR in breast and nodes. N1 includes pathology or imaging.	Consider enrollment on NSABP B-51. Off protocol: chest wall and regional nodal irradiation is recommended. It is recognized that there is controversy regarding the role of radiation in this setting. Until this question is answered by randomized data, we recommend radiation.
cT1/T2 N1 with pCR in nodes but not in the breast	Consider enrollment on NSABP B-51. Off protocol: chest wall and regional nodal irradiation is recommended. It is recognized that there is controversy regarding the role of radiation in this setting. Until this question is answered by randomized data, we recommend radiation.
cT1/T2 N1 with pCR in the breast but not in nodes	Chest wall and regional nodal irradiation is recommended.
cT3/T4 or N2/N3	Chest wall and regional nodal irradiation is recommended regardless of response to chemotherapy.

(continued)

Table 5.2 (continued)

Stage	Treatment recommendation
Lumpectomy	
pT1/T2 N0 (positive or negative for ITC) or DCIS	For patients younger than age 70, breast irradiation is recommended. For patients aged 70–75, observation is acceptable for patients with small, hormone receptor-positive, HER2-negative tumors, with good surgical margins if the patient will receive 5 years of hormonal therapy. It is recognized that there is controversy whether the age for observation should be younger than 70. As new data arise and old data mature, the age for observation will likely decrease. Breast irradiation is recommended for patients who do not fit the criteria for observation. Breast irradiation may also be given to patients who meet the criteria for observation, but express a preference for radiation treatment to decrease the risk of local recurrence. For patients aged 75–80 or older, observation is preferred unless the patient has concerning prognostic factors or she is healthy and desires radiation treatment. As patient age increases, the preference for observation becomes greater.
pT1/T2 N1mic	Breast and lower axillary irradiation is recommended. Breast-only irradiation is recommended if the patient has undergone ALND (six nodes) or if the patient is older with a small, low-grade, hormone receptor-positive, HER2-negative tumor.
pT1/T2 N1 with one node positive	Whole-breast and regional nodal irradiation is recommended. Breast-only irradiation may be considered if the patient has undergone ALND (six nodes) and is older with a small, low-grade, hormone receptor-positive, HER2-negative tumor.
pT1/T2 with two nodes positive	Whole-breast and regional nodal irradiation is recommended.
pT1/T2 N1 with three or more nodes positive	Whole-breast and regional nodal irradiation is recommended.
pT3 N0	Whole-breast and regional nodal irradiation is generally recommended. Breast-only irradiation may be considered for older patients with low- or intermediate-grade, hormone receptor-positive, HER2-negative tumors measuring 5–6 cm.
Hypofractionation	
Hypofractionation (42.56 Gy in 16 fractions) is recommended if a patient meets all of the following criteria: 1. Patient is aged 50 years or older at diagnosis 2. Pathologic stage is T1-T2 N0 and patient has been treated with breast-conserving surgery 3. Patient has not been treated with systemic chemotherapy 4. The breast size is sufficiently small such that the central axis dose is no less than 93% and no greater than 107% of the prescription dose This recommendation may be revised as additional data becomes available (RTOG 1005). Patients who do not meet the criteria for hypofractionation should receive standard fractionation (50 Gy in 2 Gy fractions).	

Table 5.2 (continued)

Stage	Treatment recommendation
Boost	
Lumpectomy patients—a boost is recommended for: • All lumpectomy patients under age 60 • Any patient with surgical margins less than 2 mm • Any patient with aggressive features: – Node positivity – ER negativity and/or PR negativity – HER2 positivity – Grade 3 For patients treated with standard fractionation, the boost may be 10–16 Gy. For patients treated with hypofractionation, the boost may be 2.66 Gy × 4–6 fractions. Mastectomy patients: a boost is not recommended for reconstructed mastectomy patients who do not have close margins. A boost is otherwise at the discretion of the treating physician.	
Accelerated partial-breast irradiation	
We accept the American Brachytherapy Society's acceptable criteria for accelerated partial-breast irradiation.	
Criteria	
Age	≥50 years old
Size	≤3 cm
Histology	All invasive subtypes and DCIS
Estrogen receptor	Positive/negative
Surgical margins	Negative
Lymphovascular space invasion	Not present
Nodal status	Negative

References

1. Polgar C, Fodor J, Major T, Sulyok Z, Kasler M. Breast-conserving therapy with partial or whole breast irradiation: ten-year results of the Budapest randomized trial. Radiother Oncol. 2013;108(2):197–202. doi:10.1016/j.radonc.2013.05.008.
2. Shah C, Vicini F, Wazer DE, Arthur D, Patel RR. The American Brachytherapy Society consensus statement for accelerated partial breast irradiation. Brachytherapy. 2013;12(4):267–77. doi:10.1016/j.brachy.2013.02.001.
3. Smith BD, Arthur DW, Buchholz TA, et al. Accelerated partial breast irradiation consensus statement from the American Society for Radiation Oncology (ASTRO). J Am Coll Surg. 2009;209(2):269–77. doi:10.1016/j.jamcollsurg.2009.02.066.
4. Fisher B, Land S, Mamounas E, Dignam J, Fisher ER, Wolmark N. Prevention of invasive breast cancer in women with ductal carcinoma in situ: an update of the national surgical adjuvant breast and bowel project experience. Semin Oncol. 2001;28(4):400–18. doi:S0093775401001531 [pii].
5. Wapnir IL, Dignam JJ, Fisher B, et al. Long-term outcomes of invasive ipsilateral breast tumor recurrences after lumpectomy in NSABP B-17 and B-24 randomized clinical trials for DCIS. J Natl Cancer Inst. 2011;103(6):478–88. doi:10.1093/jnci/djr027.
6. Donker M, Litiere S, Werutsky G, et al. Breast-conserving treatment with or without radiotherapy in ductal carcinoma in situ: 15-year recurrence rates and outcome after a recurrence, from the EORTC 10853 randomized phase III trial. J Clin Oncol. 2013;31(32):4054–9. doi:10.1200/JCO.2013.49.5077.

7. Emdin SO, Granstrand B, Ringberg A, et al. SweDCIS: radiotherapy after sector resection for ductal carcinoma in situ of the breast. Results of a randomised trial in a population offered mammography screening. Acta Oncol. 2006;45(5):536–43. doi:T673T26276376P0U [pii].
8. Cuzick J, Sestak I, Pinder SE, et al. Effect of tamoxifen and radiotherapy in women with locally excised ductal carcinoma in situ: long-term results from the UK/ANZ DCIS trial. Lancet Oncol. 2011;12(1):21–9. doi:10.1016/S1470-2045(10)70266-7.
9. Early Breast Cancer Trialists' Collaborative Group (EBCTCG), Correa C, McGale P, et al. Overview of the randomized trials of radiotherapy in ductal carcinoma in situ of the breast. J Natl Cancer Inst Monogr. 2010;2010(41):162–77. doi:10.1093/jncimonographs/lgq039.
10. Goodwin A, Parker S, Ghersi D, Wilcken N. Post-operative radiotherapy for ductal carcinoma in situ of the breast. Cochrane Database Syst Rev. 2013;11:CD000563. doi:10.1002/14651858. CD000563.pub7.
11. Silverstein MJ, Lagios MD, Craig PH, et al. A prognostic index for ductal carcinoma in situ of the breast. Cancer. 1996;77(11):2267–74. doi:10.1002/(SICI)1097--0142(19960601)77:113.0.CO;2-V [pii].
12. Silverstein MJ, Lagios MD. Treatment selection for patients with ductal carcinoma in situ (DCIS) of the breast using the University of Southern California/Van Nuys (USC/VNPI) prognostic index. Breast J. 2015;21(2):127–32. doi:10.1111/tbj.12368.
13. Wong JS, Chen YH, Gadd MA, et al. Eight-year update of a prospective study of wide excision alone for small low- or intermediate-grade ductal carcinoma in situ (DCIS). Breast Cancer Res Treat. 2014;143(2):343–50. doi:10.1007/s10549-013-2813-6.
14. McCormick B, Winter K, Hudis C, et al. RTOG 9804: a prospective randomized trial for good-risk ductal carcinoma in situ comparing radiotherapy with observation. J Clin Oncol. 2015;33(7):709–15. doi:10.1200/JCO.2014.57.9029.
15. Solin LJ, Gray R, Hughes LL, et al. Surgical excision without radiation for ductal carcinoma in situ of the breast: 12-year results from the ECOG-ACRIN E5194 study. J Clin Oncol. 2015;33(33):3938–44. doi:10.1200/JCO.2015.60.8588.
16. Veronesi U, Cascinelli N, Mariani L, et al. Twenty-year follow-up of a randomized study comparing breast-conserving surgery with radical mastectomy for early breast cancer. N Engl J Med. 2002;347(16):1227–32. doi:10.1056/NEJMoa020989.
17. Fisher B, Anderson S, Bryant J, et al. Twenty-year follow-up of a randomized trial comparing total mastectomy, lumpectomy, and lumpectomy plus irradiation for the treatment of invasive breast cancer. N Engl J Med. 2002;347(16):1233–41. doi:10.1056/NEJMoa022152.
18. Litiere S, Werutsky G, Fentiman IS, et al. Breast conserving therapy versus mastectomy for stage I-II breast cancer: 20 year follow-up of the EORTC 10801 phase 3 randomised trial. Lancet Oncol. 2012;13(4):412–9. doi:10.1016/S1470-2045(12)70042-6.
19. Arriagada R, Le MG, Rochard F, Contesso G. Conservative treatment versus mastectomy in early breast cancer: patterns of failure with 15 years of follow-up data. Institut Gustave-Roussy Breast Cancer Group. J Clin Oncol. 1996;14(5):1558–64. doi:10.1200/jco.1996.14.5.1558.
20. Sarrazin D, Le MG, Arriagada R, et al. Ten-year results of a randomized trial comparing a conservative treatment to mastectomy in early breast cancer. Radiother Oncol. 1989;14(3):177–84.
21. Liljegren G, Holmberg L, Adami HO, Westman G, Graffman S, Bergh J. Sector resection with or without postoperative radiotherapy for stage I breast cancer: five-year results of a randomized trial. Uppsala-Orebro Breast Cancer Study Group. J Natl Cancer Inst. 1994;86(9):717–22.
22. Fisher B, Bryant J, Dignam JJ, et al. Tamoxifen, radiation therapy, or both for prevention of ipsilateral breast tumor recurrence after lumpectomy in women with invasive breast cancers of one centimeter or less. J Clin Oncol. 2002;20(20):4141–9. doi:10.1200/JCO.2002.11.101.
23. Veronesi U, Marubini E, Mariani L, et al. Radiotherapy after breast-conserving surgery in small breast carcinoma: long-term results of a randomized trial. Ann Oncol. 2001;12(7):997–1003.
24. Clarke M, Collins R, Darby S, et al. Effects of radiotherapy and of differences in the extent of surgery for early breast cancer on local recurrence and 15-year survival: an overview of the randomised trials. Lancet. 2005;366(9503):2087–106. doi:S0140-6736(05)67887-7 [pii].
25. Early Breast Cancer Trialists' Collaborative Group (EBCTCG), Darby S, McGale P, et al. Effect of radiotherapy after breast-conserving surgery on 10-year recurrence and 15-year

breast cancer death: meta-analysis of individual patient data for 10,801 women in 17 randomised trials. Lancet. 2011;378(9804):1707–16. doi:10.1016/S0140-6736(11)61629-2.
26. Hughes KS, Schnaper LA, Bellon JR, et al. Lumpectomy plus tamoxifen with or without irradiation in women age 70 years or older with early breast cancer: long-term follow-up of CALGB 9343. J Clin Oncol. 2013;31(19):2382–7. doi:10.1200/JCO.2012.45.2615.
27. Fyles AW, McCready DR, Manchul LA, et al. Tamoxifen with or without breast irradiation in women 50 years of age or older with early breast cancer. N Engl J Med. 2004;351(10):963–70. doi:10.1056/NEJMoa040595.
28. Kunkler IH, Williams LJ, Jack WJ, Cameron DA, Dixon JM, PRIME II Investigators. Breast-conserving surgery with or without irradiation in women aged 65 years or older with early breast cancer (PRIME II): a randomised controlled trial. Lancet Oncol. 2015;16(3):266–73. doi:10.1016/S1470-2045(14)71221-5.
29. Whelan TJ, Olivotto IA, Parulekar WR, et al. Regional nodal irradiation in early-stage breast cancer. N Engl J Med. 2015;373(4):307–16. doi:10.1056/NEJMoa1415340.
30. Poortmans PM, Collette S, Kirkove C, et al. Internal mammary and medial supraclavicular irradiation in breast cancer. N Engl J Med. 2015;373(4):317–27. doi:10.1056/NEJMoa1415369.
31. Bartelink H, Maingon P, Poortmans P, et al. Whole-breast irradiation with or without a boost for patients treated with breast-conserving surgery for early breast cancer: 20-year follow-up of a randomised phase 3 trial. Lancet Oncol. 2015;16(1):47–56. doi:10.1016/S1470-2045(14)71156-8.
32. Romestaing P, Lehingue Y, Carrie C, et al. Role of a 10-gy boost in the conservative treatment of early breast cancer: results of a randomized clinical trial in Lyon, France. J Clin Oncol. 1997;15(3):963–8. doi:10.1200/jco.1997.15.3.963.
33. Haviland JS, Owen JR, Dewar JA, et al. The UK Standardisation of Breast Radiotherapy (START) trials of radiotherapy hypofractionation for treatment of early breast cancer: 10-year follow-up results of two randomised controlled trials. Lancet Oncol. 2013;14(11):1086–94. doi:10.1016/S1470-2045(13)70386-3.
34. Smith BD, Bentzen SM, Correa CR, et al. Fractionation for whole breast irradiation: an American Society for Radiation Oncology (ASTRO) evidence-based guideline. Int J Radiat Oncol Biol Phys. 2011;81(1):59–68. doi:10.1016/j.ijrobp.2010.04.042.
35. Hahn C, Kavanagh B, Bhatnagar A, et al. Choosing wisely: the American Society for Radiation Oncology's top 5 list. Pract Radiat Oncol. 2014;4(6):349–55. doi:10.1016/j.prro.2014.06.003.
36. Arthur DW, Vicini FA. Accelerated partial breast irradiation as a part of breast conservation therapy. J Clin Oncol. 2005;23(8):1726–35. doi:23/8/1726 [pii].
37. Fisher B, Anderson S, Fisher ER, et al. Significance of ipsilateral breast tumour recurrence after lumpectomy. Lancet. 1991;338(8763):327–31. doi:0140-6736(91)90475-5 [pii].
38. Kurtz JM, Amalric R, Brandone H, et al. Local recurrence after breast-conserving surgery and radiotherapy. Frequency, time course, and prognosis. Cancer. 1989;63(10):1912–7.
39. Fowble B. Ipsilateral breast tumor recurrence following breast-conserving surgery for early-stage invasive cancer. Acta Oncol. 1999;38(Suppl 13):9–17.
40. Freedman GM, Anderson PR, Hanlon AL, Eisenberg DF, Nicolaou N. Pattern of local recurrence after conservative surgery and whole-breast irradiation. Int J Radiat Oncol Biol Phys. 2005;61(5):1328–36. doi:S0360-3016(04)02276-X [pii].
41. Athas WF, Adams-Cameron M, Hunt WC, Amir-Fazli A, Key CR. Travel distance to radiation therapy and receipt of radiotherapy following breast-conserving surgery. J Natl Cancer Inst. 2000;92(3):269–71.
42. Kuske RR Jr. Breast brachytherapy. Hematol Oncol Clin North Am. 1999;13(3):543–58, vi–vii.
43. Vicini FA, Arthur DW. Breast brachytherapy: North American experience. Semin Radiat Oncol. 2005;15(2):108–15. doi:S1053429604001390 [pii].
44. Chen PY, Vicini FA, Benitez P, et al. Long-term cosmetic results and toxicity after accelerated partial-breast irradiation: a method of radiation delivery by interstitial brachytherapy for the treatment of early-stage breast carcinoma. Cancer. 2006;106(5):991–9. doi:10.1002/cncr.21681.

45. Shah C, Antonucci JV, Wilkinson JB, et al. Twelve-year clinical outcomes and patterns of failure with accelerated partial breast irradiation versus whole-breast irradiation: results of a matched-pair analysis. Radiother Oncol. 2011;100(2):210–4. doi:10.1016/j.radonc.2011.03.011.
46. Arthur DW, Winter K, Kuske RR, et al. A phase II trial of brachytherapy alone after lumpectomy for select breast cancer: tumor control and survival outcomes of RTOG 95-17. Int J Radiat Oncol Biol Phys. 2008;72(2):467–73. doi:10.1016/j.ijrobp.2007.12.056.
47. Strnad V, Ott OJ, Hildebrandt G, et al. 5-year results of accelerated partial breast irradiation using sole interstitial multicatheter brachytherapy versus whole-breast irradiation with boost after breast-conserving surgery for low-risk invasive and in-situ carcinoma of the female breast: a randomised, phase 3, non-inferiority trial. Lancet. 2016;387(10015):229–38. doi:10.1016/S0140-6736(15)00471-7.
48. Baglan KL, Sharpe MB, Jaffray D, et al. Accelerated partial breast irradiation using 3D conformal radiation therapy (3D-CRT). Int J Radiat Oncol Biol Phys. 2003;55(2):302–11. doi:S0360301602038117 [pii].
49. Shah C, Wilkinson JB, Lanni T, et al. Five-year outcomes and toxicities using 3-dimensional conformal external beam radiation therapy to deliver accelerated partial breast irradiation. Clin Breast Cancer. 2013;13(3):206–11. doi:10.1016/j.clbc.2012.09.020.
50. Hepel JT, Tokita M, MacAusland SG, et al. Toxicity of three-dimensional conformal radiotherapy for accelerated partial breast irradiation. Int J Radiat Oncol Biol Phys. 2009;75(5):1290–6. doi:10.1016/j.ijrobp.2009.01.009.
51. Liss AL, Ben-David MA, Jagsi R, et al. Decline of cosmetic outcomes following accelerated partial breast irradiation using intensity modulated radiation therapy: results of a single-institution prospective clinical trial. Int J Radiat Oncol Biol Phys. 2014;89(1):96–102. doi:10.1016/j.ijrobp.2014.01.005.
52. Olivotto IA, Whelan TJ, Parpia S, et al. Interim cosmetic and toxicity results from RAPID: a randomized trial of accelerated partial breast irradiation using three-dimensional conformal external beam radiation therapy. J Clin Oncol. 2013;31(32):4038–45. doi:10.1200/JCO.2013.50.5511.
53. Lei RY, Leonard CE, Howell KT, et al. Four-year clinical update from a prospective trial of accelerated partial breast intensity-modulated radiotherapy (APBIMRT). Breast Cancer Res Treat. 2013;140(1):119–33. doi:10.1007/s10549-013-2623-x.
54. Livi L, Meattini I, Marrazzo L, et al. Accelerated partial breast irradiation using intensity-modulated radiotherapy versus whole breast irradiation: 5-year survival analysis of a phase 3 randomised controlled trial. Eur J Cancer. 2015;51(4):451–63. doi:10.1016/j.ejca.2014.12.013.
55. Vaidya JS, Wenz F, Bulsara M, et al. Risk-adapted targeted intraoperative radiotherapy versus whole-breast radiotherapy for breast cancer: 5-year results for local control and overall survival from the TARGIT-A randomised trial. Lancet. 2014;383(9917):603–13. doi:10.1016/S0140-6736(13)61950-9.
56. Ragaz J, Olivotto IA, Spinelli JJ, et al. Locoregional radiation therapy in patients with high-risk breast cancer receiving adjuvant chemotherapy: 20-year results of the British Columbia randomized trial. J Natl Cancer Inst. 2005;97(2):116–26. doi:97/2/116 [pii].
57. Overgaard M, Hansen PS, Overgaard J, et al. Postoperative radiotherapy in high-risk premenopausal women with breast cancer who receive adjuvant chemotherapy. Danish Breast Cancer Cooperative Group 82b trial. N Engl J Med. 1997;337(14):949–55. doi:10.1056/NEJM199710023371401.
58. Overgaard M, Jensen MB, Overgaard J, et al. Postoperative radiotherapy in high-risk postmenopausal breast-cancer patients given adjuvant tamoxifen: Danish Breast Cancer Cooperative Group DBCG 82c randomised trial. Lancet. 1999;353(9165):1641–8. doi:S0140-6736(98)09201-0 [pii].
59. Danish Breast Cancer Cooperative Group, Nielsen HM, Overgaard M, Grau C, Jensen AR, Overgaard J. Study of failure pattern among high-risk breast cancer patients with or without postmastectomy radiotherapy in addition to adjuvant systemic therapy: long-term results from the Danish Breast Cancer Cooperative Group DBCG 82 b and c randomized studies. J Clin Oncol. 2006;24(15):2268–75. doi:JCO.2005.02.8738 [pii].

60. EBCTCG (Early Breast Cancer Trialists' Collaborative Group), McGale P, Taylor C, et al. Effect of radiotherapy after mastectomy and axillary surgery on 10-year recurrence and 20-year breast cancer mortality: meta-analysis of individual patient data for 8135 women in 22 randomised trials. Lancet. 2014;383(9935):2127–35. doi:10.1016/S0140-6736(14)60488-8.
61. Recht A, Comen EA, Fine RE, et al. Postmastectomy radiotherapy: an American Society of Clinical Oncology, American Society for Radiation Oncology, and Society of Surgical Oncology focused guideline update. J Clin Oncol. 2016;34(36):4431–42. doi:10.1200/JCO.2016.69.1188.
62. Huang EH, Tucker SL, Strom EA, et al. Postmastectomy radiation improves local-regional control and survival for selected patients with locally advanced breast cancer treated with neoadjuvant chemotherapy and mastectomy. J Clin Oncol. 2004;22(23):4691–9. doi:22/23/4639 [pii].
63. Mamounas EP, Anderson SJ, Dignam JJ, et al. Predictors of locoregional recurrence after neoadjuvant chemotherapy: results from combined analysis of National Surgical Adjuvant Breast and Bowel Project B-18 and B-27. J Clin Oncol. 2012;30(32):3960–6. doi:10.1200/JCO.2011.40.8369.

Part II

Representative Cases: Diagnosis, Management and Radiologic Pathologic Correlation of Common Breast Lesions/Tumors

Fibroepithelial Lesions

6

Valentina Robila, Priti A. Shah, and Michael O. Idowu

Fibroadenoma is a common benign breast mass and is the most common solid mass in women under 30; 15–20% of women have multiple, including bilaterally [1, 14]. If palpable, it can be a discrete, firm, mobile mass and may wax and wane in size and tenderness with cyclical hormonal changes [10]. Fibroadenomas measuring ≥8 cm in greatest length are referred to as giant fibroadenomas and can be seen in adolescents [10, 12, 14].

Mammographically, a fibroadenoma most commonly has a round or oval shape, low density, and circumscribed margins (Fig. 6.1) [10]. As women get older, and hormone levels decrease, these masses may hyalinize, resulting in decreased size, increased radiographic density, and sometimes the development of large, coarse, chunky "popcorn"-like calcifications (Fig. 6.2). However, as mentioned elsewhere in this handbook, even large, dense calcifications may start out fine and faint and if imaged at that stage may pose a diagnostic dilemma for the radiologist, since not all masses with calcifications can be classified as fibroadenomas. Moreover, sometimes the soft tissue mass is not evident radiographically, and so a group of developing calcifications may be the only finding of a fibroadenoma (Fig. 6.3), warranting biopsy for confirmation.

The sonographic appearance of a fibroadenoma is typically analogous to the mammographic. It is oval, has an orientation parallel to the skin and chest wall (horizontal, traveling along tissue planes rather than disrupting them), uniform

V. Robila, MD, PhD • M.O. Idowu, MD, MPH (✉)
Department of Pathology, Virginia Commonwealth University Health (VCU HEALTH), Richmond, VA, USA
e-mail: valentina.robila@vcuhealth.org

P.A. Shah, MD
Department of Radiology, Breast Imaging Section, Virginia Commonwealth University Health (VCU HEALTH), Richmond, VA, USA
e-mail: priti.shah@vcuhealth.org

M.O. Idowu et al. (eds.), *Diagnosis and Management of Breast Tumors*,
DOI 10.1007/978-3-319-57726-5_6

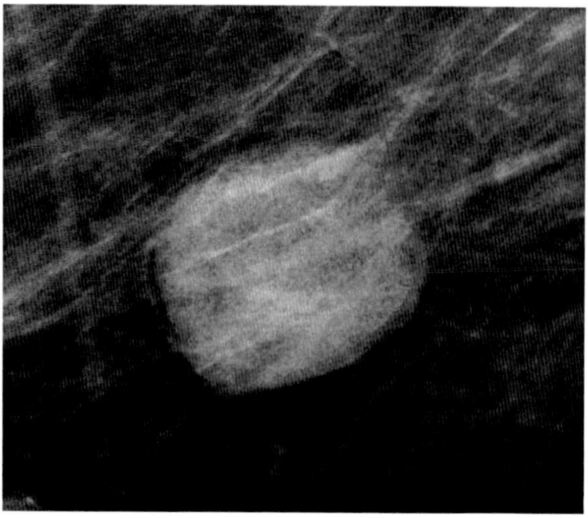

Fig. 6.1 Biopsy-proven fibroadenoma. Spot compression mammographic view demonstrates an oval, low to equal density mass with circumscribed margins

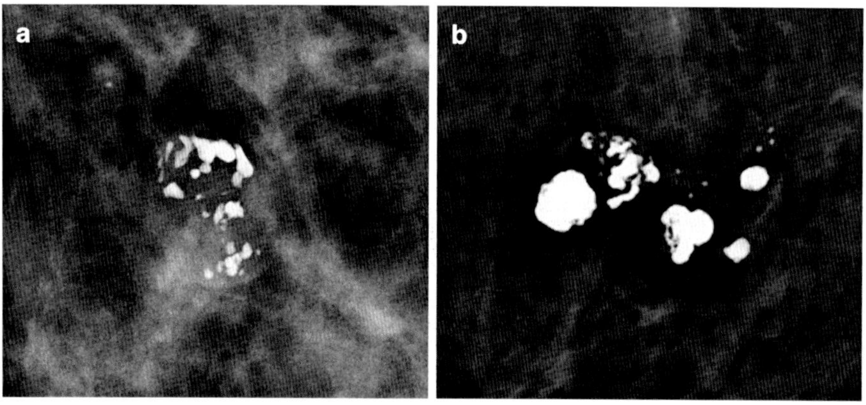

Fig. 6.2 Hyalinizing fibroadenoma, two different patients (**a**) and (**b**). Coarse, "chunky," "popcorn"-type dystrophic calcifications form in the stroma and can be seen on standard (non-magnified) mammographic views

hypoechogenicity, and circumscribed margins (Fig. 6.4) [1–3, 10]. In some cases, thin internal echogenic fibrous septa may be seen. If hyalinized but without the characteristic large calcifications to define it radiographically, it may appear more hypoechoic, or nearly anechoic, and demonstrate posterior acoustic shadowing at ultrasound. If even partially calcified, there may be intense shadowing. If not hyalinized, its appearance in both modalities may be indistinguishable from that of a phyllodes tumor; the latter might be higher in echogenicity with slit-like anechoic spaces (Fig. 6.5) [10–12]. Phyllodes tumors have malignant potential, so the distinction is important. Although the classic teaching is that phyllodes are "large" masses, size should not be the sole criteria for exclusion or inclusion in a differential diagnosis.

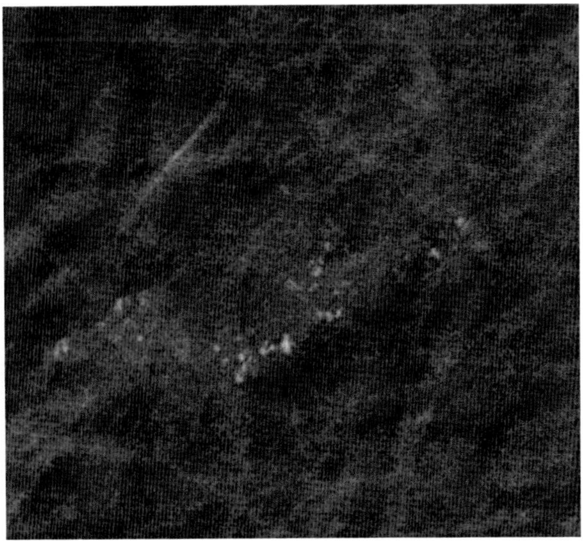

Fig. 6.3 Biopsy-proven hyalinizing fibroadenoma. Spot compression magnification view in a 48-year-old woman recalled for these new fine, pleomorphic calcifications. These were biopsied under stereotactic guidance as no associated mass was identified by imaging

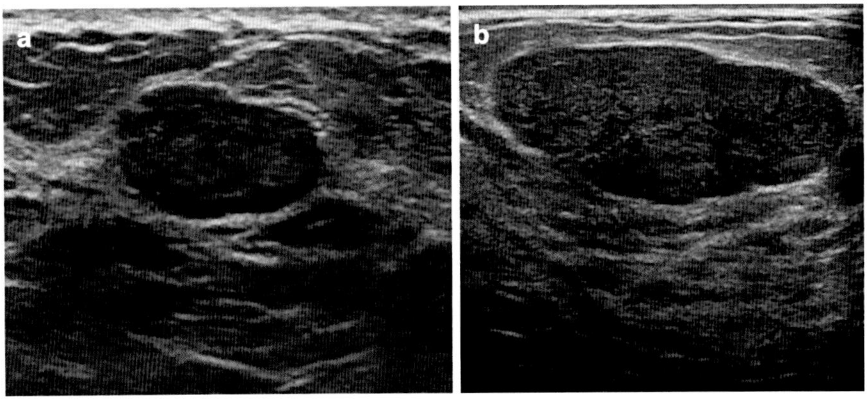

Fig. 6.4 Biopsy-proven fibroadenomas in two patients. (**a**) The typical ultrasound appearance is that of an oval, horizontally oriented hypoechoic mass with circumscribed margins. The patient in (**b**) is 25 years old and has six similar appearing masses bilaterally

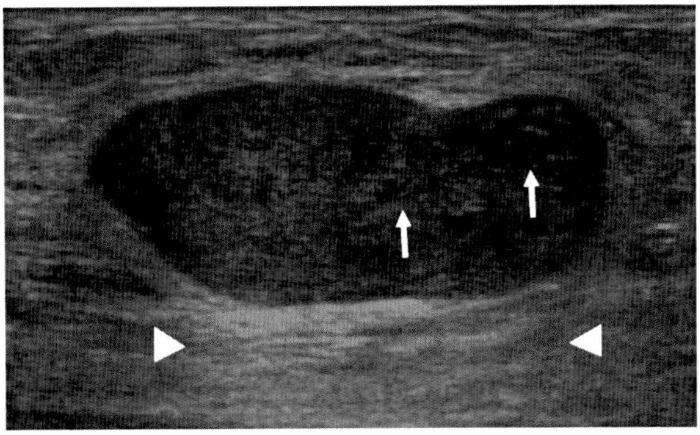

Fig. 6.5 Biopsy-proven low-grade phyllodes tumor. Slightly higher in echogenicity than a fibroadenoma on ultrasound, with internal cystic slit-like spaces (*arrows*) and posterior acoustic enhancement (*between arrowheads*)

According to the original prospective works and reviews by Sickles [4, 5, 6], if a non-palpable mass with circumscribed margins and no calcifications is identified after mammographic work-up from a baseline screening, it may be managed with periodic radiographic follow-up (assigned a BI-RADS 3 category assessment, with one short interval follow-up at 6 months, and then yearly), for a total of 2–3 years. After this, in the absence of significant growth or suspicious change, it may be deemed benign with no further follow-up. With support from later work focused on ultrasound, it is now recommended to include sonographic findings to support this recommendation for "watching and waiting," or to rely only on ultrasound features in young patients for whom mammography is not done [3, 7, 8]. The data shows that the likelihood of malignancy is <2% (and in some studies, <1%) for an oval, hypoechoic mass with circumscribed margins, parallel orientation, and no posterior acoustic shadowing. Furthermore, palpability no longer excludes such masses from short-term follow-up, which makes sense, since the size and location in the breast (closer to the skin), relative to breast size and composition, do not incur additional likelihood of malignancy. If a mass looks like a fibroadenoma and has no suspicious imaging features, our practice is to discuss this with the patient and recommend a 6-month follow-up but also offer her the options of a needle biopsy or excisional biopsy if depending on the patient's comfort level [3–9].

Classically, at follow-up, if the lesion has increased in volume by >20%, biopsy should be undertaken. However one must take into consideration the context of the patient: for example, these may normally grow in concert with breast development in adolescents and young women, or in pregnancy. If at follow-up there have been changes in morphology or margins suspicious for malignancy, biopsy is also warranted. Needle biopsy (rather than excisional biopsy) is the method of choice as it is less invasive and can be done right then, and the diagnosis may change the operative plan if surgery is in fact needed.

For core needle biopsy-proven fibroadenomas, some advocate an ultrasound follow-up in 6 months to ensure that a phyllodes tumor was not missed due to sampling error; if the lesion is truly a phyllodes, it would be expected to grow significantly in 6 months and thereby "declare itself." Given the rarity of this occurring in our practice, we do not routinely recommend nor perform ultrasound follow-up for biopsy-proven fibroadenomas. Unless symptomatic, resection of a biopsy proven fibroadenoma is not typically warranted.

In some instances, a core biopsy sample is insufficient in distinguishing between a fibroadenoma and a phyllodes tumor. It is paramount that the physician performing the core biopsy be familiar with the nuances in the language of pathologists. Such a core biopsy may be reported as a "fibroepithelial lesion, phyllodes not excluded," in which case an excisional biopsy may be needed for definitive results. The surgeon, also recognizing that a phyllodes tumor is possible based on this wording, would allow for wider margins at excision to ensure its entire removal given its propensity for recurrence.

Complex fibroadenomas are also most often indistinguishable from fibroadenomas by imaging. Findings suggestive of the former may include associated round, punctate, or amorphous calcifications radiographically and cystic spaces ≤3 mm sonographically. Although these lesions can increase a patient's risk for developing breast cancer later on, since they themselves are not premalignant, we do not routinely recommend excision when a core biopsy yields a complex fibroadenoma.

Although not indicated for the work-up of a fibroadenoma, MRI characteristics can help narrow the differential diagnosis when done for other reasons. *In premenopausal women, fibroadenomas have increased T2 signal and enhancement that is either homogeneous or interrupted by nonenhancing septa* (Fig. 6.6). In postmenopausal women, these may have decreased T2 signal and not enhance, highlighting the hormonal influences on these benign tumors (Fig. 6.7). Phyllodes tumors, given their increased cellularity, may have more heterogeneous enhancement and T2 signal [11, 12, 14].

A discussion of fibroadenomas would be remiss without mentioning tubular and lactational adenomas. Both are benign and may be indistinguishable from each other and fibroadenomas on imaging; lactational adenomas may also have areas of increased echogenicity on ultrasound related to increased lipid (milk) content (Fig. 6.8). A lactational adenoma may be suspected starting in the third trimester of pregnancy. There is controversy as to whether it arises de novo or transforms from preexisting fibroadenoma with the hormonal effects of pregnancy [13].

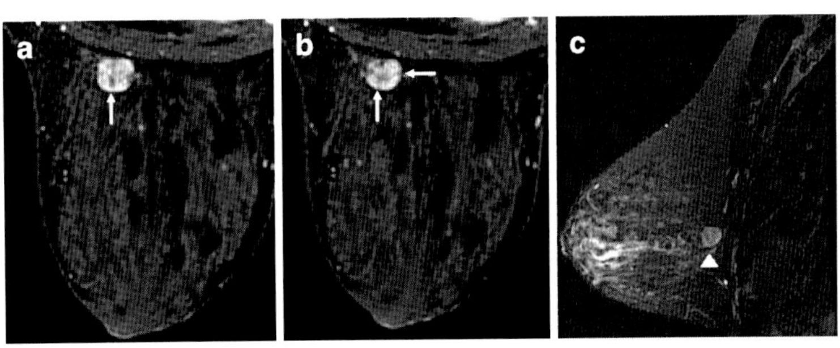

Fig. 6.6 MRI appearance of fibroadenoma in a premenopausal patient. (**a** and **b**) Axial post-contrast images at 1 mm intervals through the left breast show a round, enhancing mass with circumscribed margins and nonenhancing internal fibrous septa (*arrows*). (**c**) The mass is intermediately hyperintense on non-contrast T2-weighted sequences (*arrowhead*). This patient is 27 years old and is undergoing annual MRI due to a personal history of breast cancer

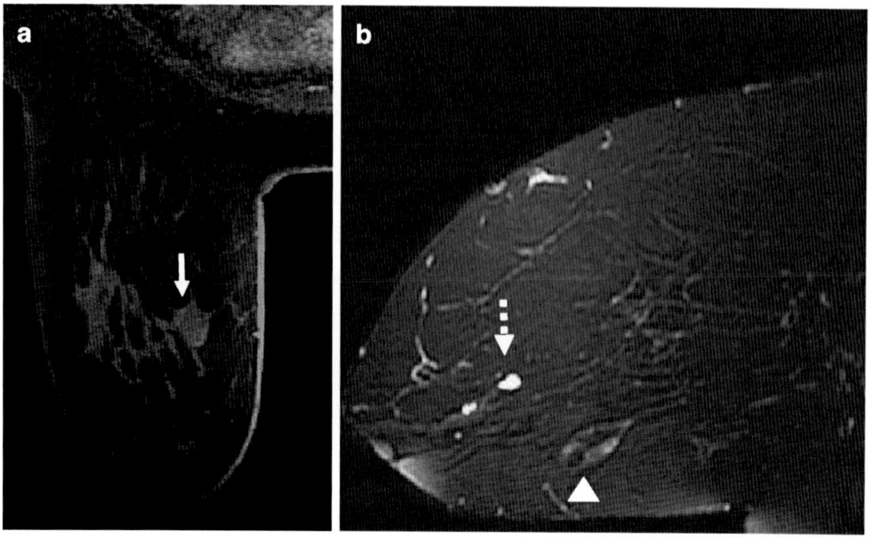

Fig. 6.7 MRI appearance of fibroadenoma in a postmenopausal patient. (**a**) Axial post-contrast images at 1 mm intervals through the left breast show a round, non-enhancing mass with circumscribed margins (*arrow*). Cardiac and internal mammary vascular enhancement posteriorly confirms the presence of intravenous contrast. (**b**) The mass is hypointense centrally, with intermediate signal peripherally, on non-contrast T2 weighted sequences (*arrowhead*); scattered subcentimeter cysts are noted (*dashed arrow*). This is a 56-year-old woman undergoing MRI for a biopsy-proven ipsilateral cancer (not shown).

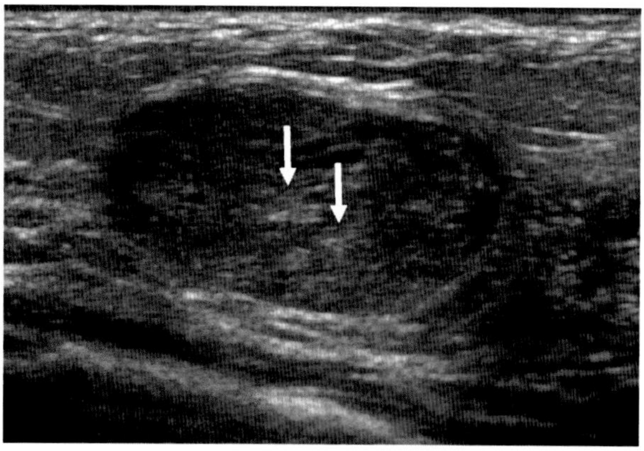

Fig. 6.8 Lactational adenoma. This may appear similar to a fibroadenoma on ultrasound but may also have areas of increased echogenicity representing lipid content (milk, *arrows*)

Chapter 2 of this text contains some discussion on the pathologic approach to diagnosis of fibroepithelial lesions. Selected radiologic–pathologic correlation of fibroepithelial lesions is highlighted in the following cases:

Case 1

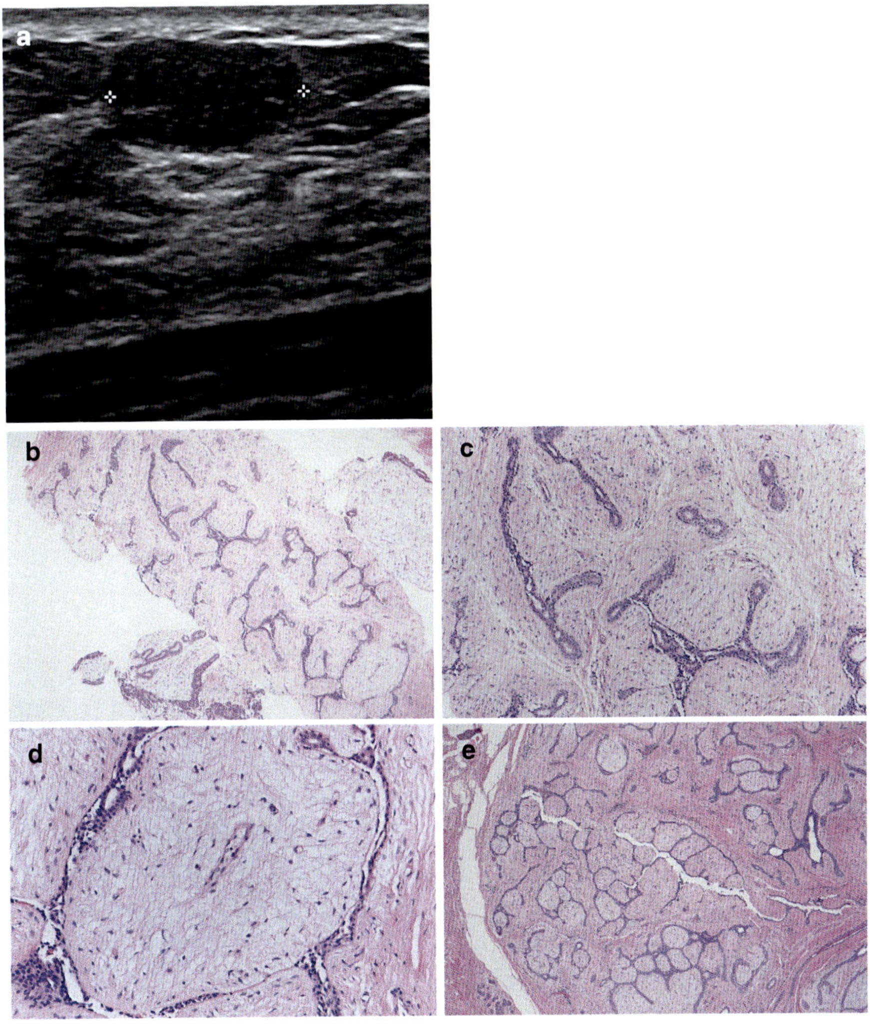

Fibroadenoma. (**a**) 17-year-old woman presenting with a "lump." Ultrasound shows an oval, hypoechoic to isoechoic mass with circumscribed margins. This is a typical appearance of a fibroadenoma and so the lesion was assigned a BI-RADS 3 with recommendation for short-interval follow-up. Ultrasound-guided core needle was done at the patient's request, followed by surgical excision. (**b**) Needle-core biopsy shows fibroadenoma. (**c** and **d**) The growth pattern is intracanalicular, in which the stroma proliferation compresses the ducts to slit-like lumens or invaginates the epithelium. Low stromal cellularity and absence of atypia are noted on high power view. (**e**) The diagnosis on excision was fibroadenoma with focal myxoid features. Note the lesion's well circumscribed margin on surgical excision

Case 2

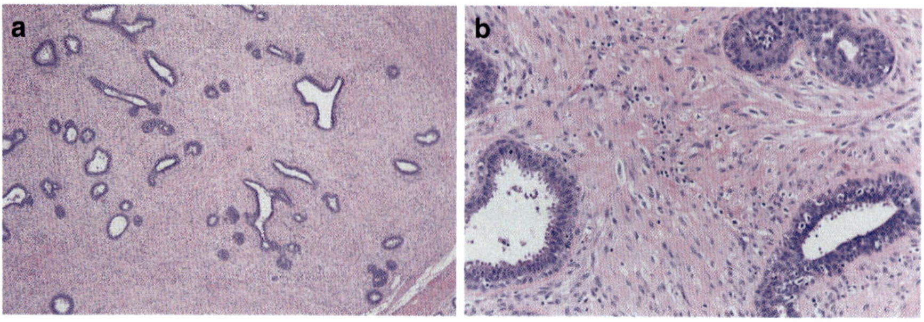

Fibroadenoma with pericanalicular growth pattern. (**a** and **b**) The glands maintain their round or oval shapes. There is no clinical significance associated with either pericanalicular and intracanalicular growth patterns

Case 3

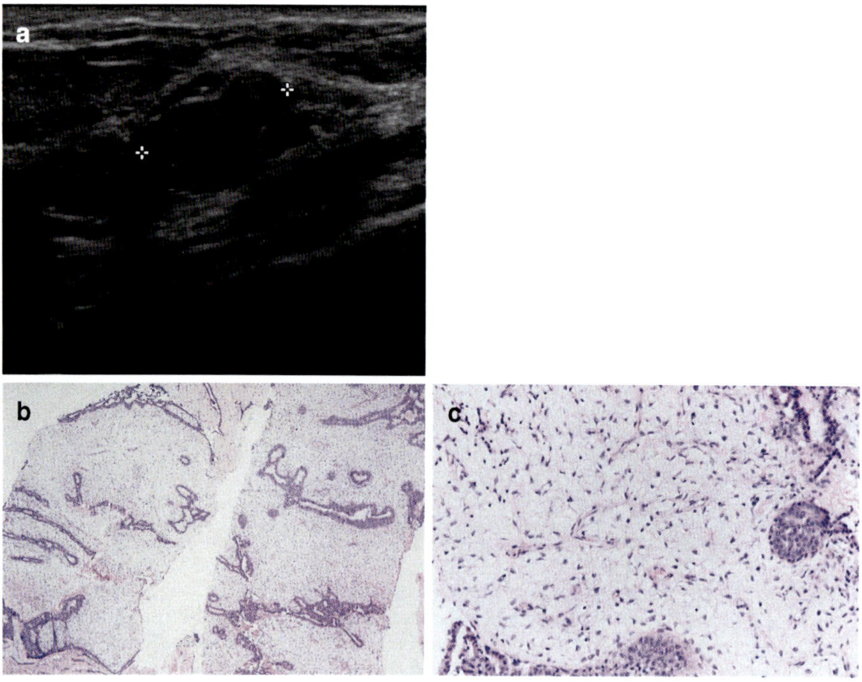

Fibroadenoma with myxoid stroma. (**a**) Oval mass with circumscribed margins in this 50-year old patient was nearly anechoic, but solid, on ultrasound. (**b** and **c**) Needle-core biopsy shows fibroadenoma with myxoid stroma. Myxoid fibroadenoma may be associated with Carney's syndrome

Case 4

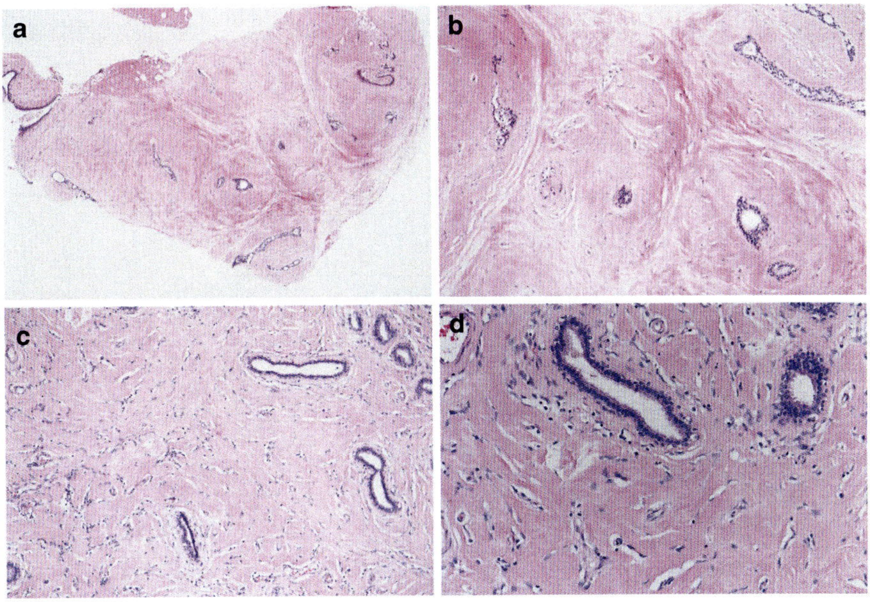

Stromal changes in fibroadenoma. (**a** and **b**) Fibroadenoma with marked stromal fibrosis and atrophic epithelium. (**c** and **d**) Pseudoangiomatous stromal hyperplasia in a fibroadenoma. The benign stromal changes are of no clinical significance

Case 5

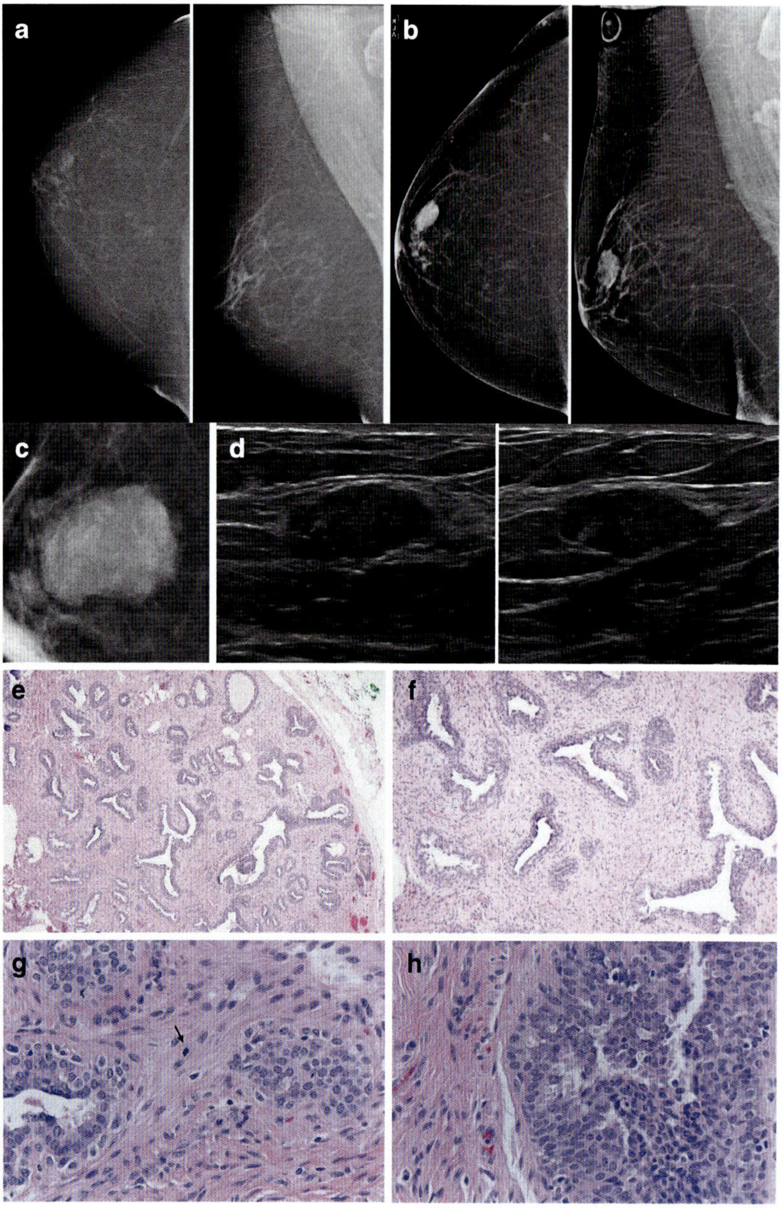

Cellular fibroadenoma. (**a**) Images of the right breast from this (now 62 year old) patient's last screening mammogram 8 years ago were normal. (**b**) Current screening study shows a new mass anteriorly. (**c**) The mass is equal density with circumscribed margins on a spot compression view. (**d**) Orthogonal ultrasound images show a hypoechoic mass with mostly circumscribed and some microlobulated margins (posteriorly). The diagnosis rendered on needle core biopsy was fibroepithelial lesion. (**e**) The low power view of the excision specimen shows a fibroepithelial lesion with a well circumscribed border. (**f**) Moderate stromal cellularity are noted. Stromal condensation around ducts is not definitely identified. (**g**) The stromal nuclei show mild atypia and rare mitoses (*arrow*), up to 1/ 10hpf. Overall, the histological features are consistent with a cellular fbroadenoma. (**h**) The lesion is focally involved by usual ductal hyperplasia

Case 6

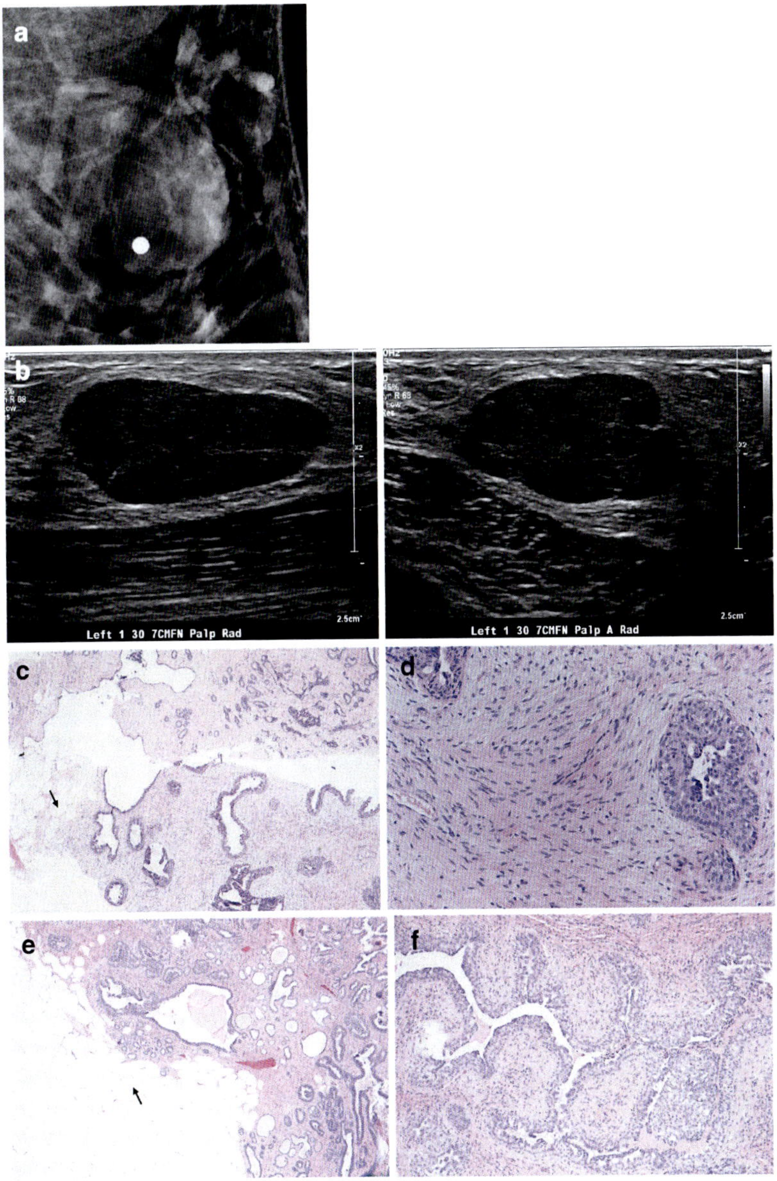

Fibroepithelial lesion, fibroadenoma vs. low grade phyllodes. (**a**) Low-density mass with circumscribed margins; this mass was palpable as denoted by the metallic BB skin marker. (**b**) Targeted ultrasound shows characteristics of a fibroadenoma: oval, orientation parallel to the skin, circumscribed margins, and hypoechoic. But since the mass was new in this 44-year-old, biopsy was undertaken. (**c** and **d**) Needle-core biopsy shows a fibroepithelial lesion with ill-defined borders (*arrow*). There is moderate stromal cellularity with mild atypia, but no mitoses seen. (**e**) The lesion's invasive border (*arrow*) and stroma with similar characteristics are also apparent in excision. (**f**) Prominent leaf-like architecture is seen, with stromal condensation around the ducts. The overall findings favor a benign phyllodes tumor. Focal epithelial hyperplasia is seen

Case 7

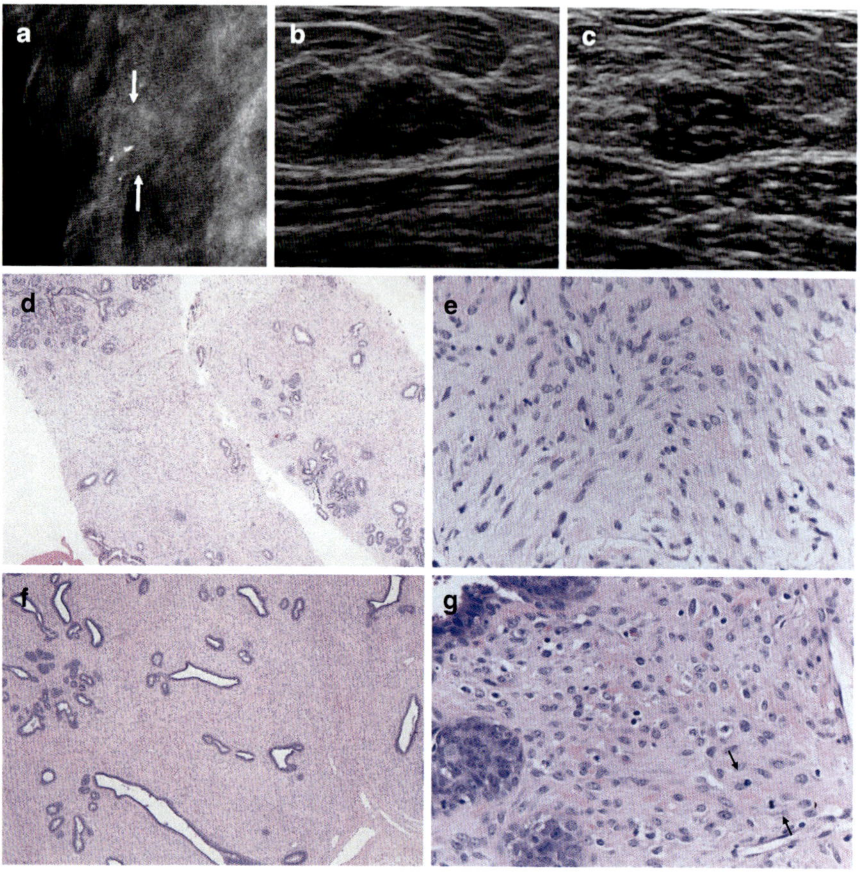

Fibroepithelial lesion with increased stroma cellularity. (**a**) Spot compression view of a mass with circumscribed margins (*between arrows*) and calcifications superimposed on dense breast tissue in a 44-year-old woman, worked up from a screening mammogram. (**b** and **c**) Orthogonal ultrasound images show a hypoechoic mass with slit-like anechoic spaces and circumscribed margins. (**d**) Needle-core biopsy shows a fibroepithelial lesion with pericanalicular growth pattern and focal stromal overgrowth. (**e**) Stroma is moderately cellular with mild atypia. (**f**) Similar areas of stromal expansion are seen on excision. (**g**) The stroma is moderately cellular, with mild atypia and up to 5 mitoses/10hpf (*arrows*). The findings are consistent with low grade phyllodes tumor

Case 8

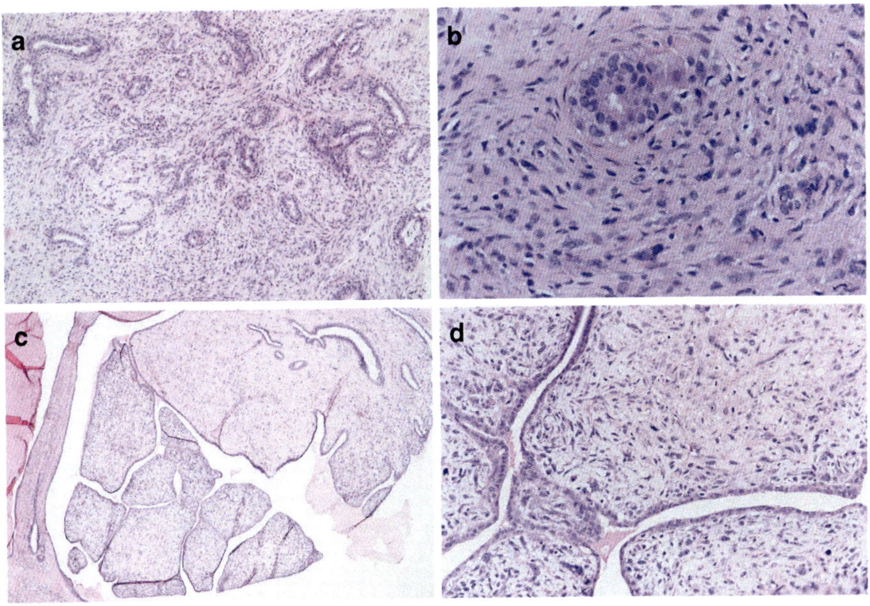

Malignant phyllodes tumor. The imaging (not shown) was significant for a mass highly suggestive of malignancy. (**a** and **b**) Needle-core biopsies show a fibroepithelial lesion with moderate to high stromal cellularity and occasional stromal cells with moderate atypia (*arrow*), consistent with phyllodes tumor. (**c** and **d**) Malignant phyllodes tumor is diagnosed on excision. Prominent leaf-like architecture, and peri-ductal stromal condensation with highly pleomorphic cells are seen

Case 9

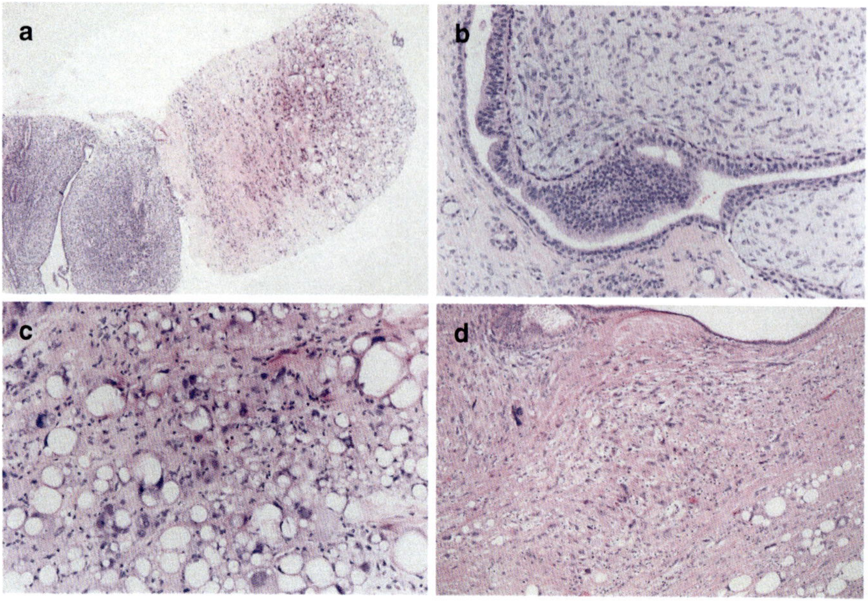

Malignant phyllodes tumor with liposarcomatous differentiation. (**a**) The core needle biopsy shows a biphasic tumor, with sharp transition between the two components. (**b**) Phyllodes tumor component with moderate to high stromal cellularity and occasional stromal cells with marked atypia. (**c**) Liposarcomatous component. (**d**) On excision, the tumor was classified as malignant phyllodes tumor with elements of liposarcoma.

References

1. Fornage BD, Lorigan JG, Andry E. Fibroadenoma of the breast: sonographic appearance. Radiology. 1989;172:671–5. doi:10.1148/radiology.172.3.2549564. Accessed 25 Feb 2017.
2. Stavros AT, Thickman D, Rapp CL, et al. Solid breast nodules: use of sonography to distinguish between benign and malignant lesions. Radiology. 1995;196:123–34. doi:10.1148/radiology.196.1.7784555. Accessed 25 Feb 2017.
3. Hong AH, Rosen EL, Soo MS, Baker JA. BI-RADS for sonography: positive and negative predictive values of sonographic features. AJR Am J Roentgoenol. 2005;184(4):1260–5. doi:10.2214/ajr.184.4.01841260. Accessed 25 Feb 2017.
4. Sickles EA. Periodic mammographic follow-up of probably benign lesions: results in 3,184 consecutive cases. Radiology. 1991;179:463–8.
5. Sickles EA. Nonpalpable, circumscribed, noncalcified solid breast masses: likelihood of malignancy based on lesion size and age of patient. Radiology. 1994;192:439–42. doi:10.1148/radiology.192.2.8029411.
6. Sickles EA. Management of probably benign breast lesions. Radiol Clin North Am. 1995;33:1123–30.
7. Graf O, Helbich TH, Hopf G, et al. Probably benign breast masses at US: is follow-up an acceptable alternative to biopsy? Radiology. 2007;244(1):87–93. doi:10.1148/radiol.2441060258.

Papillary Lesions

7

Priti A. Shah, Valentina Robila, and Michael O. Idowu

From the radiologist's perspective, benign papillary lesions can be divided into those that are symptomatic versus asymptomatic, those that are central (subareolar) versus peripheral, or those that are solitary versus multiple. There is some overlap; it is most commonly the solitary, central papilloma that is symptomatic rather than multiple or peripheral ones; however both central and peripheral solitary lesions may be incidental findings that can be followed.

If symptomatic, a central papilloma may "declare itself" with spontaneous nipple discharge; intraductal papilloma is the most common cause of this symptom, accounting for about 50% of patients [1]. This discharge is characteristically described by the patient as noted on the inside of her bra cup or night clothes or "leaking" from the nipple after a warm bath or shower [1]. This history must be specifically elicited and distinguished from discharge seen on expression only (e.g., during a breast exam, mammogram, or intimacy); discharge seen only with expression is normal and warrants no further evaluation. The character of the discharge is of less importance: a spectrum of appearances—including clear, serous, milky, greenish, and grayish—may be considered physiologic. Lastly, it is discharge from a single duct that is more often associated with a papilloma, rather than that from multiple ducts. The latter may be physiologic. Single versus multiple duct discharge is usually clarified with physical examination.

Although some clinicians may send discharge fluid for cytology or hemoccult testing, these studies are controversial and generally considered inadequate as stand-alone

P.A. Shah, MD (✉)
Department of Radiology, Breast Imaging Section, Virginia Commonwealth University Health (VCU HEALTH), Richmond, VA, USA
e-mail: priti.shah@vcuhealth.org

V. Robila, MD, PhD • M.O. Idowu, MD, MPH
Department of Pathology, Virginia Commonwealth University Health (VCU HEALTH), Richmond, VA, USA
e-mail: valentina.robila@vcuhealth.org

M.O. Idowu et al. (eds.), *Diagnosis and Management of Breast Tumors*,
DOI 10.1007/978-3-319-57726-5_7

practices in predicting malignancy due to poor accuracy [2]. Up to a 50% false-negative rate has been reported for cytologic analysis. Over 50% of patients with spontaneous discharge as the presenting sign of their malignancy have non-bloody discharge, and hemoccult testing of discharge is negative in almost one-third of patients with cancer. Moreover, as malignancy is the cause of spontaneous discharge in only about 10% of patients, even true-negative cytology and hemoccult testing do not aid in the diagnosis the underlying cause—most commonly, a papilloma or duct ectasia [2, 3].

In diagnostic breast imaging, ductography (galactography) or sonography may be used, in conjunction with mammography, in the work-up of spontaneous, single duct discharge. A ductogram is done by insertion of a blunt-tipped needle (we use a 30G sialography needle) into the secreting duct orifice and gentle injection of a few drops (0.2–0.4 mL) of radiopaque contrast. Special mammographic views of the subareolar region are then done, and these may show a dilated duct and/or an intraductal filling defect rather than the normal smooth caliber branches tapering posteriorly (Figs. 7.1 and 7.2). These filling defects may be only millimeters in size. Irregularities in the duct contour may suggest DCIS (Fig. 7.3). The false-negative rate of ductography is about 15%, and it is usually well tolerated; the main complication is pain or a "burning" sensation from a too-forceful injection. The only absolute contraindication is an acute abscess or mastitis [4].

Alternatively, ultrasound may be used to identify a subareolar mass (Fig. 7.4); however, one must be cautious in attributing the discharge to it if palpation of the mass does not reproduce the discharge (a "trigger point" as described by Haagensen) [5]. The elegance of the ductogram is that it has the potential to isolate the culprit duct and specifically localize the lesion for a more conservative surgical excision, particularly in the setting of multiple dilated ducts or duct ectasia [1, 4, 6, 7].

Sonographically, a papillary lesion commonly appears as a complex solid and cystic mass with circumscribed margins (Fig. 7.5); a solid mass in the subareolar

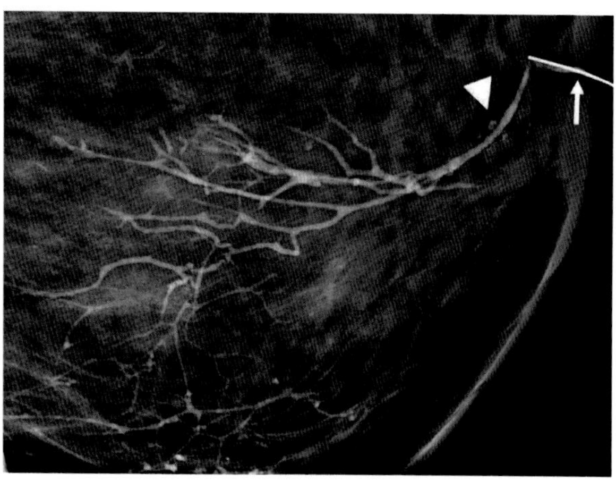

Fig. 7.1 Normal ductogram. A 30G blunt-tipped needle (*arrow*) is inserted into a duct orifice and drops of radiopaque contrast are injected, after which, magnified mammographic images of the subareolar region are taken. The opacified duct is smooth, normal in caliber, and tapers normally as it branches and courses into the remainder of the segment. Tiny outpouchings of contrast anteriorly reflect filling of the lobules (*arrowhead*)

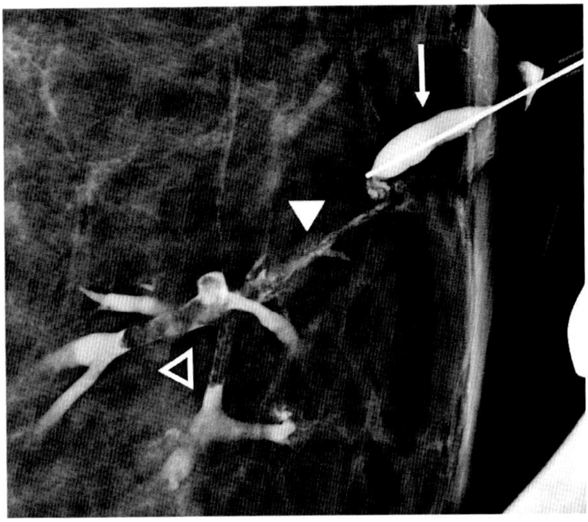

Fig. 7.2 Abnormal ductogram—done for a 64-year-old woman with spontaneous nipple discharge. This duct is abnormally dilated anteriorly (*arrow*) and narrows abruptly (*arrowhead*). A filling defect (*open arrowhead*) traverses a branch point. Excisional biopsy done for symptomatic relief yielded a papilloma

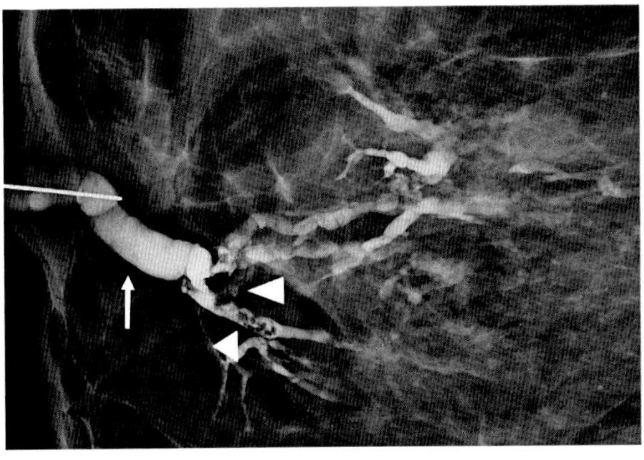

Fig. 7.3 Abnormal ductogram: Ductal carcinoma in situ—in a 77-year-old patient. The opacified duct is dilated (*arrow*) and abruptly changes caliber rather than tapering smoothly. Intraductal filling defects (*arrowheads*) and caliber irregularities (alternating areas of sacculation and narrowing) are highly suggestive of malignancy

region may also suggest this histology based on its location, particularly if it can be seen within a duct (intraductal). If seen radiographically without ductography, papillomas can be round to oval with circumscribed or spiculated margins and may have associated calcifications [1, 8, 9].

MRI is also being increasingly studied as a diagnostic tool in the evaluation of spontaneous discharge, with the advantage that it is noninvasive; cannulation and intraductal injection of contrast are avoided since MRI utilizes the intrinsic fluid

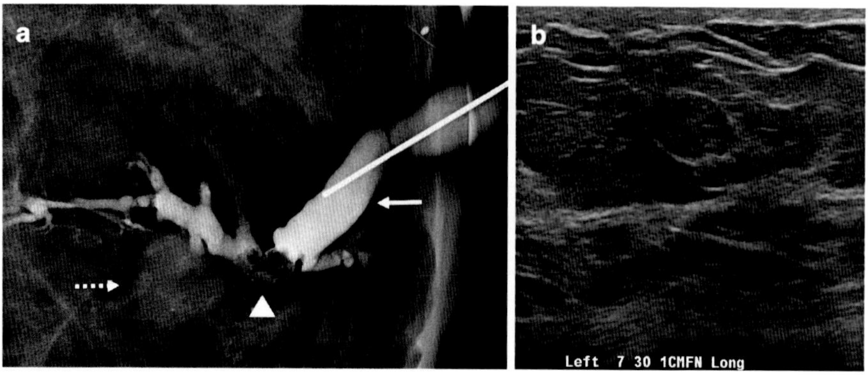

Fig. 7.4 Papillomas—(**a**) Ductogram shows a dilated duct (*arrow*) and intraductal filling defect (*arrowhead*), posterior to which a soft tissue mass (*dashed arrow*) is seen associated with a branch of the same duct. (**b**) That mass was identified and biopsied sonographically, and both lesions were excised for treatment of spontaneous nipple discharge

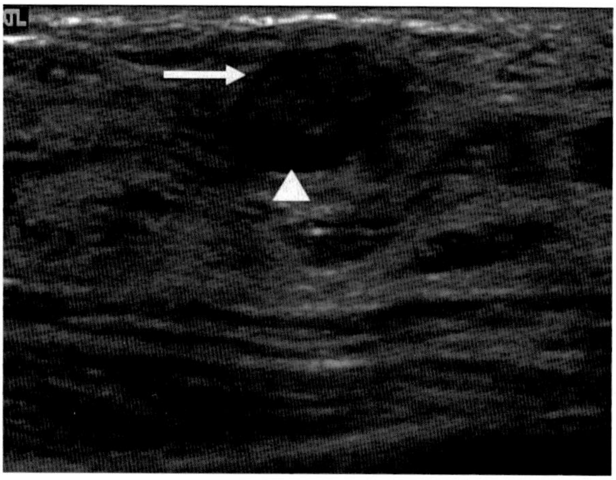

Fig. 7.5 Papilloma—Ultrasound of the subareolar region in a 25-year-old presenting with a palpable "lump" shows a complex mass with solid (*arrow*) and cystic (*arrowhead*) components and circumscribed margins

signal of ducts on T2-weighted images. However, as with sonography, this may be less specific as it demonstrates all major subareolar ducts, not isolating the "culprit" duct contemporaneously with eliciting of discharge. Intravenous gadolinium contrast can increase sensitivity and specificity, since duct ectasia or intraductal debris may not enhance; however, it may not help in distinguishing between benign and malignant papillary lesions since both of these can enhance. Also, given the tiny size of most papillomas, and duct lumens, the use of specialized microscopic coils is advocated in improving image resolution over conventional MRI imaging [10–13]. At this time, all of this may be time- and cost-prohibitive given the more accessible and efficient methods of conventional ductography and sonography [5].

We refer patients for excisional biopsy of lesions found at ductography for alleviation of their symptoms (spontaneous discharge can become quite frustrating) and for confirmation of histology. A preoperative ductogram is done in the morning of surgery to guide the surgeon and the pathologist. After re-cannulating the duct, injecting a combination of radiopaque dye and methylene blue, radiographs are repeated and sent to the operating room with the patient for surgical planning.

Some papillomas are found incidentally at mammography or sonography in asymptomatic patients. We do not routinely recommend excision of core needle biopsy-proven solitary papillomas without atypia in these patients if there is radiologic-pathologic concordance, rather, we follow these patients. This has been controversial as previous data suggested a high rate of upstaging to malignancy on excision of papillomas. However, solitary papillomas without atypia are in fact not associated with an increased risk of malignancy; the upgrade rate has been documented as low as 2.3%—and as high as 36%; however some of the latter studies do not account for radiological-pathological congruence [14–19]. In our own patients, there was an 8.3% rate of malignancy in excised papillomas without associated atypia, compared to a 30–40% of those with atypia [15]. It is widely accepted that papillary lesions associated with atypia on core needle biopsy (termed as such, or as atypical papillomas) require excision, even if solitary. Papillomas that are associated with an increased risk of malignancy, even if atypia is not identified concurrently, are those classified as multiple peripheral papillomas, the appearance, diagnosis, and work-up of which are different than the solitary or central.

Multiple peripheral papillomas may be seen on imaging as similar appearing masses in a segmental or ductal distribution. Patients are typically asymptomatic. Biopsy for tissue diagnosis of representative lesions, if possible at two opposite extents, is sufficient. Excision is usually recommended due to the likelihood of malignancy.

Papillary carcinomas are further divided histologically as invasive or in situ. Typically larger and faster growing than benign papillomas, these may exhibit lager cystic spaces amidst solid components under ultrasound (Fig. 7.6) [1]. As with all papillary lesions, the presence of a fibrovascular core histologically makes these susceptible to bleeding following a needle biopsy.

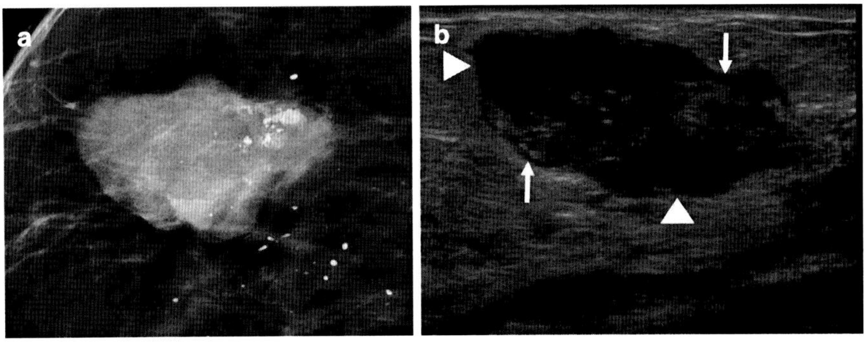

Fig. 7.6 Papillary carcinoma—(**a**) Spot tangential view of a palpable "lump" in an 84-year-old woman shows an equal density mass with circumscribed margins and coarse calcifications. (**b**) Correlative ultrasound demonstrates complex solid (*arrows*) and cystic (*arrowheads*) mass. Intraductal disease was seen on core needle biopsy and invasive ductal carcinoma at lumpectomy. Intraductal and invasive papillary carcinoma are indistinguishable on imaging

Chapter 2 of this text contains some discussion on the pathology approach to diagnosis of papillary lesions. Selected radiologic-pathologic correlation of papillary lesions is highlighted below.

Case 1

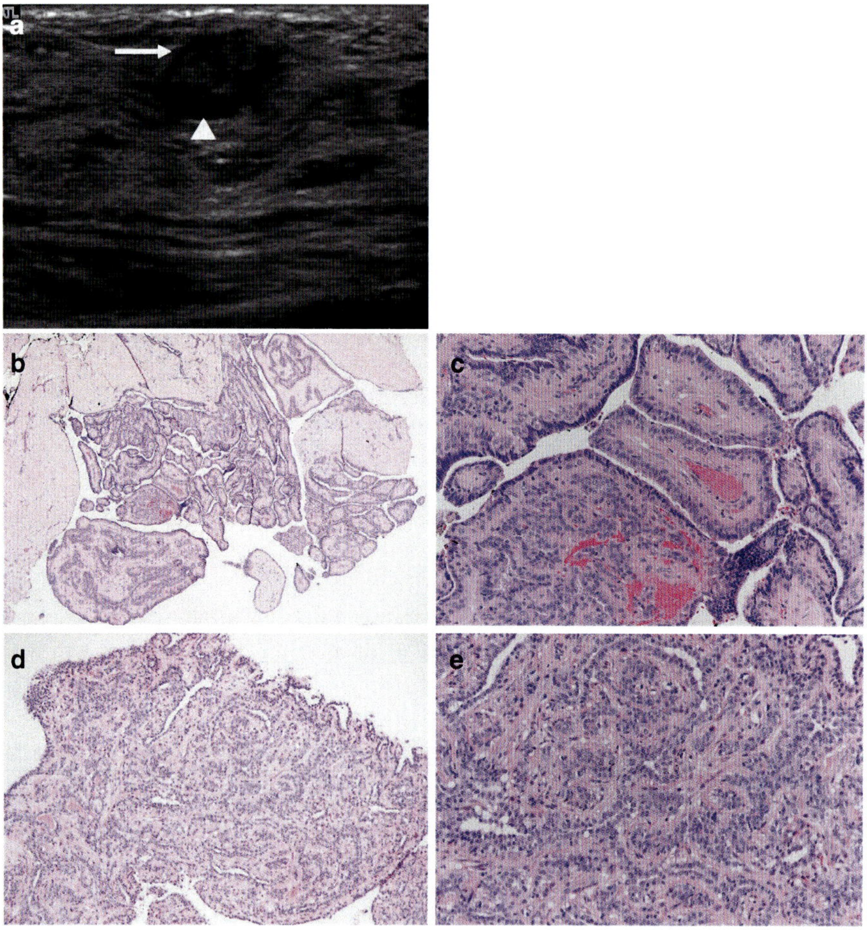

Intraductal papilloma—(**a**) Ultrasound of the subareolar region in a 25-year-old presenting with a palpable "lump" shows a complex mass with solid (*arrow*) and cystic (*arrowhead*) components and circumscribed margins. (**b**) The needle core biopsy shows a portion of the cyst wall around a papilloma. The mass is composed papillae with an arborizing pattern. (**c**) Epithelial cells, cuboidal or columnar, and myoepithelial cells are lining the fibrovascular cores. (**d**, **e**) The papillary fronds in this case appear fused with apparent solid appearance

Case 2

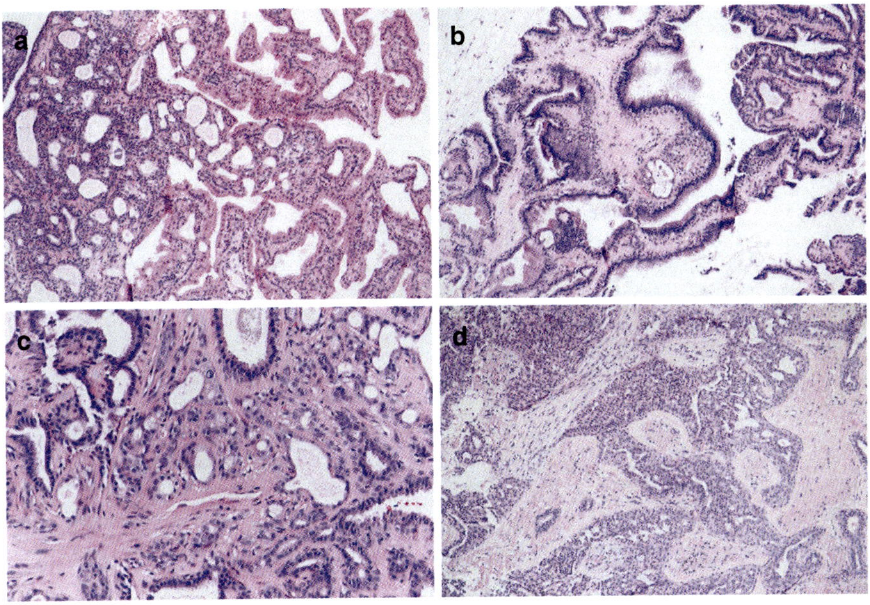

Benign changes in papillary lesions. (**a**) Papilloma with apocrine metaplasia. (**b** and **c**) Hyalinization of the vascular cores and adenosis type glands in the stroma. (**d**) Epithelial hyperplasia of the usual type and sclerosis

Case 3

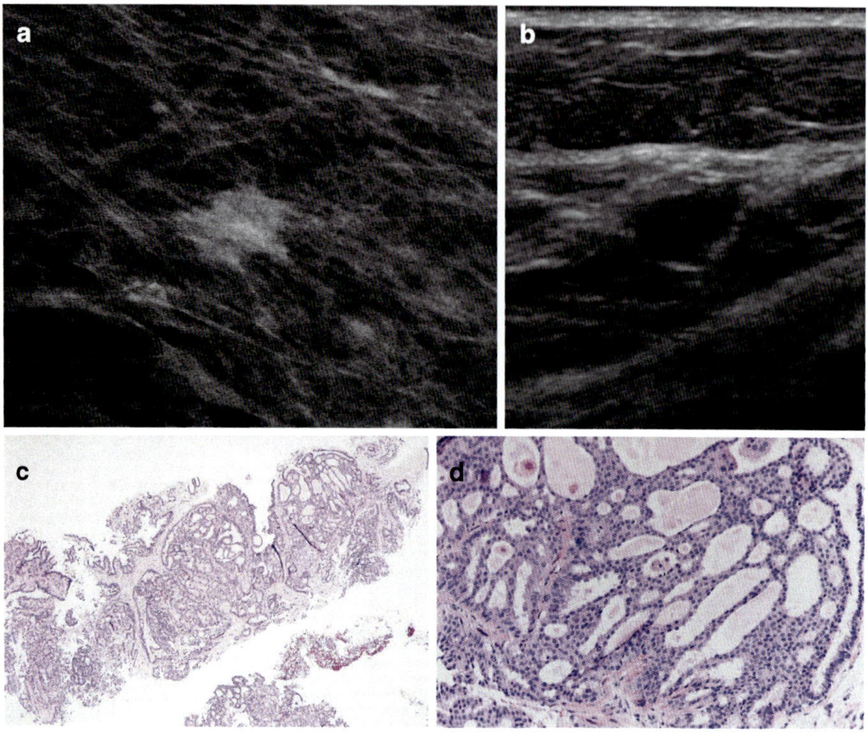

Atypical papilloma (papilloma with ADH or papilloma with DCIS). (**a**) Spot compression view of a screening detected irregular mass with indistinct margins in a 68-year-old woman. (**b**) Targeted sonography reveals an oval mass with nearly circumscribed margins. Given the mammographic appearance, and that the lesion was new, this was considered BI-RADS 4 lesion and core biopsy was done. (**c**) Needle core biopsies show a papilloma with epithelial hyperplasia. (**d**) At higher magnification, note the area of atypia, with round, uniform cells, oriented around microlumens. If such area is less than 3.0 mm, it is termed papilloma with ADH; if greater than or equal to 3 mm it is termed papilloma with DCIS. Excision of the lesion confirmed the atypical papilloma

Case 4

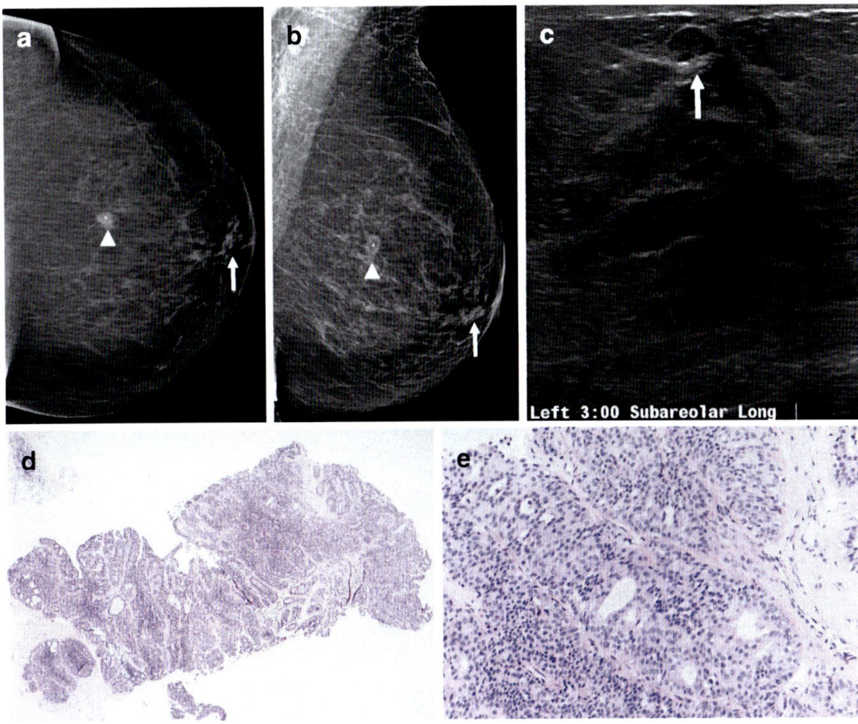

Atypical subareolar papilloma. (**a–c**, *arrows*) 63-year-old woman with a biopsy-proven cancer (*arrowheads*) and an additional subareolar mass. (**d**) Needle core biopsies show a papilloma with florid usual ductal hyperplasia. (**e**) Focal atypical ductal hyperplasia is also noted, consistent with atypical papilloma

Case 5

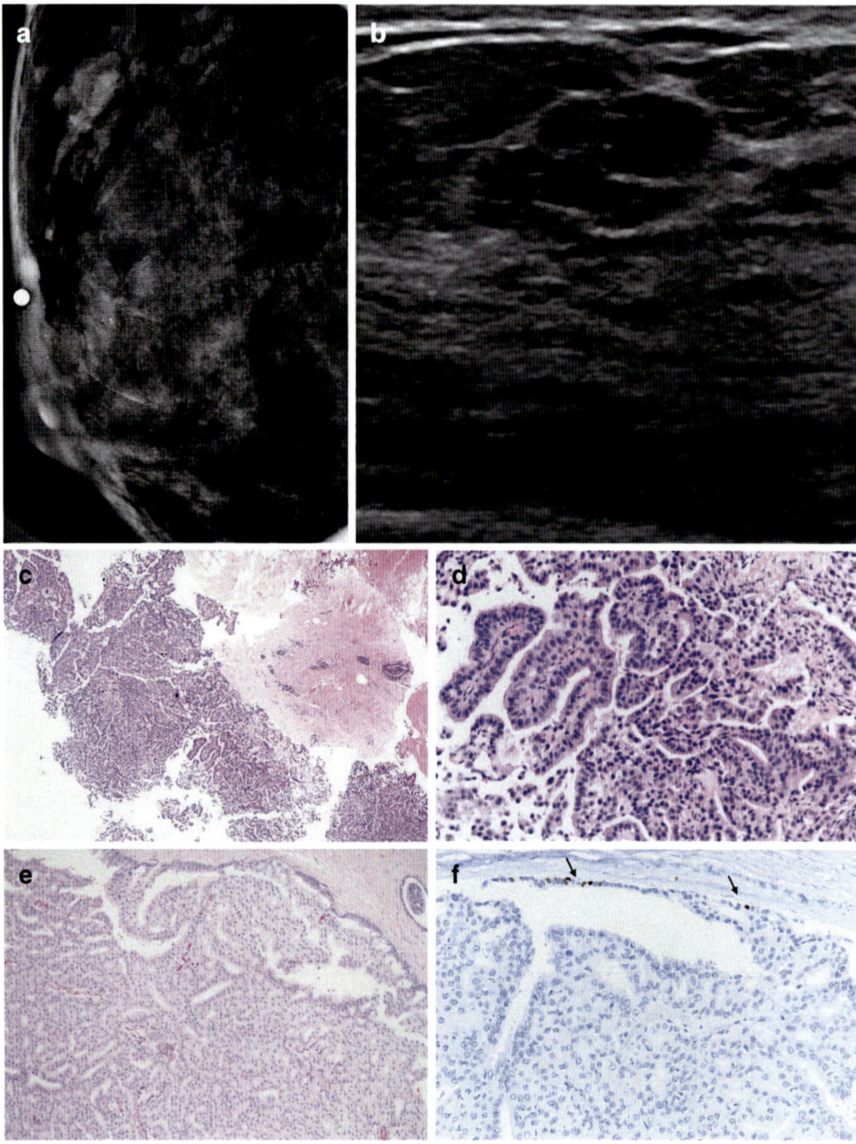

Papillary carcinoma in situ. (**a**) Spot tangential mammographic view demonstrates multiple palpable lobulated subareolar masses deep to the metallic BB in this 50-year-old patient. (**b**) Ultrasound showed cystic masses with intervening dilated ducts (not shown). Biopsy of this, the largest mass, is done. (**c**) Needle core biopsies show a portion of fibrous wall and the intra-cystic papillary epithelial proliferation. (**d**) The uniform hyperchromatic epithelial cells with nuclei oriented perpendicular to the axis, the apparent lack of myoepithelial cells and scant stroma favor papillary carcinoma, at least in situ. (**e**) Excision showed papillary DCIS. Note the intraductal proliferation of uniform cells around very thin fibrovascular stalks. (**f**) Rare p63- positive myoepithelial cells (*arrow*) are seen only at the periphery of the lesion

Case 6

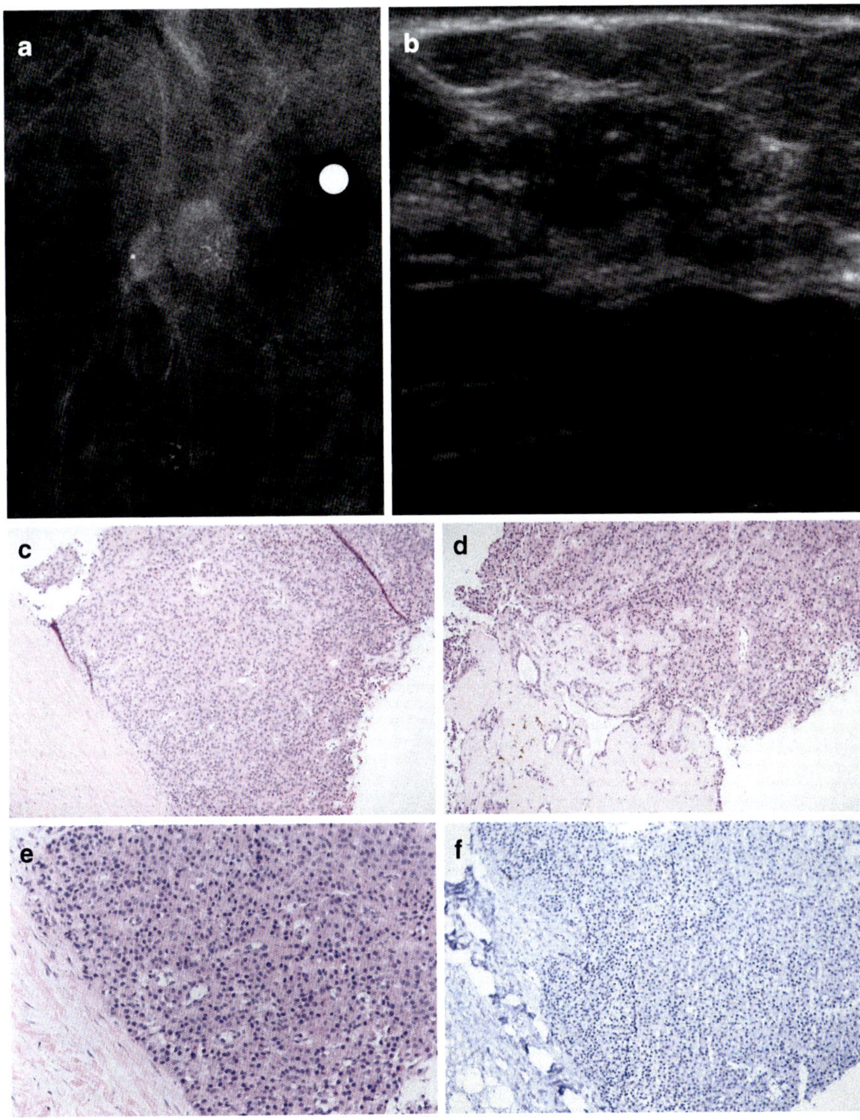

Papillary carcinoma in situ. (**a**) 59-year-old woman with a palpable mass containing calcifications and adjacent grouped calcifications. (**b**) Irregular mass (rather than the calcifications) was chosen for biopsy to increase likelihood of sampling invasive disease and thereby upstaging disease prior to definitive treatment. (**c**, **d**) Needle core biopsies show an intraductal proliferation with focal area of stromal hyalinization. (**e**) The epithelial proliferation creates a predominant solid appearance. The presence of rare thin fibrovascular cores suggest a papillary carcinoma. (**f**) The p63 stain is negative for myoepithelial cells within the lesion but focally positive for rare myoepithelial cells at the periphery consistent with papillary carcinoma in situ

Case 7

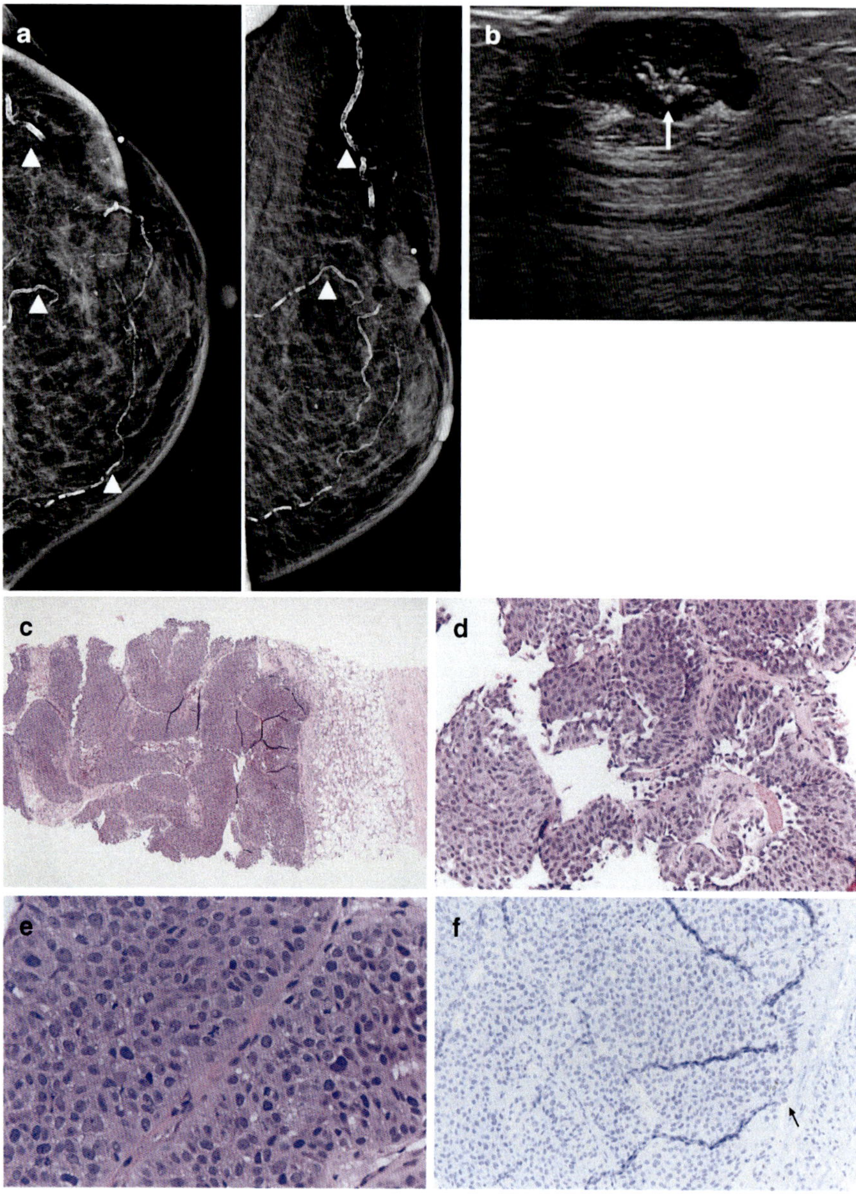

Papillary carcinoma. (**a**) 77-year-old woman with a palpable mass containing calcifications at prior lumpectomy site, marked on skin with metallic BB. Overlying skin retraction is from surgical scarring. Vascular calcifications were incidentally noted (*arrowheads*). (**b**) Lobulated complex solid and cystic mass seen on ultrasound; echogenic foci are calcifications (*arrow*). (**c** and **d**) Needle core biopsies show carcinoma with solid areas arranged around arborizing, thin fibrovascular cores and collagenized stroma. Tissue fragmentation is sometimes noted. (**e**) The epithelial cells have distinct borders, amphophilic cytoplasm, round nuclei with moderate pleomorphism, and mitoses. (**f**) The p63 stain highlights rare myoepithelial cells only at the periphery of the lesion (*arrow*)

Case 8

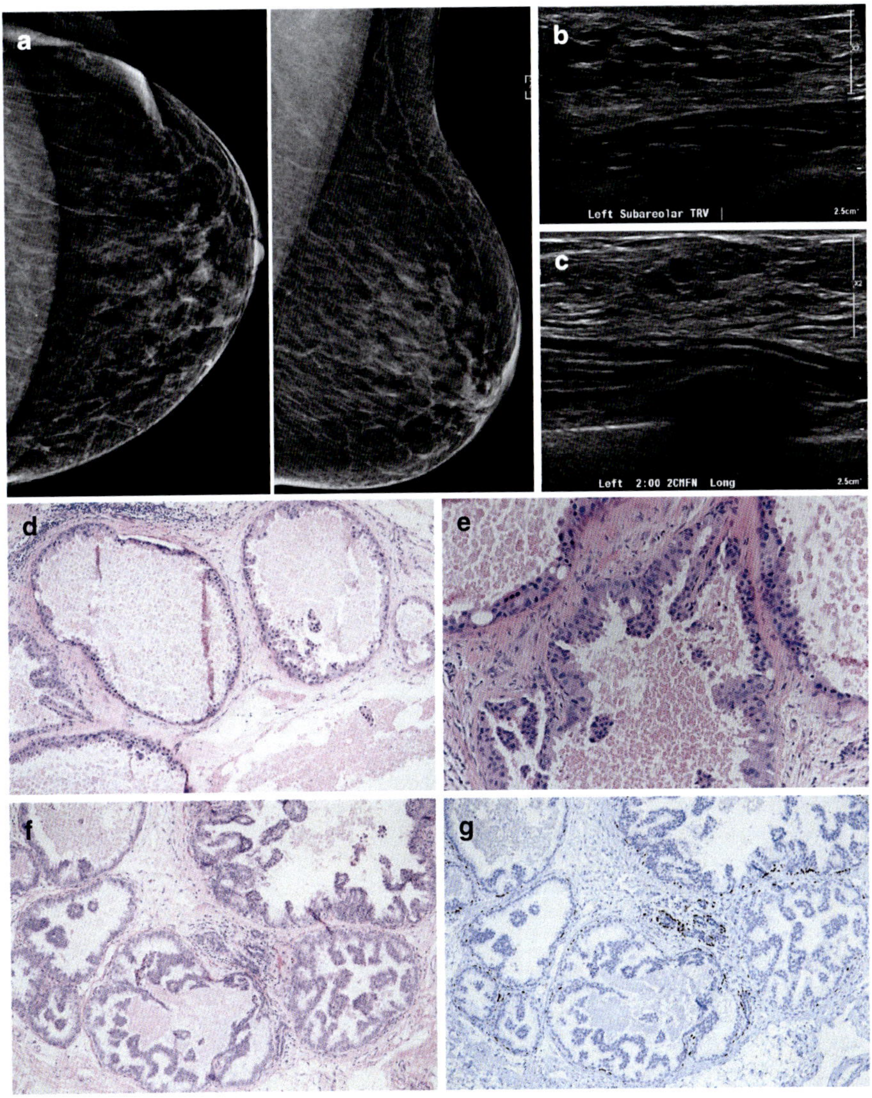

Ductal carcinoma in situ, micropapillary type. (**a**) CC and MLO screening mammographic views of the left breast in a 70-year-old woman demonstrate increased density in the retroareolar region; this was a developing asymmetry when compared with prior exams. (**b**) Targeted ultrasound showed duct ectasia; a mass (**c**) was targeted for core needle biopsy. (**d–e**) Needle core biopsy shows dilated ducts with small proliferations of uniform cells and central necrosis. At higher magnification, note the intraductal epithelial projections which are narrower at the base than apex consisting of uniform cells with no fibrovascular core (micropapillary architecture). The findings are consistent with micropapillary intraductal carcinoma. (**f**) Excision of the lesion showed similar histologic findings. (**g**) The p63 stain highlights the preserved peripheral myoepithelial cells

References

1. Cardenosa G. Clinical breast imaging, the essentials. Philadelphia, PA: Wolters Kluwer; 2015.
2. Moriarty AT, Schwartz MR, Laucirica R, Booth CN, et al. Cytology of spontaneous nipple discharge—is it worth it? performance of nipple discharge preparations in the College of American Pathologists Interlaboratory Comparison Program in Nongynecologic Cytopathology. Arch Pathol Lab Med. 2013;137:1039–42.
3. Morrogh M, Park A, Elkin EB, King TA. Lessons learned from 416 cases of nipple discharge of the breast. Am J Surg. 2010;200(1):73–80.
4. Cardenosa G, Doudna C, Eklund GW. Ductography of the breast: technique and findings. AJR Am J Roentgenol. 1994;162:1081–7.
5. Haagensen DC. Diseases of the breast. 3rd ed. Philadelphia, PA: WB Saunders; 1986.
6. Tabar L, Dean PB, Pentek Z. Galactography: the diagnostic procedure of choice for nipple discharge. Radiology. 1983;149:31–8. doi:10.1148/radiology.149.1.6611939. Accessed 26 Feb 2017.
7. Peters J, Thalhammer A, Jacobi V, Vogl TJ. Galactography: an important and highly effective procedure. Eur Radiol. 2003;13:1744–7. doi:10.1007/s00330-002-1739-x. Accessed 26 Feb 2017.
8. Pisano ED, Braeuning MP, Burke E. Case 8: solitary intraductal papilloma. Radiology. 1999;210(3):795–8.
9. Cardenosa G, Eklund GW. Benign papillary neoplasms of the breast: mammographic findings. Radiology. 1991;181:751–5.
10. Orel SG, Dougherty CS, Reynolds C, et al. MR imaging in patients with nipple discharge: initial experience. Radiology. 2000;216(1):248–54. doi:10.1148/radiology.216.1.r00jn28248.
11. Rovno HD, Siegelman ES, Reynolds C, et al. Solitary intraductal papilloma: findings at MR imaging and MRI galactography. AJR Am J Roentgenol. 1999;172:151–5. doi:10.2214/ajr.172.1.9888758.
12. Kanemaki Y, Kurihara Y, Itoh D. MR mammary ductography using a microscopy coil for assessment of intraductal lesions. AJR Am J Roentgenol. 2004;182(5):1340–2. doi:10.2214/ajr.182.5.1821340. Accessed 25 Feb 2017.
13. Nhattara N, Kanemaki Y, Kurihara Y, et al. Intraductal papilloma: features on MR ductography using a microscopic coil. AJR Am J Roentgenol. 2006;186(1):44–7. doi:10.2214/AJR.04.1600. Accessed 25 Feb 2017.
14. Pareja F, Corben AD, Brennan SB, et al. Breast intraductal papillomas without atypia in radiologic-pathologic condordant core needle biopsies: rate of upgrade to carcinoma at excision. Cancer. 2016;122(18):2819–27. doi:10.1002/cncr.30118. Accessed 25 Feb 2017.
15. Khan S, Diaz A, Archer KJ, Lehman RR, Mullins TC, Cardenosa G, Bear HD. Abstract P5-08-37: intraductal papillomas: risk of cancer, immediate and delayed. Cancer Res. 2016;76(Suppl 4). P5-08-37. doi:10.1158/1538-7445.SABCS15-P5-08-37. Accessed 25 Feb 2017.
16. Agoff SN, Lawton TJ. Papillary lesions of the breast with and without atypical ductal hyperplasia: can we accurately predict benign behavior from core needle biopsy? Am J Clin Pathol. 2004;122(3):440–3. doi:10.1309/NAPJMB0GXKJC6PTH. Accessed 25 Feb 2017.
17. Rizzo M, Lund MJ, Oprea G, et al. Surgical follow up and clinical presentation of 142 papillary lesions diagnosed by ultrasound guided core needle biopsy. Ann Surg Oncol. 2008;15:1040–7. doi:10.1245/s10434-007-9780-2. Accessed 25 Feb 2017.
18. Swapp RE, Glazebrook KN, Jones KN, et al. Management of benign intraductal solitary papilloma diagnosed on core needle biopsy. Ann Surg Oncol. 2013;20:1900–5. doi:10.1245/s10434-012-2846-9. Accessed 25 Feb 2017.
19. Holley SO, Appleton CM, Farria DM, et al. Pathologi outcomes of nonmalignant papillary breast lesions diagnosed at imaging-guided core needle biopsy. Radiology. 2012;265:379–84. doi:10.1148/radiol.12111926. Accessed 25 Feb 2017.

Proliferative and in situ Ductal and Lobular Breast Lesions

8

Priti A. Shah and Valentina Robila

Clinically speaking, proliferative lesions may be divided into three broad categories: those that are benign and warrant no further intervention, "high-risk" lesions that either are associated with an increased risk of being upstaged to malignancy at excision *or* increase a patient's lifetime risk, and those that are malignant, requiring excision with clear margins and likely further treatment such as radiation and/or adjuvant chemotherapy.

Benign Proliferative Lesions

Some benign proliferative lesions commonly fall under the umbrella of fibrocystic changes (FCC), a wide spectrum of entities best described in detail histologically. Some people use the term "fibrocystic disease", however, this is in a way a misnomer, since it is not a disease to be diagnosed or treated; rather, fibrocystic changes are those that breast tissue undergo in response to mostly physiologic and hormonal influences throughout a lifetime and, accordingly, are unequivocally benign [1, 5].

Although a "grab bag" of terms, specific entities under the umbrella of FCC have certain predictable appearances on imaging that may allow us to avoid unnecessary follow-ups or biopsies [5]. Some examples are presented below.

- *Cysts*—since mammography does not discern between solid and fluid-filled masses, a cyst is best diagnosed at ultrasound. However, the low density and

P.A. Shah, MD (✉)
Department of Radiology, Breast Imaging Section, Virginia Commonwealth University Health (VCU HEALTH), Richmond, VA, USA
e-mail: priti.shah@vcuhealth.org

V. Robila, MD, PhD
Department of Pathology, Virginia Commonwealth University Health (VCU HEALTH), Richmond, VA, USA
e-mail: valentina.robila@vcuhealth.org

M.O. Idowu et al. (eds.), *Diagnosis and Management of Breast Tumors*,
DOI 10.1007/978-3-319-57726-5_8

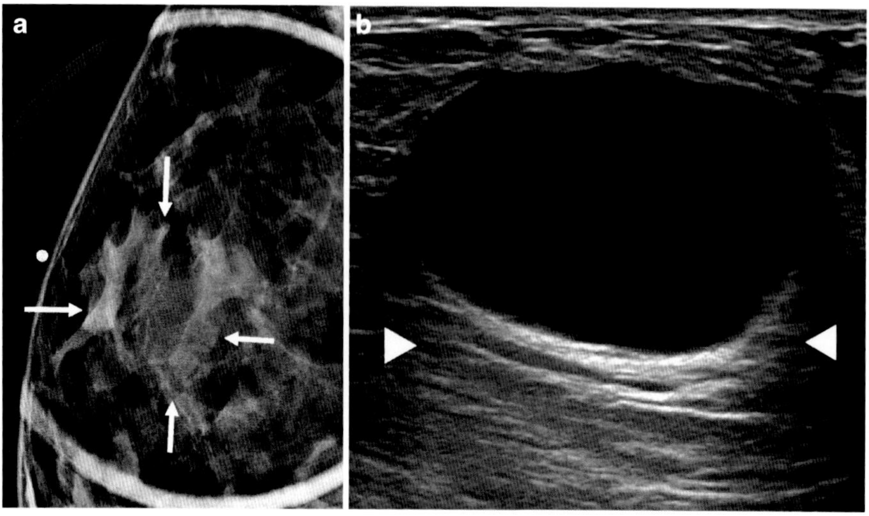

Fig. 8.1 Cyst (**a**) Spot tangential compression mammographic view of a palpable "lump" reported by this 45-year-old patient (the site of which is marked with a metallic BB on the skin) shows an equal density mass (*between arrows*) with partially circumscribed and obscured margins. (**b**) Targeted ultrasound demonstrates a cyst, defined as such because it is anechoic with circumscribed margins, has barely perceptible walls, and demonstrates posterior acoustic enhancement (*between arrowheads*). This is benign and warrants no further intervention if the patient is otherwise asymptomatic

circumscribed margins of a mass on X-ray may portend this diagnosis, and its absence of internal echoes ("anechoic"), barely perceptible walls, and increased transmission of sound waves posteriorly sonographically ("enhancement") is confirmatory (Fig. 8.1). As cysts are benign and may fluctuate in size or disappear as a result of hormonal influences, and 30–80% of cysts may recur once drained, we do not typically recommend aspiration or excision of simple cysts unless they cause significant discomfort [2, 3, 18]. It has been observed that injection of air into the cyst after drainage may be associated with decreased recurrence rates [3, 18].

- *Apocrine metaplasia*—The diagnosis is suggested mammographically by groups of calcifications that appear round or amorphous ("smudgy") on a craniocaudal (top to bottom) view, but curvilinear (concave up) or linear on a lateral (side to side) view (Fig. 8.2). This change in appearance is pathognomonic for milk of calcium and is due to the layering or sedimentation of calcium in suspension in the fluid of micro- or macrocysts. When viewed in the side-to-side projection, the calcifications appear like a meniscus, mimicking a "teacup." Sonographically, apocrine metaplasia may present as clustered microcysts with thin septa (Fig. 8.2) [2].
- *Sclerosing adenosis, ductal hyperplasia (without atypia), columnar cell changes*—may appear as grouped or diffusely distributed punctate or amorphous calcifications (Fig. 8.3), sometimes with associated masses. Typically, for most morphologies of calcifications, more diffuse and bilateral calcifiations are more likely to reflect benign fibrocystic changes [14]. If isolated, new, or increasing, work-up, follow-up, and/or biopsy may be warranted for confirmation.

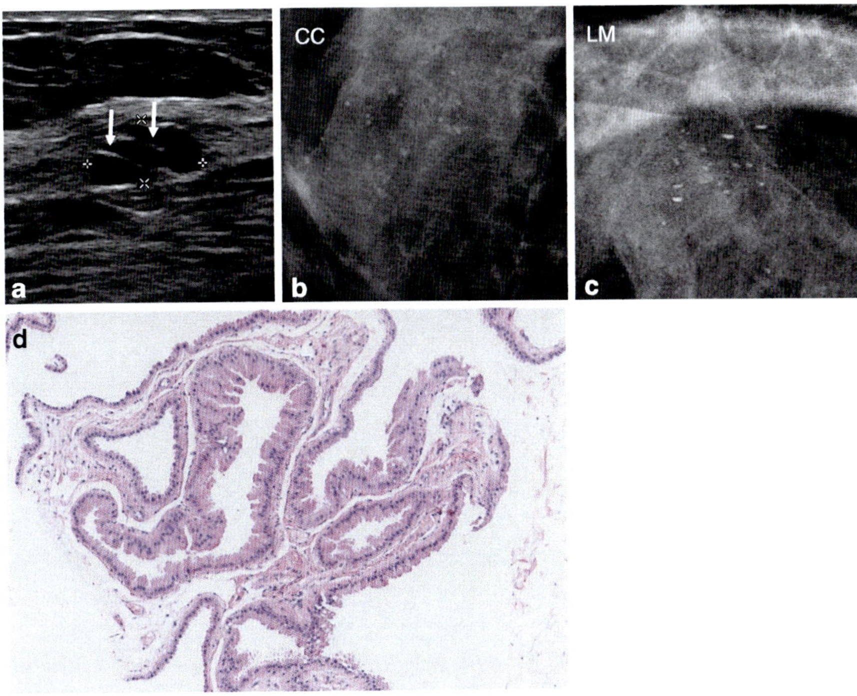

Fig. 8.2 Clustered cysts/apocrine metaplasia (**a**) Clusters of microcysts separated by thin septa (*arrows*) seen at ultrasound. (**b** and **c**) Different patient with milk of calcium seen mammographically; the change in form of calcifications from amorphous on the craniocaudal view to linear or curvilinear in the lateral-medial projection is pathognomonic for this benign process. (**d**) Cysts lined by apocrine cells, with ample eosinophilic cytoplasm and uniform nuclei. Apocrine metaplasia is often associated with calcium oxalate (not shown), best seen with polarization

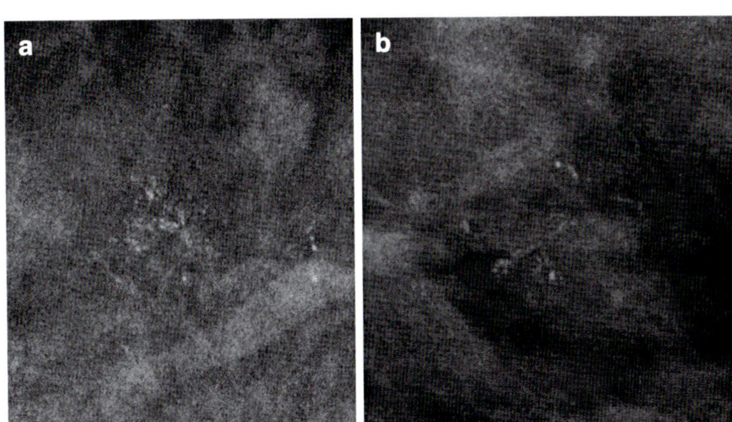

Fig. 8.3 Benign amorphous calcifications, spot compression magnification views. (**a**) Biopsy in this 46-year-old yielded fibrocystic change including sclerosing adenosis, columnar cell change, and pseudoangiomatous stromal hyperplasia. (**b**) Calcifications were associated with benign breast tissue on histology in this 53-year-old

- *Duct ectasia*—may appear as large (>2–3 mm), rod-like, solid, linear and branching calcifications mammographically (Fig. 8.4); these are intraductal and the result of inspissated secretions (and therefore debunk the mammography myth that all linear/intraluminal calcifications signify DCIS). On ultrasound, one may see dilated, fluid-filled ducts that taper normally.
- *Periductal/stromal fibrosis*—associated calcifications may appear linear or "jagged," since they are extraductal (Fig. 8.5) if in the walls of the ducts, there may

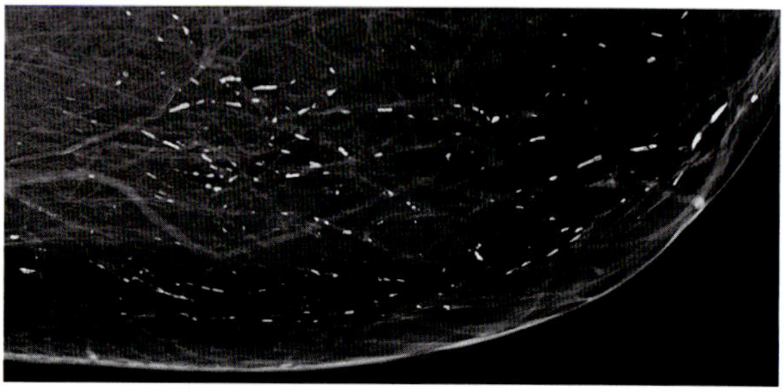

Fig. 8.4 Duct ectasia, plasma cell mastitis. Large rod-like calcifications are intraductal, the result of inspissated secretions

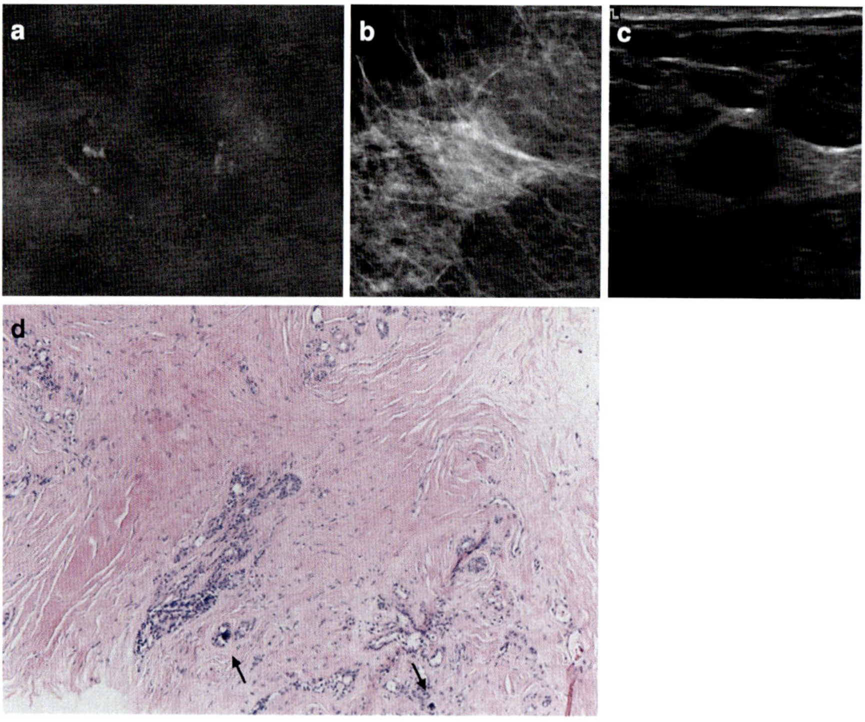

Fig. 8.5 Stromal fibrosis. (**a**) Coarse heterogenous and linear calcifications in a 50-year-old woman. (**b**) A round mass with indistinct margins on baseline screening mammogram and subsequent targeted ultrasound (**c**) in a 59-year-old. The mass appeared nearly anechoic (cystic), but when aspiration yielded no fluid (not shown), core biopsy of this solid mass was undertaken. (**d**) The needle core biopsy shows diffuse stromal fibrosis and focal microcalcifications (*arrows*)

be a central linear lucency. Stromal fibrosis may present as an oval or irregular hypoechoic mass sonographically (Fig. 8.5).

High-Risk Lesions

These entities incur increased future lifetime risk, or have potential to be upstaged to malignancy at excision. Management is controversial. Whether or not these lesions are excised, patients may undergo additional screening and/or (endocrine) chemopreventive measures based on their cumulative lifetime risk of breast cancer. If resected, susbsequent radiation treatment is not indicated for these lesions (unless upstaged to cancer at surgery).

- *Atypical ductal hyperplasia (ADH)/flat epithelial atypia (FEA)*—most commonly diagnosed in the work-up of calcifications (often punctate, amorphous). These entities can coexist in a spectrum of proliferative changes from (usual) hyperplasia to low-grade DCIS; upstage rates to malignancy ranging from 11 to 62% [6, 7, 10, 19]. We recommend excision as definitive treatment. Patients with ADH are considered at intermediate risk (15–20% lifetime risk) for future breast cancer [8].
- *Lobular neoplasia*: atypical lobular hyperplasia (ALH), lobular carcinoma in situ (LCIS)–these are proliferative processes of the lobules and are most commonly incidental findings on imaging-guided core needle biopsies; in other words, they have no associated radiological appearance or "classic" finding. Despite the name (another unfortunate misnomer), LCIS is considered a risk factor for future malignancy (in either breast) rather than a malignancy (or pre-malignancy) itself [9, 20, 21]. Historically, its management has therefore been one of the most controversial in breast health, ranging from no action to surgical excision. Our practice is mixed, but several of us recommend excision after a core biopsy yielding LCIS.
- *Radial scar/complex sclerosing lesion*—may be diagnosed at core biopsy of architectural distortion, with or without calcifications, seen mammographically (Fig. 8.6). These are distinguished by size, with radial scar less than 1cm in size, and complex sclerosing lesion larger than 1cm. The former may be found incidentally on histology; even if larger than 1cm, these lesions are usually not palpable and may be sonographically occult. Despite the word "scar," these are unrelated to prior trauma. Distorted ducts with a central fibroelastoic core are seen histologically. As up to 50% of these can be associated with atypia or upstaged to intraductal or invasive carcinoma, excisional biopsy is recommended; however if found incidentally microscopically for an otherwise benign process, some advocate follow up alone [5, 11, 12, 13].

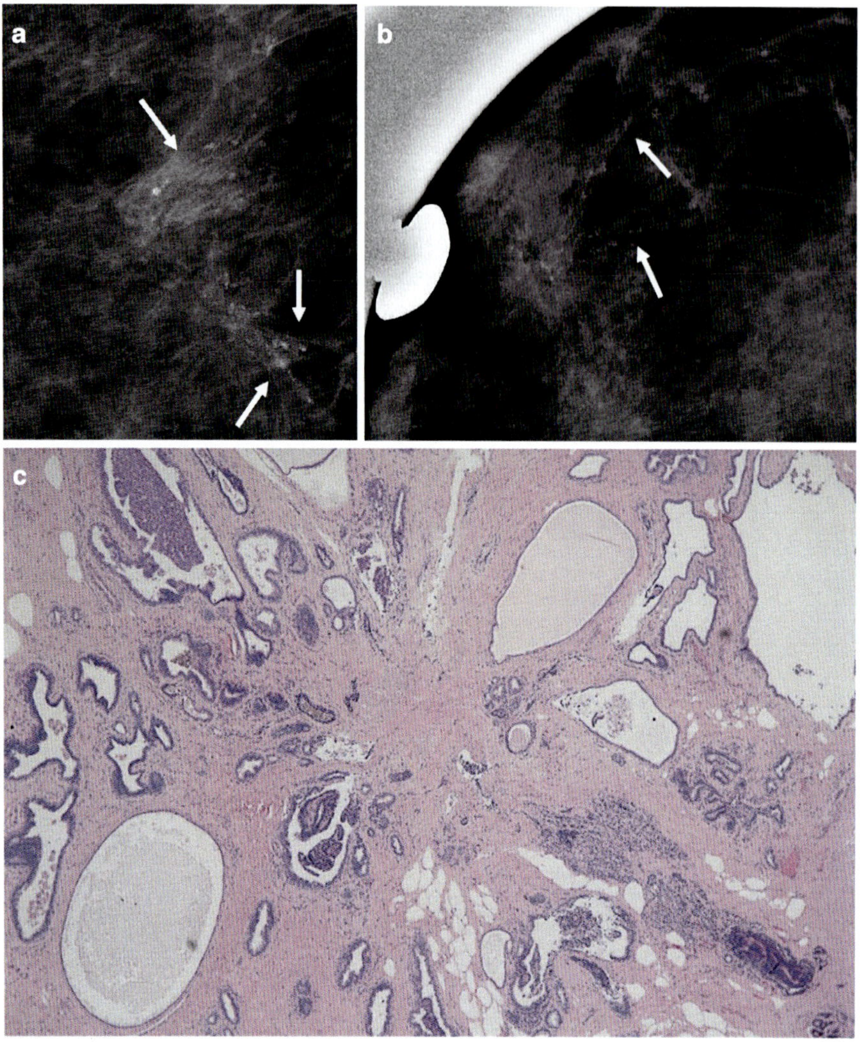

Fig. 8.6 Complex sclerosing lesion/radial scar. 54-year-old woman recalled from screening mammogram (**a**) CC and (**b**) MLO spot compression magnification views confirming architectural distortion ("straightening" of parenchymal contours, *arrows*) and associated amorphous calcifications. The distortion was biopsied under stereotactic guidance as no ultrasound correlate could be identified. (**c**) Needle core biopsy shows a complex sclerosing lesion. Note the central scar with entrapped benign glands. The radiating ductal structures show dilation and focal usual ductal hyperplasia

Ductal Carcinoma In Situ

As mentioned in Chap. 1, the introduction of a routine, annual screening mammography program drastically increased the diagnoses of ductal carcinoma in situ (DCIS) in the United States. This "epidemic" was due to the ability to detect with mammography microcalcifications associated with this process. As its name implies, the neoplastic cells in DCIS are contained within the duct lumen, bound by the myoepithelium. As these cells multiply, outgrow their vascularity, and undergo necrosis, this cellular debris calcifies. Since the calcifications form amidst irregular cells and debris, they too are small and irregular ("fine and pleomorphic" by the BI-RADS lexicon); still confined to the duct, the calcifications themselves may be linear in shape or "line up," following the ductal distribution, visible as fine linear and branching forms mammographically (Fig. 8.7). Of the BI-RADS morphology descriptors for calcifications, these have the highest likelihood of malignancy (53–81%) [14] and are associated with higher nuclear grade and comedonecrosis. Lower grades may manifest with punctate or amorphous forms (Fig. 8.7); it is also

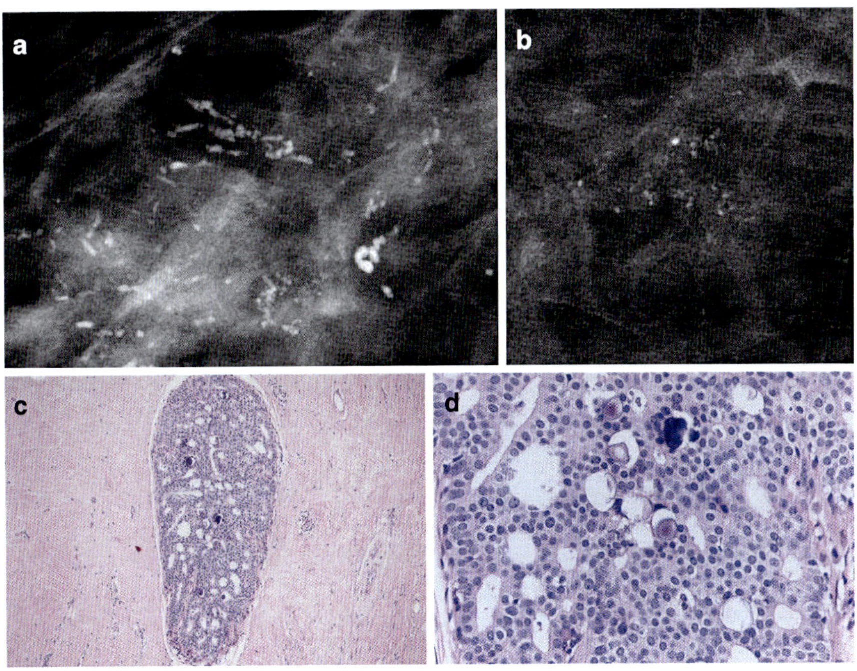

Fig. 8.7 (**a**) Fine linear or fine-linear branching calcifications are the "buzzwords" for DCIS (typically high nuclear grade, with comedonecrosis and resultant "casting" of the ducts), as in this 69-year-old woman. (**b**) Grouped fine pleomorphic calcifications, as in this 63-year-old patient, suggest a lower histologic grade of DCIS. (**c**) Ductal carcinoma in situ. Note the dilated duct filled with uniform cells forming "punched out" spaces, characteristic of cribriform architecture. (**d**) The nuclei are small, round, uniform with inconspicuous nucleoli, characteristic of low grade DCIS. Mitoses are not identified. Note the associated microcalcifications

important to note that not all DCIS calcifies; and though less common, other radiographic findings may include ductal dilation, parenchymal asymmetry, architectural distortion, or a mass. DCIS may also be found histologically in the absence of radiological findings.

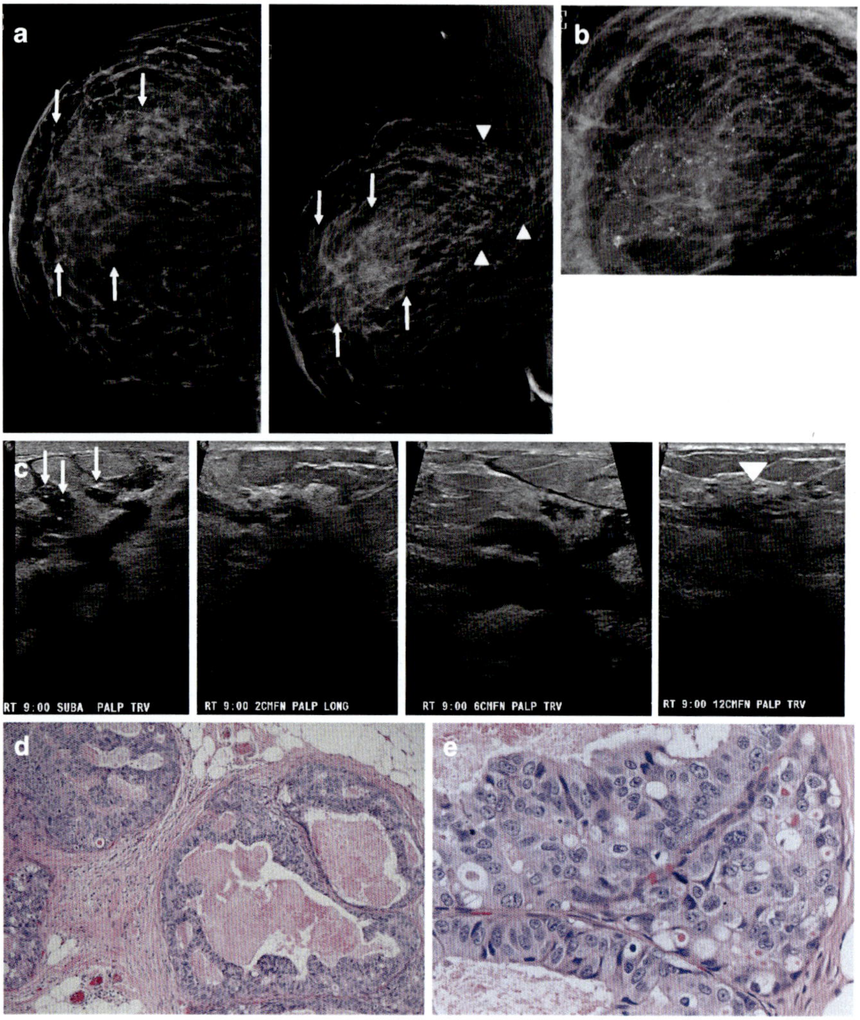

Fig. 8.8 Extensive ductal carcinoma in situ, nuclear grade 3, with comedonecrosis. (**a**) Standard CC and MLO views of the right breast show increased density and segmentally distributed calcifications in the outer central aspect, anterior half (*arrows*). and increased trabecular markings extending to the pectoralis major suggestive of edema (*arrowheads*). This 32-year-old had reported pain and "swelling"; on physical exam there was bulging and peau d'orange change laterally with nipple retraction and discharge on expression. (**b**) Spot compression magnification view better shows the calcifications as fine and pleomorphic with amorphous, coarse, heterogeneous, and linear forms. (**c**) Multiple ultrasound images along the 9 o'clock axis from the subareolar region posteriorly show dilated ducts containing echogenic foci (calcifications, *arrows*). An irregular mass (*arrowhead*) with indistinct margins is also seen, suggestive of invasive disease. (**d**) Ductal carcinoma in situ, high nuclear grade. The intraductal proliferation is associated with extensive central necrosis. (**e**) The epithelial cells show high grade pleomorphic nuclei with coarse chromatin and prominent nucleoli

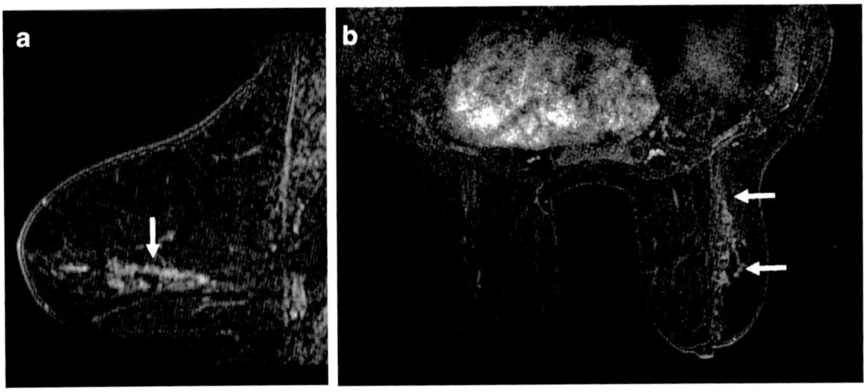

Fig. 8.9 Non-mass enhancement, ductal carcinoma in situ. (**a**) Sagittal and (**b**) axial images post contrast subtraction MRI images demonstrate clumped and linear enhancement (*arrows*) in the right breast, extending toward the nipple

Sonographically, malignant-type calcifications may be identified if using careful technique; their conspicuity is increased in the setting of dilated ducts (Fig. 8.8). Intraductal soft tissue filling defects may also be seen. However, ultrasound is not routinely used in the work-up of calcifications suggestive of DCIS unless there is an associated finding (ductal dilation, asymmetry, distortion, or mass) that would suggest invasive disease and therefore be a target for ultrasound-guided biopsy.

Lower-grade DCIS may not enhance on MRI as avidly as higher grades. As expected given the absence of a mass on mammogram or ultrasound, enhancement may be in a "non-mass" configuration, for example, clumped and linear in a segmental fashion, or in clustered rings representing ductal wall enhancement, following the ductal distribution (Fig. 8.9) [15].

Paget disease of the nipple, albeit rare, may have no imaging correlate in up to 50% of patients; when visible, findings include those of DCIS and/or invasive disease (such as duct ectasia, distortion, non-mass enhancement, mass, or focal asymmetry), and possibly thickening, retraction, and abnormal MRI enhancement of the nipple itself [16, 17].

References

1. Love SM, Gelman RS, Silen W. Fibrocystic disease of the breast—a nondisease? N Engl J Med. 1982;307:1010–4. doi:10.1056/NEJM198210143071611. Accessed 13 Feb 2017.
2. Cardenosa G. Clinical breast imaging, the essentials. Philadelphia, PA: Wolters Kluver; 2015.
3. Gizienski TA, Harvey JA, Sobel AH. Breast cyst recurrence after postaspiration injection of air. Breast J. 2002;8(1):34–7.
4. Ikeda DM. Breast imaging: the requisites. Philadelphia, PA: Elsevier Mosby; 2004.
5. Guray M, Sahin AA. Benign breast diseases: classification, diagnosis, management. Oncologist. 2006;11(5):435–49. doi:10.1634/theoncologist.11-5-435. Accessed 25 Feb 2017.
6. Tkaczuk KH, Kesmodel SB, Feibenberg SJ. Handbook of breast cancer and related breast disease. New York, NY: Springer Publishing Company; 2017.

7. Sinn HP, Elsawaf Z, Helmchen B. Early breast cancer precursor lesions: lessons learned from molecular and clinical studies. Breast Care. 2010;5:218–26. doi:10.1159/000319624. Accessed 28 May 2017.
8. American College of Radiology. ACR appropriateness criteria: breast cancer screening. https://acsearch.acr.org/docs/70910/Narrative/. Accessed 13 Feb 2017.
9. Berg WA, Mrose HE, Ioffe OB. Atypical lobular hyperplasia or lobular carcinoma in situ at core-needle breast biopsy. Radiology. 2001;218(2):503–9. doi:10.1148/radiology.218.2.r01fe32503. Accessed 13 Feb 2017.
10. Mina L, Storniolo AM, Douglas H, et al. Breast cancer prevention and treatment. Switzerland: Springer International Publishing; 2016.
11. Adler DD, Helvie MA, Oberman HA, Ikeda DM, Bhan AO. Radial sclerosing lesions of the breast: mammographic features. Radiology. 1990;176(3):737–40. doi:10.1148/radiology.176.3.2389032. Accessed 19 Feb 2017.
12. Smetherman DH, Gowharji LF. Clinical images: radial scar of the breast. Oschner J. 2015;15(3):219–22.
13. Dominguez A, Durando M, Mariscotti G, et al. Breast cancer risk associated with the diagnosis of radial scar (RS): retrospective analysis in 10 years of experience. Radiol Med. 2015;120:377–85. doi:10.1007/s11547-014-0456-2. Accessed 23 Feb 2017.
14. Sickles EA, D'Orsi CJ, Bassett LW. ACR BI-RADS® mammography. In: ACR Bi-RADS Atlas, editor. Breast imaging reporting and data system. Reston, VA: American College of Radiology; 2013.
15. Rosen EL, Smith-Foley SA, DeMartini WB, et al. BI_RADS MRI enhancement characteristics of ductal carcinoma in situ. Breast J. 2007;13(6):545–50. doi:10.1111/j.1524-4741.2007.00513.x. Accessed 23 Feb 2017.
16. Lim HS, Jeong SJ, Lee JS, et al. Paget disease of the breast: mammographic, US, and MR imaging findings with pathologic correlation. Radiographics. 2011;31(7):1973–87. doi:10.1148/rg.317115070. Accessed 23 Feb 2017.
17. Ikeda DM, Helvie MD, Frank TS, et al. Paget disease of the nipple: radiologic-pathologic correlation. Radiology. 1993;189:89–94.
18. Vargas HI, Vargas MP, Gonzalez KD, Eldrageely K, Khalkhali I. Outcomes of sonography-based management of breast cysts. Am J Surg. 2004;188(4):443–7.
19. Youk JH, Kim EK, Kim MJ. Atypical ductal hyperplasia diagnosed at sonographically guided 14-gauge core needle biopsy of breast mass. Am J Roentgenol. 2009;192(4):1135–41.
20. Salvadori B, Bartoli C, Zurrida S, Delledonne V, Squicciarini P, Rovini D, Barletta L. Risk of invasive cancer in women with lobular carcinoma in situ of the breast. Eur J Cancer Clin Oncol. 1991;27(1):35–7.
21. Page DL, Kidd TE, Dupont WD, Simpson JF, Rogers LW. Lobular neoplasia of the breast: higher risk for subsequent invasive cancer predicted by more extensive disease. Hum Pathol. 1991;22(12):1232–9.

Invasive Carcinomas

9

Hetal Vachhani, Priti A. Shah, Valentina Robila, and Michael O. Idowu

There are several histologic subtypes of invasive carcinoma of the breast, including, but not limited to the following: invasive carcinoma of no special type (commonly known as invasive ductal carcinoma); invasive lobular carcinoma; tubular carcinoma; carcinoma with medullary features (sometimes called medullary carcinoma); and metaplastic carcinoma. Invasive (or infiltrating) ductal carcinoma (IDC) accounts for the majority (approximately 75%) of breast cancers, with invasive lobular carcinoma (ILC) accounting for 5–15%. Ultimately, management and prognosis are based on size, grade, predictive marker status, molecular phenotype, tumor biology, nodal status, and distant metastasis.

More aggressive, rapidly growing high nuclear grade IDCs, often triple negative cancers, tend to be expansile, round, or oval masses on imaging, mimicking some benign masses. They may be dense radiographically with nearly circumscribed margins; sonographically they may be nearly anechoic but should not be

H. Vachhani, MD (✉)
Division of Hematology Oncology, Department of Internal Medicine, Massey Cancer Center, Virginia Commonwealth University Health (VCU HEALTH), Richmond, VA, USA
e-mail: hetal.vachhani@vcuhealth.org

P.A. Shah, MD
Department of Radiology, Breast Imaging Section, Virginia Commonwealth University Health (VCU HEALTH), Richmond, VA, USA
e-mail: priti.shah@vcuhealth.org

V. Robila, MD, PhD • M.O. Idowu, MD, MPH
Department of Pathology, Virginia Commonwealth University Health (VCU HEALTH), Richmond, VA, USA
e-mail: valentina.robila@vcuhealth.org; michael.idowu@vcuhealth.org

M.O. Idowu et al. (eds.), *Diagnosis and Management of Breast Tumors*,
DOI 10.1007/978-3-319-57726-5_9

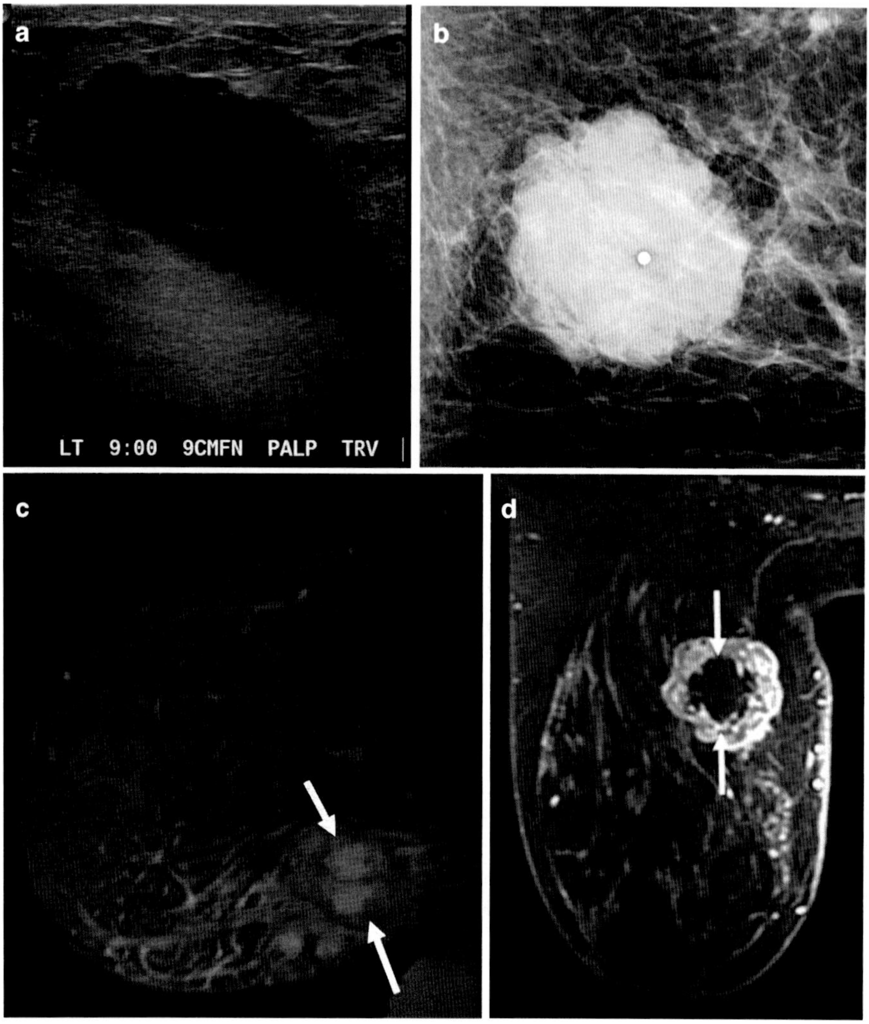

Fig. 9.1 Invasive ductal carcinoma, high nuclear grade. (**a**) Ultrasound shows a nearly anechoic, "cystic" appearing mass; however, its microlobulated borders and density mammographically (**b**) portend a more suspicious etiology in this 42-year-old woman. A metallic BB placed on the overlying skin indicates this is palpable to the patient. (**c**) Pre-contrast sagittal T2-weighted (fluid-sensitive) MRI image shows increased signal around the mass (peritumoral edema) and centrally in the mass (*between arrows*) that corresponds absence of enhancement on axial post-contrast imaging (**d**), reflecting central necrosis

mistaken for a cyst (Fig. 9.1). On MRI, these masses may demonstrate heterogeneous or peripheral enhancement, sometimes with central nonenhancement and T2 hyperintensity ("fluid" signal) that may reflect central necrosis, and peritumoral edema. In contrast, low nuclear grade IDCs more commonly present as ill-defined masses with spiculated margins or architectural distortion; the spicules are indicative of its slower, more infiltrative growth pattern, "creeping" along tissue planes and disrupting ligaments (Fig. 9.2). Some of the "mass" on imaging may be part of a fibrotic or a desmoplastic reaction, rather than viable tumor. While low-grade carcinomas enhance on MRI, contrast uptake may be non-mass (i.e., it does not conform to the definition of a mass; it may be a "region" of enhancement) in appearance and less avid than that of a higher-grade tumor. Malignant-type calcifications seen radiographically in association with a mass suspicious for IDC may reflect associated ductal carcinoma in situ; these may extend a distance away from the mass such that additional biopsy may be needed

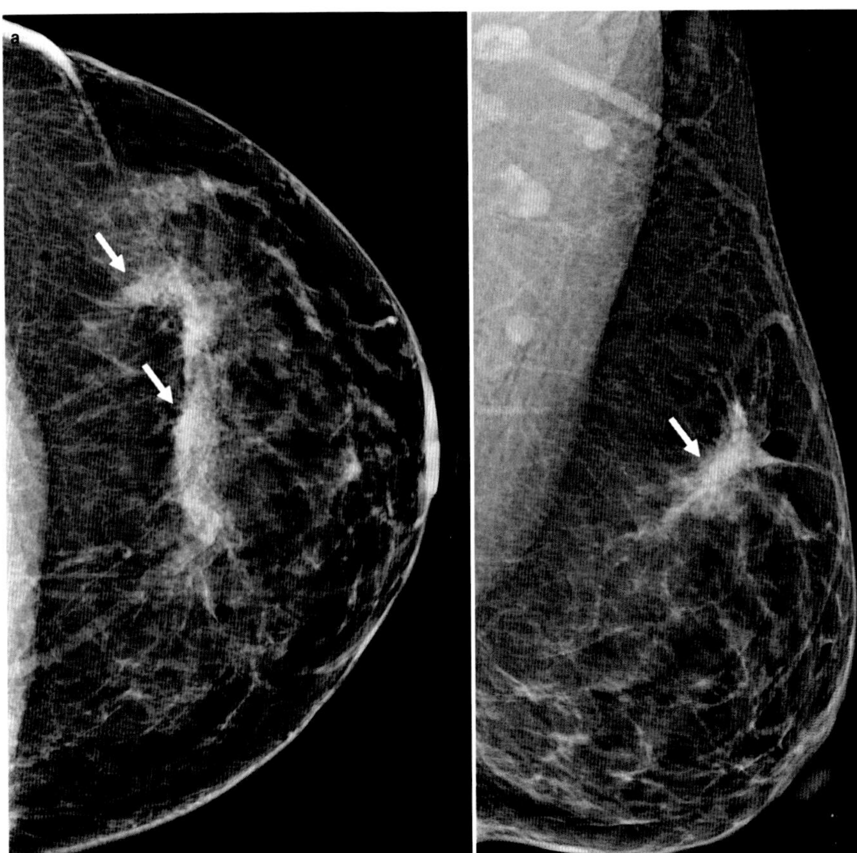

Fig. 9.2 Invasive ductal carcinoma, low nuclear grade. (**a**) Screening mammogram in this 41-year-old woman shows architectural distortion (*arrows*) in the upper central aspect of the left breast—"straightening" of the parenchymal lines. (**b**) On ultrasound of the upper inner and outer quadrants, multiple areas of ill-defined hypoechogenicity and disruption of tissue planes are seen, without an expansile mass. (**c**) Post-contrast axial MRI image demonstrates non-mass enhancement occupying the majority of the parenchyma in the upper quadrants (*arrow*); the normal right breast is shown for comparison

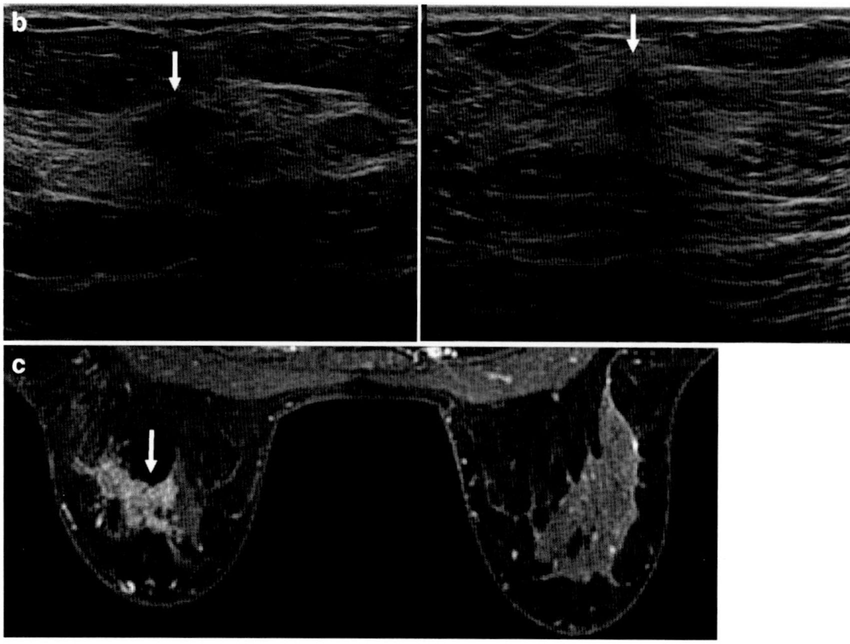

Fig. 9.2 (continued)

to confirm extent of disease for surgical planning (malignant-type calcifications themselves are not seen on MRI).

Mucinous and papillary carcinomas, seen more commonly in postmenopausal women, are less aggressive and metastasize less frequently than IDC, providing for a better prognosis. This may seem counterintuitive as these masses are classically described as "large" and expansile; however, their size comes from their internal matrix. On imaging, these are typically round or oval lobulated masses, and their echogenicity can help predict their histology (Figs. 9.3 and 9.4). Mucinous carcinomas tend to be iso- to slightly hyperechoic and are slow growing. Papillary carcinomas are typically complex solid and cystic and may grow more rapidly depending in part on the cystic component but may also be spiculated and solid. The mucin and fluid in these masses, respectively, also contribute to T2 hyperintensity (fluid signal) on MRI. Additionally, non-enhancing septa may be seen in mucinous cancers, compared with the enhancing solid portions of the vascular papillary carcinoma. Although these may present as large masses, the imaging features should supersede size when trying to confirm radiologic-pathologic concordance; all cancers have a starting point and may be found in early stages when still small. Papillary carcinomas are further described in the chapter "Papillary Lesions." Tubular carcinomas tend to be small (< 1 cm) masses with spiculated margins, or areas of distortion, and are also slow growing. Histologically they may be associated with radial scars or complex sclerosing lesions, which is why excision is recommended for these high-risk lesions if found on imaging-guided core biopsy.

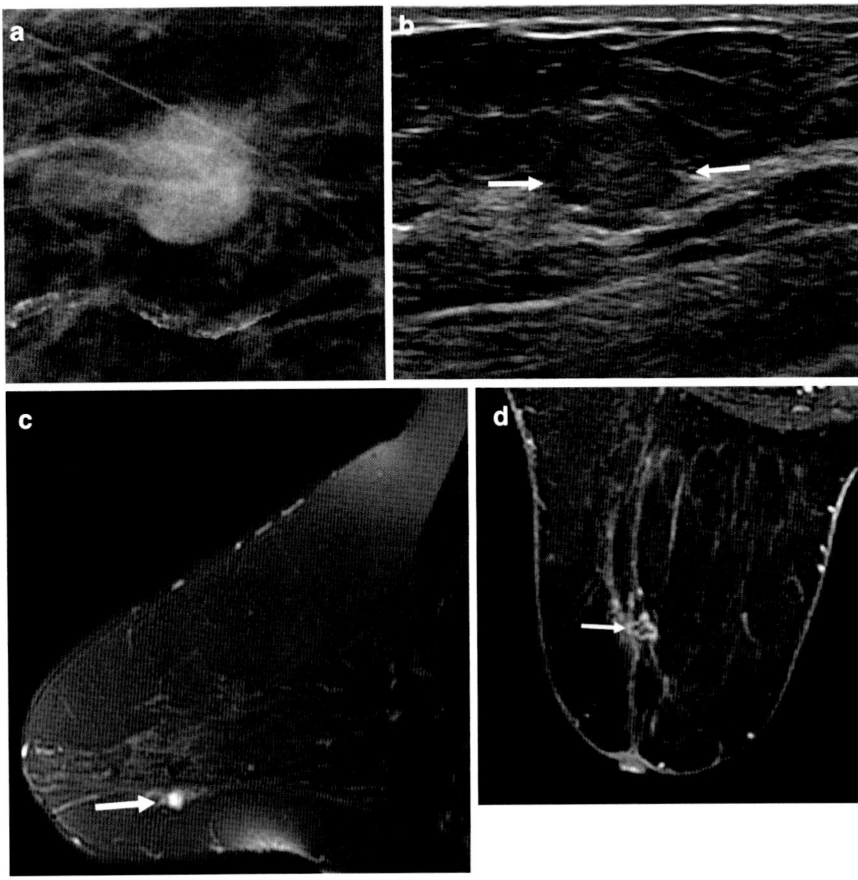

Fig. 9.3 Mucinous carcinoma in an 80-year-old woman. (**a**) Spot compression view after screening callback shows a round equal-density mass with mostly circumscribed and some indistinct margins. (**b**) On ultrasound this was an iso- to slightly hyperechoic mass (*between arrows*), relative to subcutaneous fat. (**c**) Pre-contrast sagittal T2-weighted (fluid-sensitive) MRI image shows a mass of increased signal intensity (*arrow*) that corresponds to a peripherally enhancing mass on post-contrast images. (**d**) The central portion of the mass is mucin, which itself does not enhance

Metaplastic carcinomas are rapidly growing masses with a worse prognosis, with axillary or distant (including hematogenous) metastases possible at the time of diagnosis (Fig. 9.5). By imaging they may be indistinguishable from a high nuclear grade IDC NOS, but histologically they are comprised of glandular, squamous or mesenchymal elements.

Invasive lobular carcinoma (ILC), which represents about 10% of all breast cancers, is more common in postmenopausal women and is slow growing. Radiographically, ILC may appear as an area of architectural distortion,

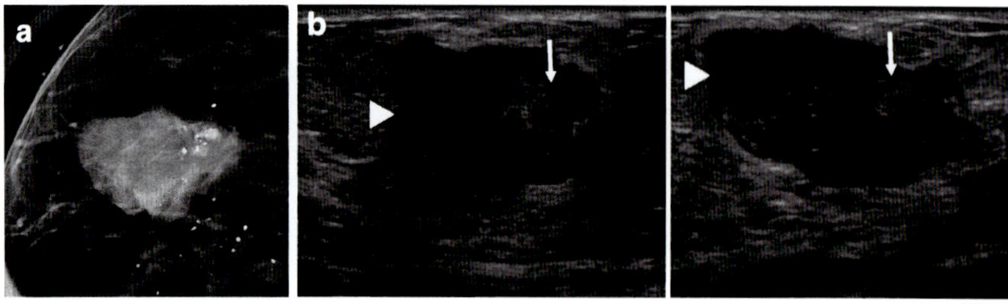

Fig. 9.4 Papillary carcinoma in an 84-year-old woman. (**a**) Spot tangential mammographic view shows an equal-density oval mass with circumscribed and lobulated margins and associated and adjacent coarse calcifications. (**b**) Orthogonal ultrasound images demonstrate a complex solid (*arrows*) and cystic (*arrowheads*) mass. The solid portion was targeted for ultrasound-guided needle biopsy. Although at core biopsy a papillary lesion with involvement by ductal carcinoma in situ was identified, invasive disease was found at lumpectomy. Intraductal and invasive papillary carcinoma may be indistinguishable on imaging

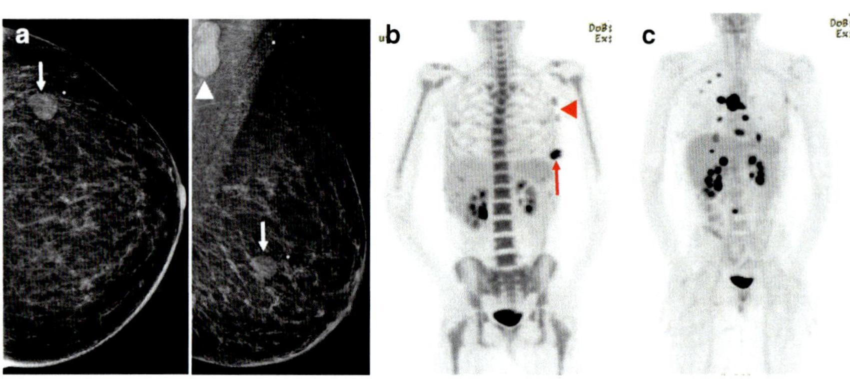

Fig. 9.5 Metaplastic carcinoma. (**a**) A 50-year-old woman presenting with a palpable mass in the outer central aspect of the left breast (*arrows*) and palpable axillary adenopathy (*arrowhead*). (**b**) 3-D maximum intensity projection reconstructions from a PET/CT scan show persistent disease in the breast (*arrow*) and to a lesser degree in the axilla (*arrowhead*) 7 months into chemotherapy and (**c**) progression of metastases at 11 months despite mastectomy, axillary dissection, and additional chemotherapy

developing asymmetry, or mass with spiculated margins, rather than an expansile mass, alluding to its more indolent, "single-file" cell growth pattern. Also because of its histology, ILC may be planar, seen better in one plane (classically the craniocaudal projection) than the orthogonal. Sonographically, these may be quite ill-defined masses with disruption of tissue planes and intense posterior acoustic shadowing, or vague areas of architectural distortion (Fig. 9.6). One uncommon exception is pleomorphic ILC, an aggressive subtype that manifests as an expansile mass, and is treated like a high nuclear grade IDC (Fig. 9.7). ILC may also present with diffuse changes (edema) in the background of an enlarging or shrinking breast.

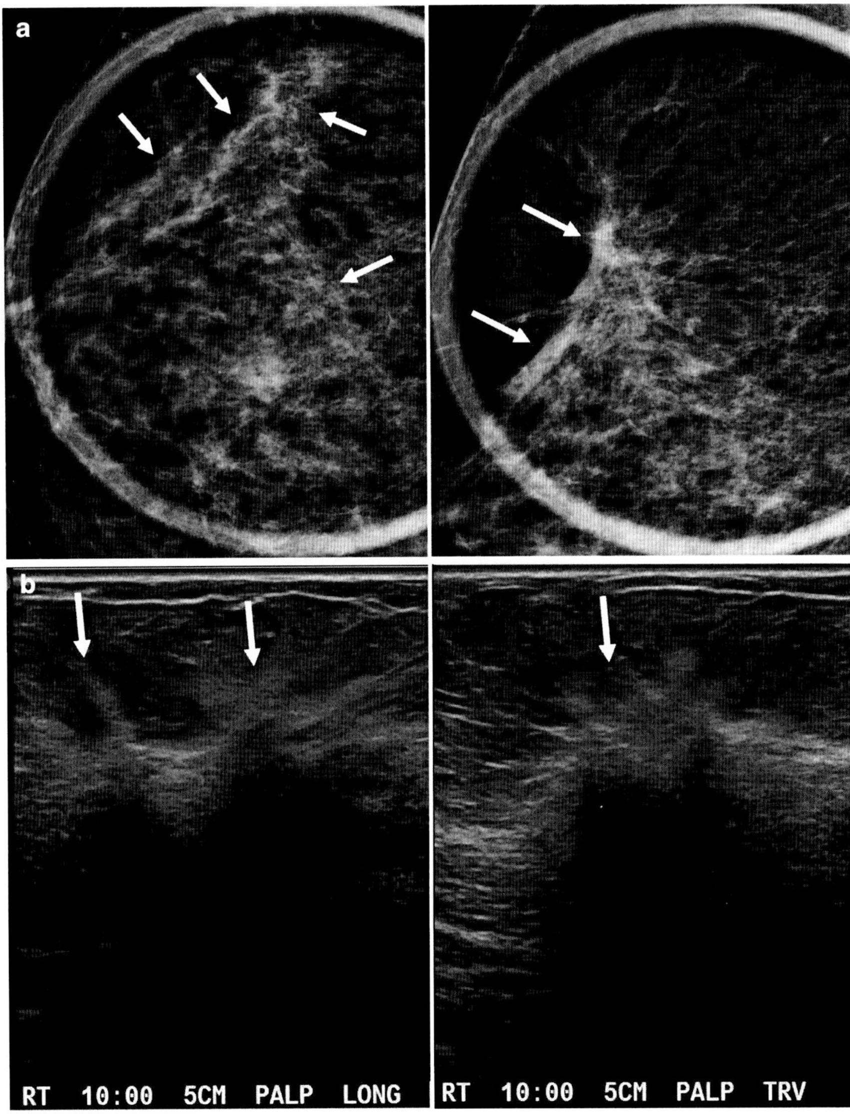

Fig. 9.6 Invasive lobular carcinoma. (**a**) Spot compression CC and MLO views done in a 68-year-old woman recalled from a screening mammogram show architectural distortion, "straightening" of the parenchymal lines (*arrows*). (**b**) Sonographically, ill-defined hypoechoic to nearly anechoic tissue with echogenic peaks (*arrows*) that disrupt tissue planes, and posterior acoustic shadowing, all confirmed in orthogonal planes, reflects the distortion seen radiographically

In patients in whom a suspicious mass is seen mammographically, sonography allows for further characterization and biopsy guidance, as well as the opportunity to evaluate the axilla for evidence of lymph node metastasis. As with calcifications, biopsy of the mass can be done with a needle under imaging

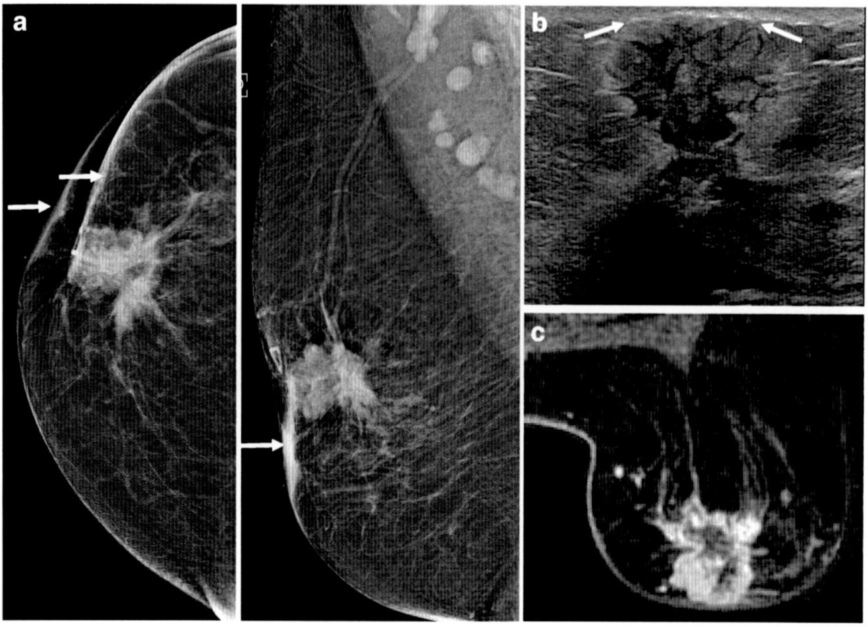

Fig. 9.7 Invasive lobular carcinoma, pleomorphic type. (**a**) Diagnostic mammogram in a 65-year-old woman with a "lump." There is skin thickening and retraction overlying the mass (*arrows*). (**b**) Skin involvement is confirmed on ultrasound, as this heterogeneous mass is inseparable from the deep dermal layer (*arrows*). (**c**) Post-contrast axial MRI image showing an irregular mass with thick rim enhancement extending to the skin. Lobular carcinoma rarely presents as an expansile mass, except for this aggressive subtype that clinically mimics a grade 3 invasive ductal carcinoma

guidance, or surgically. However, the former is preferred in the majority of cases as it is far less invasive, does not require sedation or special patient preparation (e.g., withholding of anticoagulation), costs less, and can allow for appropriate staging and surgical planning prior to definitive treatment. A metallic clip placed in the mass at the time of biopsy is most useful if the treatment plan includes neoadjuvant chemotherapy that will shrink the lesion to the point that it is occult on preoperative imaging or wire/seed localization; in our experience, in patients in whom lumpectomy (partial or segmental mastectomy) is a first-line treatment because of smaller lesion size (or patient preference), the tumor is still visible on imaging for preoperative localization on or shortly before the day of surgery regardless of a clip. Ultrasound-guided core-needle biopsy (or fine needle aspiration) of axillary adenopathy can be also done in the same setting as for the primary breast mass, providing the surgeon and oncologist additional information with regard to staging. A positive lymph node can also be marked with a clip so that surgical excision can be confirmed with a specimen radiograph.

Once a diagnosis of breast cancer is confirmed by imaging-guided core-needle biopsy, MRI may be used to evaluate the extent of disease to aid in treatment planning. The sensitivity of MRI is higher than that of mammography or ultrasound, some reporting as high as 100% for invasive cancer, and the cancer detection rate is nearly double that of mammography and ultrasound combined, resulting in detection of additional disease that changes management in up to 20% of patients, most commonly shifting from breast-conserving treatment (BCT; lumpectomy and radiation) to mastectomy. This includes finding multifocal or multicentric disease in up to 10–25% and contralateral disease in up to 6%. However, the use of MRI remains controversial because there is also data showing that this test does not significantly improve re-excision or local recurrence rates, suggesting that surgical planning is adequately guided by mammography and ultrasound and that any "undetected" or residual disease after lumpectomy may be treated by subsequent breast radiation and systemic adjuvant chemotherapy without negatively impacting survival. Moreover, by current data, the conversion rate of lumpectomy to mastectomy based on additional MRI findings seems to outnumber the recurrence rates in patients who undergo BCT without a preoperative MRI. Therefore, some have suggested that the additional MRI findings may not lead to future "biologically significant" disease.

These arguments are somewhat counterintuitive for many reasons encountered in day to day practice, one being the principle of confirming the extent of disease suspected on routine imaging, namely, mammographically or sonographically. For example, if a patient has several centimeters of segmentally distributed suspicious calcifications, the accepted practice is to biopsy 2 sites, the two extremes in terms of location, that are far enough away from each other to "prove" that all of the involved and intervening tissue must be resected. Or if multiple separate, suspicious masses are seen on sonography, biopsy of more than 1 is typically done to prove multifocal or multicentric disease, and guide excision, if a patient desires breast conservation treatment. So if we are actively seeking out and biopsying additional disease to develop a complete, definitive treatment plan, one could argue that an MRI, which is more sensitive, is in keeping with this practice of establishing extent of disease. Many use the aforementioned argument that MRI-detected disease is not biologically significant; however, one could also counter that MRI-detected disease *is* biologically significant because its detection relies on properties unique to cancer: neovascularity and vascular permeability (tumor characteristics that result in the rapid, avid uptake of contrast). Iaconni et al. reported that MRI-detected multicentric disease was invasive in 76% of their studied patients, and larger than 1 cm or the index cancer in up to 25%, suggesting biological relevance.

Moreover, patients are routinely taken back to the operating room for re-excision in the case of positive surgical margins, regardless of the use of preoperative MRI. If the disease potentially "left behind" that would be found by MRI is of no consequence, treated effectively with radiation and chemotherapy, at no detriment to survival, why incur the additional cost, risk, and recovery of another surgery for re-excision of disease "left behind" in the setting of positive margins?

In this vein, surgical practices and breast-conserving treatment plans are evolving, such as more precise excisions with smaller volumes (margins) of tissue removed, multiple lumpectomies for multicentric disease (previously, multicentric disease was a contraindication to BCS), advanced oncoplastic reconstructive techniques, accelerated partial breast irradiation (versus whole breast irradiation), and use of recurrence risk assessment scores that may obviate the need for adjuvant chemotherapy. Therefore, the case could be made for using the most sensitive methods to accurately measure disease burden and exclude other sites of cancer preoperatively, thereby allowing for a more precise, patient-specific treatment plan before definitive surgery. Needless to say, these issues do not address the impact of preoperative MRI on detection of contralateral disease that could be treated simultaneously as the index lesion.

To address some of the controversies and conflicting data, at this time a multicenter, randomized controlled trial is in place to determine the effect of preoperative MRI with regard to staging and local regional control, with attention also on cost-effectiveness, quality of life, re-excision rates, and disease-free survival, among many other objectives.

In the meantime, in practice, while some advocate breast MRI should be done in all newly diagnosed patients, practice variations (and preferences of patients, surgeons, and oncologists) may focus efforts for MRIs in patients with cancer who are high risk, have dense breast tissue, and have triple negative disease or DCIS (given that it can be discontinuous and uncalcified), or ILC (which, due to its ill-defined appearance, can be underestimated with regard to size even on ultrasound and can have up to 30% risk of synchronous or contralateral disease). Additional suspicious lesions found on MRI should be worked up with a biopsy to help determine if the patient is still a candidate for breast conservation treatment.

Chapter 2 of this text contains some discussion on the pathology approach to diagnosis of invasive carcinomas. All invasive carcinomas of the breast must be staged based on the most current AJCC Cancer Staging Manual. Selected radiologic-pathologic correlation of invasive carcinomas is highlighted below.

Case 1

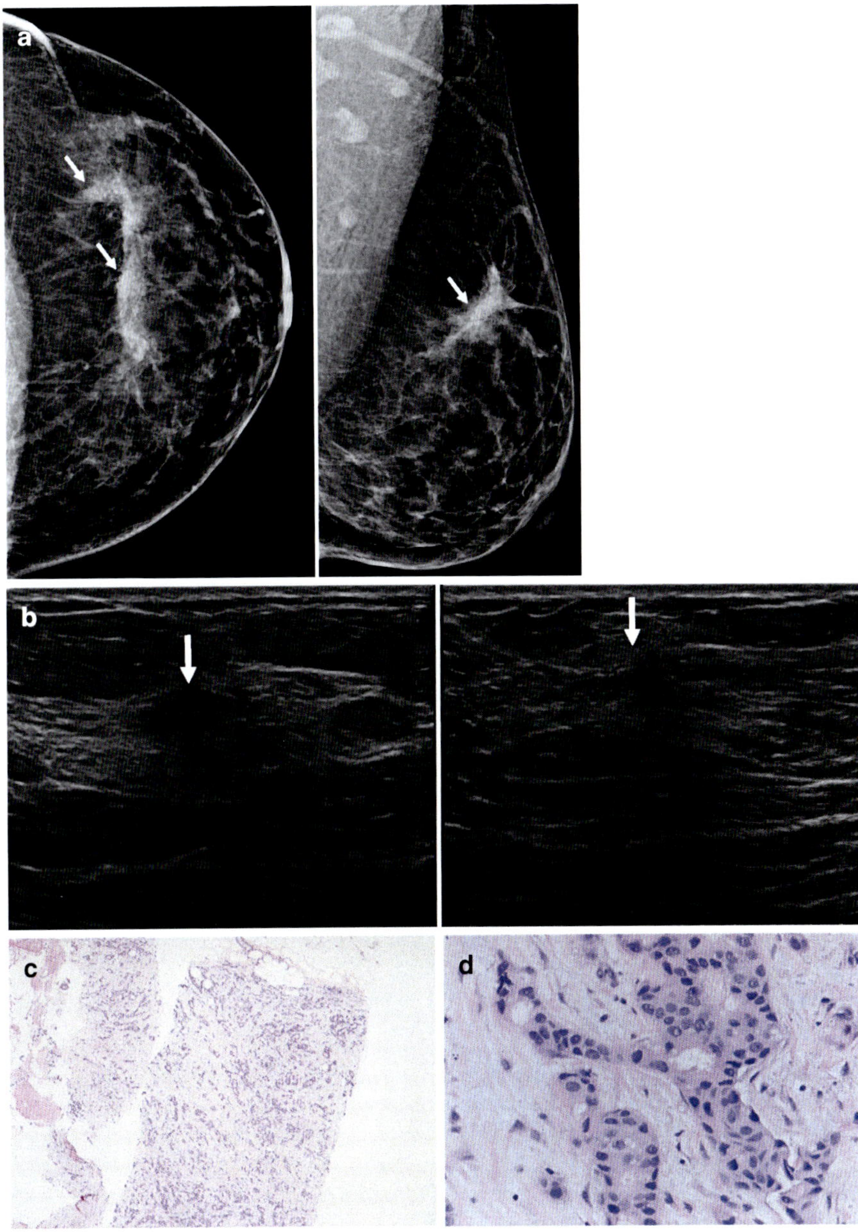

Invasive ductal carcinoma, low nuclear grade. (**a**) Screening mammogram in a 41-year-old woman shows architectural distortion (*arrows*) in the upper central aspect of the left breast—"straightening" of the parenchymal lines. (**b**) On ultrasound of the upper inner and outer quadrants, multiple areas of ill-defined hypoechogenicity and disruption of tissue planes are seen, without an expansile mass. (**c**) Invasive ductal carcinoma. Epithelial cells in nests, cords, and tubules infiltrate a desmoplastic stroma. (**d**) The low-grade nuclei show minimal pleomorphism and uniform chromatin

Case 2

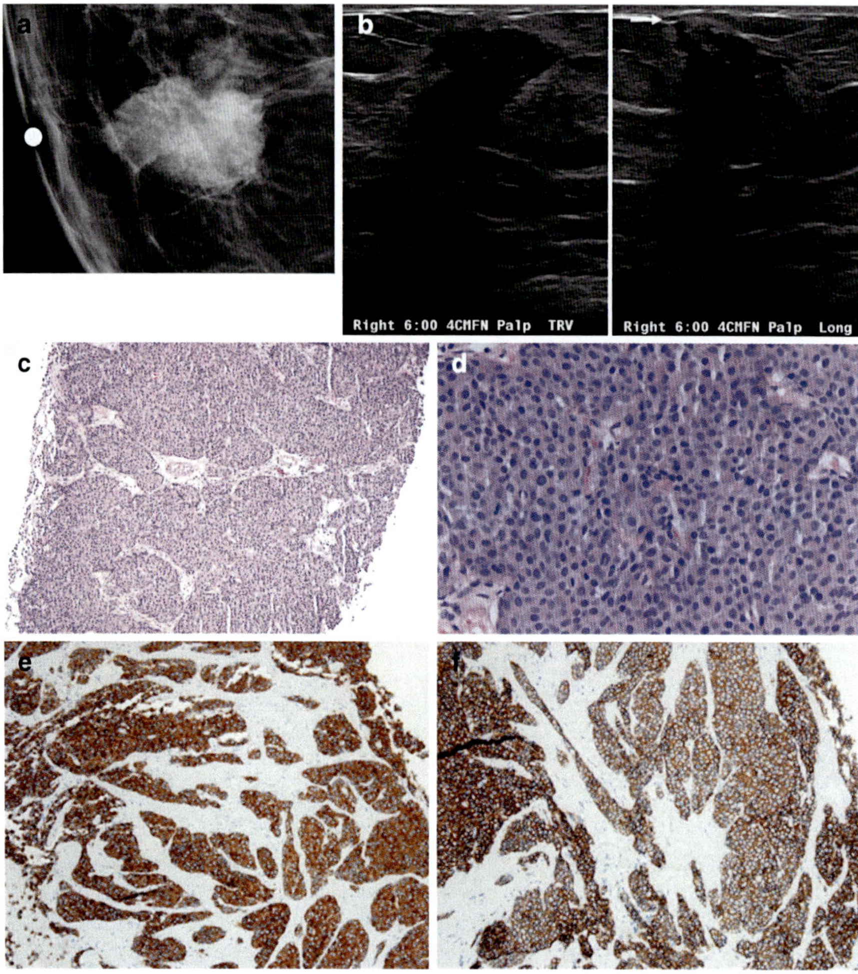

Invasive ductal carcinoma, low nuclear grade with neuroendocrine differentiation. (**a**) Spot tangential view of a palpable "lump" (marked on skin with a metallic BB) in a 62-year-old woman. The mass is irregular, with high density and with indistinct and spiculated margins. (**b**) Orthogonal ultrasound images show similar features. In addition, there is disruption of normal tissue planes and the mass approaches the skin (*arrow*). (**c** and **d**) Core-needle biopsy with infiltrating cells in solid nests/insular pattern with focal peripheral palisading, low nuclear grade, and fine chromatin. Necrosis is not identified. (**e**) The cells are diffusely positive for synaptophysin. (**f**) Expression of E-cadherin is preserved. The p63 stain was negative (*not pictured*)

Invasive ductal carcinoma, high nuclear grade. (**a**) A 54-year-old woman with a palpable (designated by metallic BB) nodular asymmetry in the upper outer quadrant of the right breast, which corresponds to an irregular, nearly anechoic but solid mass with angular and indistinct margins on ultrasound (**b**) and an irregular mass with heterogeneous enhancement on MRI (**c**, *arrow*). (**d**) Epithelial cells in small solid nests and cords infiltrate the desmoplastic stroma. (**e**) The high grade nuclei show pleomorphism and visible nucleoli

Case 3

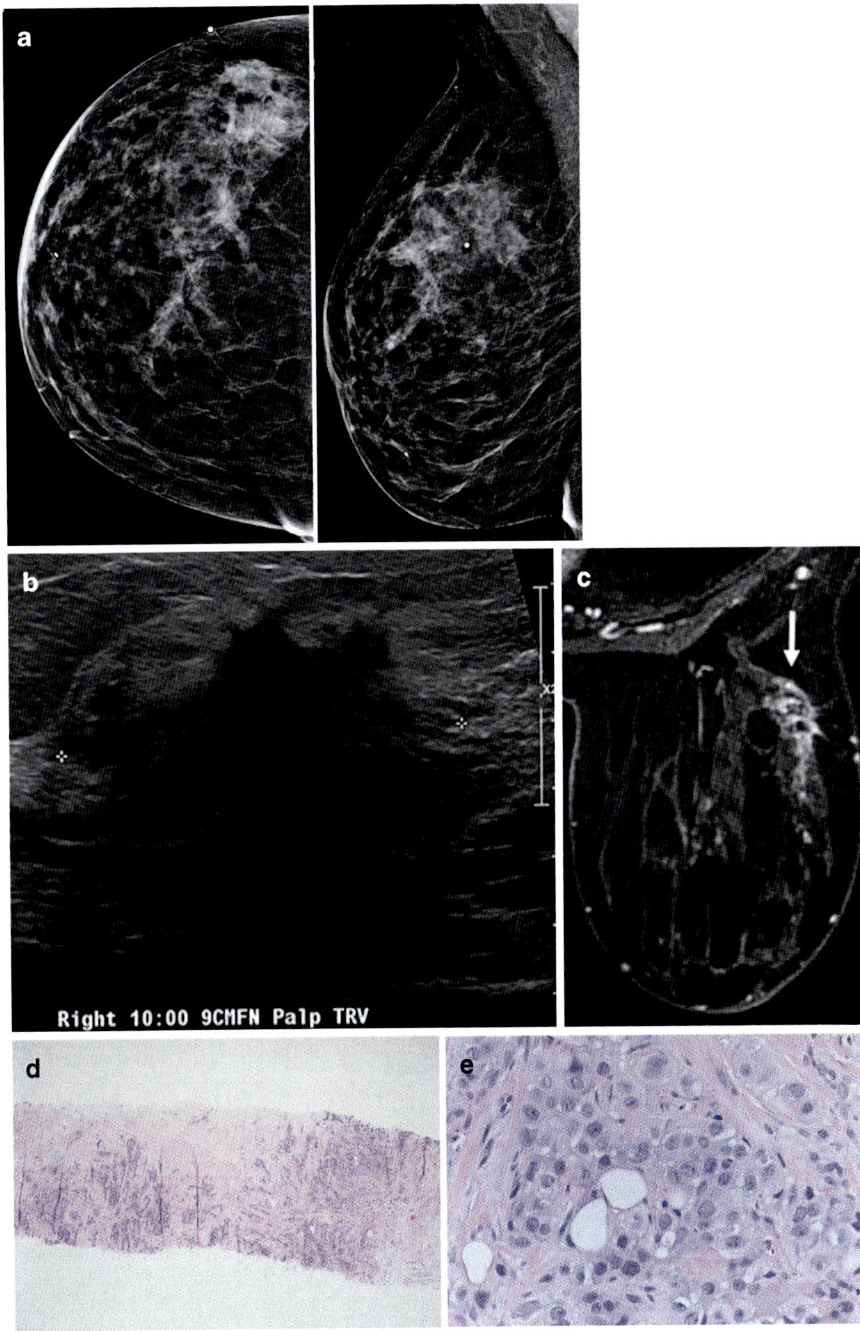

Case 4

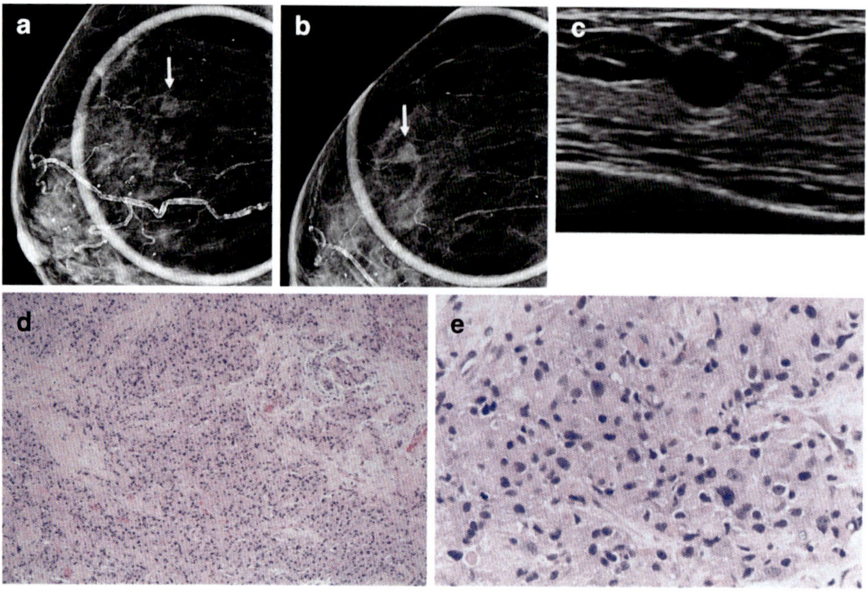

Invasive ductal carcinoma, intermediate nuclear grade with apocrine features. (**a**) CC and (**b**) MLO spot compression views of a mass (*arrow*) in the right breast in a 62-year-old woman with known locally advanced left breast cancer (not shown). (**c**) Targeted ultrasound shows a nearly anechoic mass. Because it is not clearly a cyst, biopsy is done. (**d** and **e**) Note the cells with abundant granular, eosinophilic cytoplasm, and mildly pleomorphic round nuclei with prominent nucleoli

Invasive ductal carcinoma, intermediate nuclear grade, with mucinous features/mucinous carcinoma. (**a**) An 80-year-old woman with a history of right lumpectomy and radiation for breast cancer, with new subcentimeter round mass with partially circumscribed and indistinct margins found in the left breast on annual mammogram. (**b**) Targeted ultrasound shows an isoechoic to slightly hyperechoic mass (*between arrows*) with circumscribed margins. (**c**) Central nonenhancement on the MRI with corresponding increased T2 (fluid) signal (**d**) reflects mucin (*arrows*). (**e** and **f**) Core-needle biopsies show nests of epithelial cells in pool of extracellular mucin, consistent with mucinous carcinoma. (**g** and **h**) Mucinous carcinoma in the excision specimen shows epithelial cells in in pool of extracellular mucin. A pure mucinous carcinoma must composed of more than 90% mucinous carcinoma, making the diagnosis difficult sometimes on core needle biopsy as the entire lesion is cannot be evaluated

Case 5

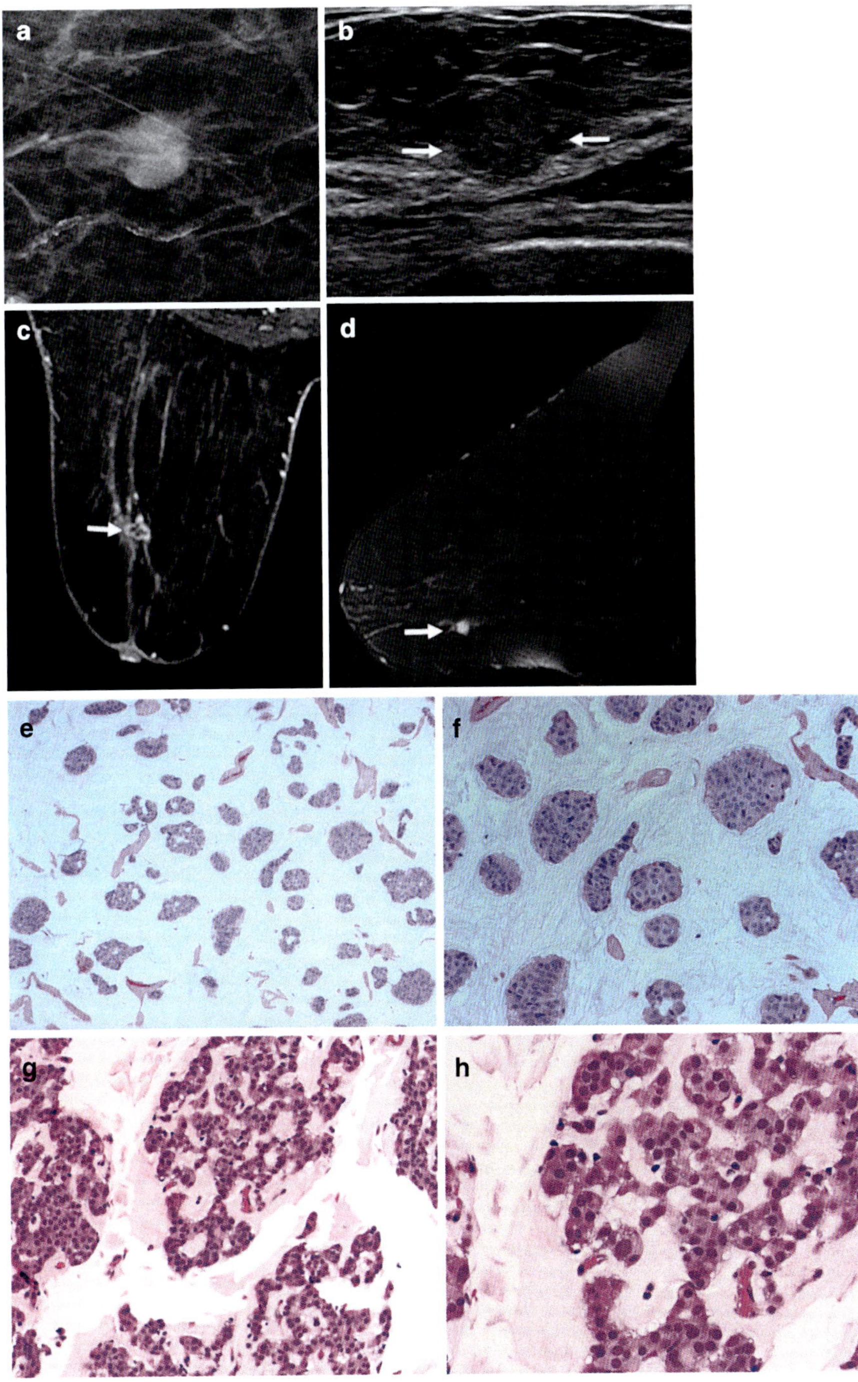

Case 6

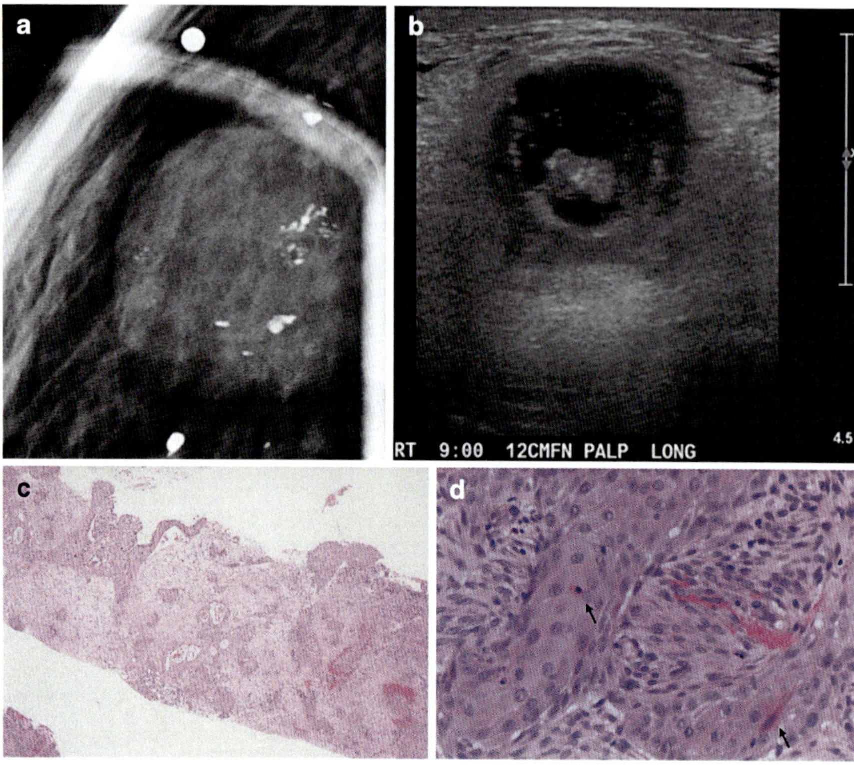

Invasive carcinoma with squamous features. (**a**) A palpable mass with mostly circumscribed margins and coarse calcifications is marked with an overlying metallic BB in this 87-year-old woman. (**b**) Complex solid and cystic mass is seen sonographically; ultrasound-guided biopsy targeted the solid (*deeper*) portion. (**c** and **d**) Invasive carcinoma shows extensive squamous features. This is a variant of metaplastic carcinoma

Case 7

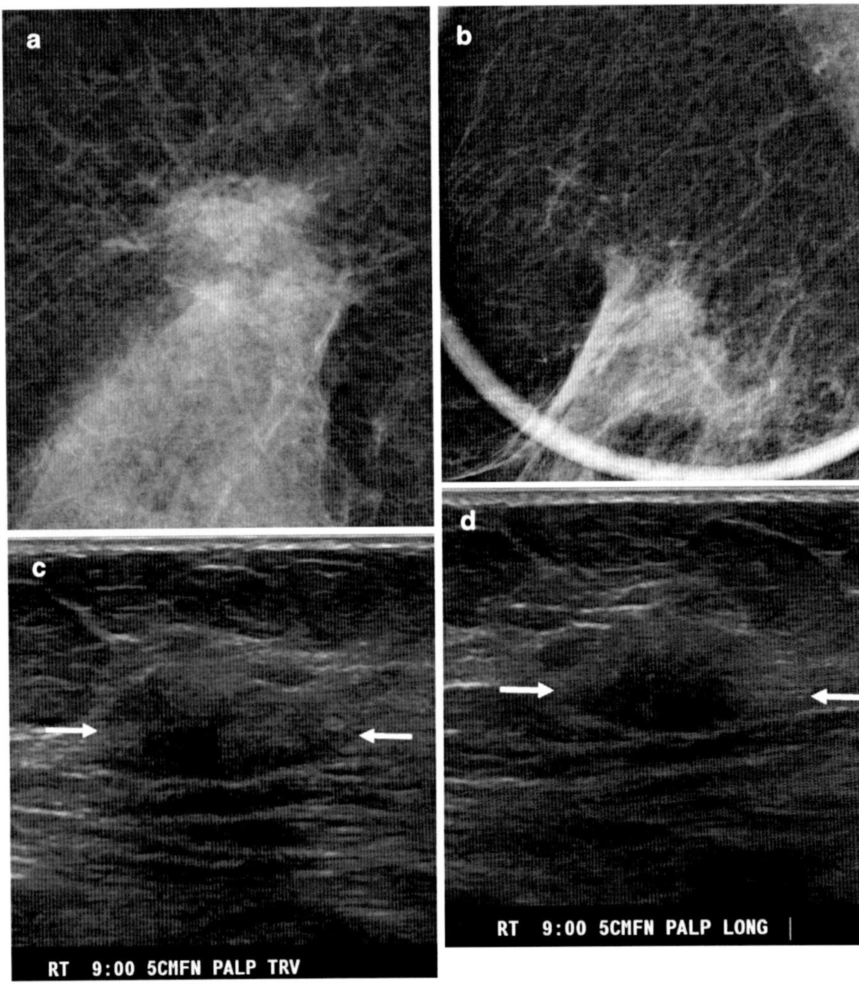

Invasive ductal carcinoma, with lobular features. (**a** and **b**) CC and MLO spot compression views of a screening detected mass in a 64-year-old woman. The irregular mass is developing at the edge of the parenchyma in the right breast and has spiculated margins. (**c** and **d**) Orthogonal ultrasound images confirm an irregular mass (*arrows*) with indistinct margins and heterogeneous echogenicity and that disrupts tissue planes. (**e** and **f**) Core-needle biopsies show invasive carcinoma, with cells infiltrating as nests, as well as individual cells in linear distribution. (**g**) Similar histological features are seen in the excision specimen. (**h**) The e-cadherin stain is diffusely positive, arguing against invasive lobular carcinoma

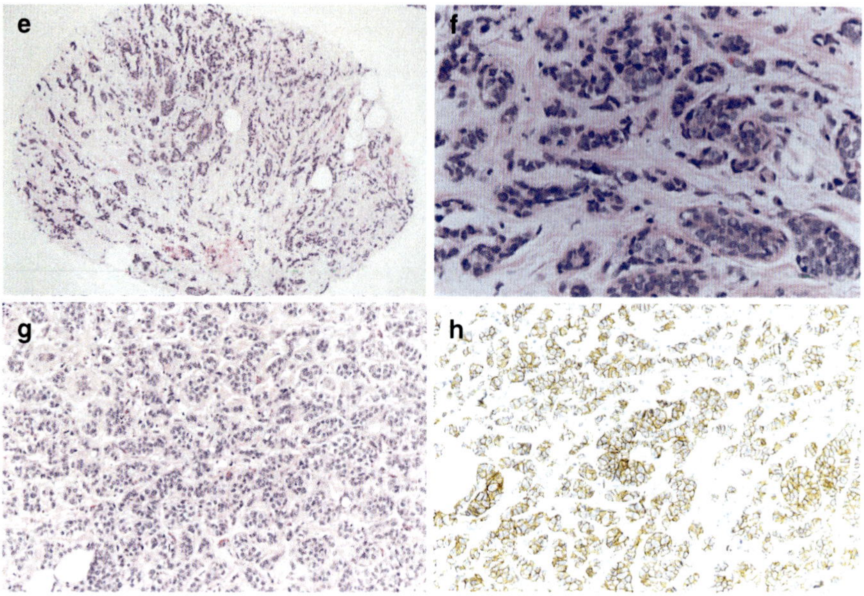
e
f
g
h

Case 8

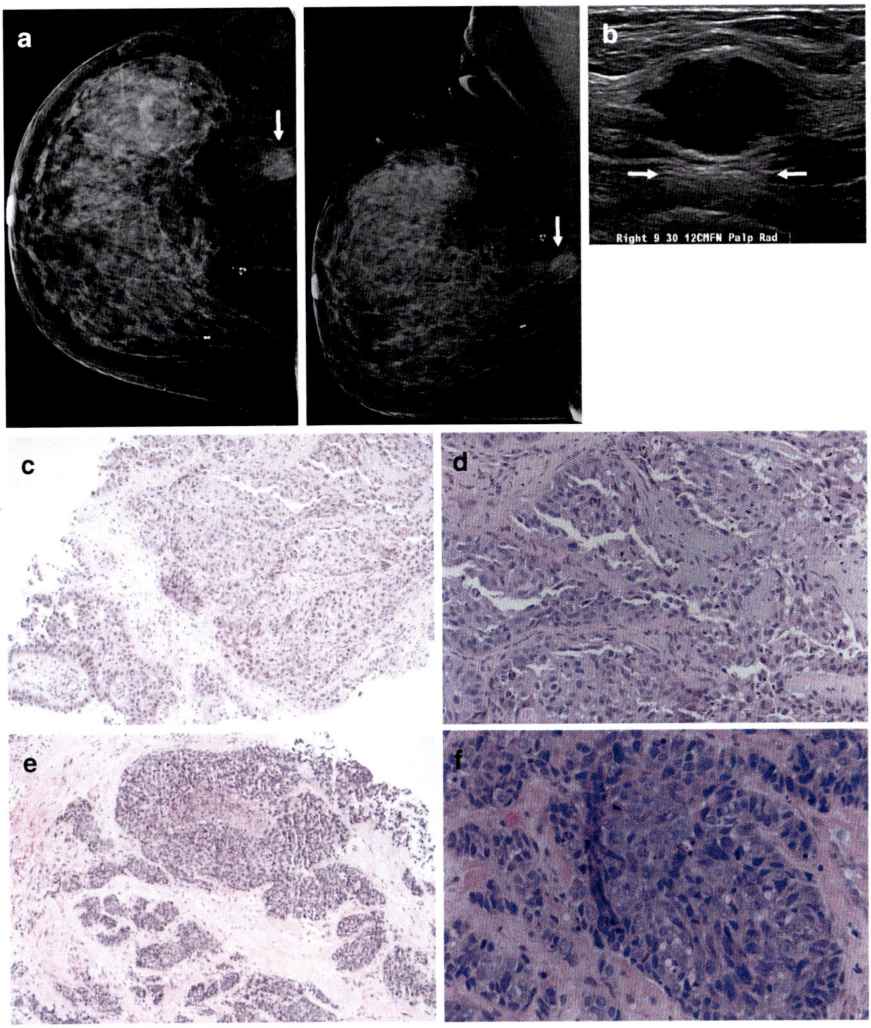

Invasive ductal carcinoma, high nuclear grade. (**a**) A 65-year-old woman with a round mass (*arrows*) in the retroglandular fat detected on screening mammogram. (**b**) Ultrasound shows an irregular, hypoechoic mass with mostly circumscribed and few indistinct margins. Posterior acoustic enhancement (*between arrows*) is nonspecific; this should not be mistaken for a complicated cyst. (**c** and **d**) Core biopsy: invasive ductal carcinoma, high nuclear grade, with papillary architecture. (**e** and **f**) Histologic variant of IDC, high nuclear grade with invasive ductal carcinoma consisting of solid nests of tumor cells with pleomorphic nuclei with coarse chromatin and prominent nucleoli

Case 9

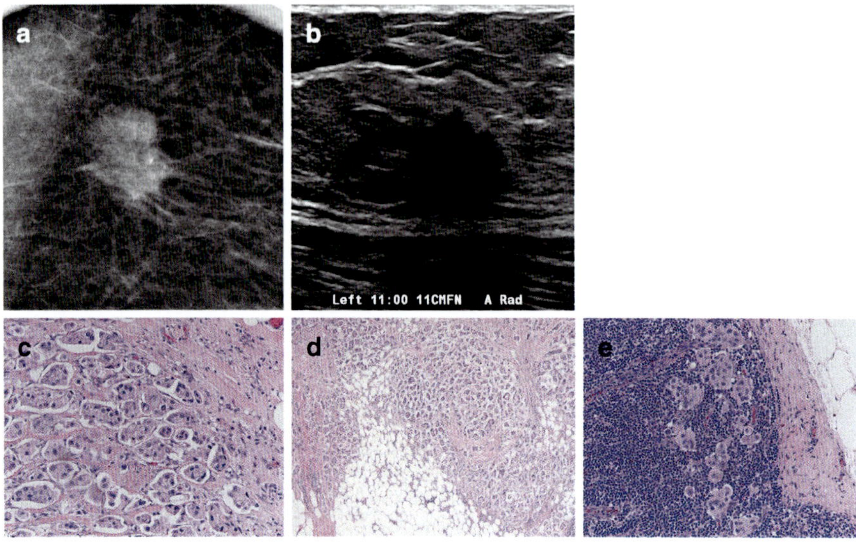

Invasive ductal carcinoma, high nuclear grade (micropapillary type). (**a**) Spot compression view of a screening detected irregular mass with partially circumscribed and spiculated margins, in a 51-year-old woman. The mass is just anterior to the pectoralis major. (**b**) Similar features are seen on ultrasound. (**c**) Needle core biopsy shows invasive ductal carcinoma with micropapillary architecture: with morular-like or nest of cells without fibrovascular core, surrounded by empty stromal spaces. The empty stromal spaces are likely fixation artifact and not lymphatic spaces. (**d**) Same micropapillary features are seen in the surgical excision specimen. (**e**) This variant of invasive carcinoma is often associated with lymph node metastasis

Case 10

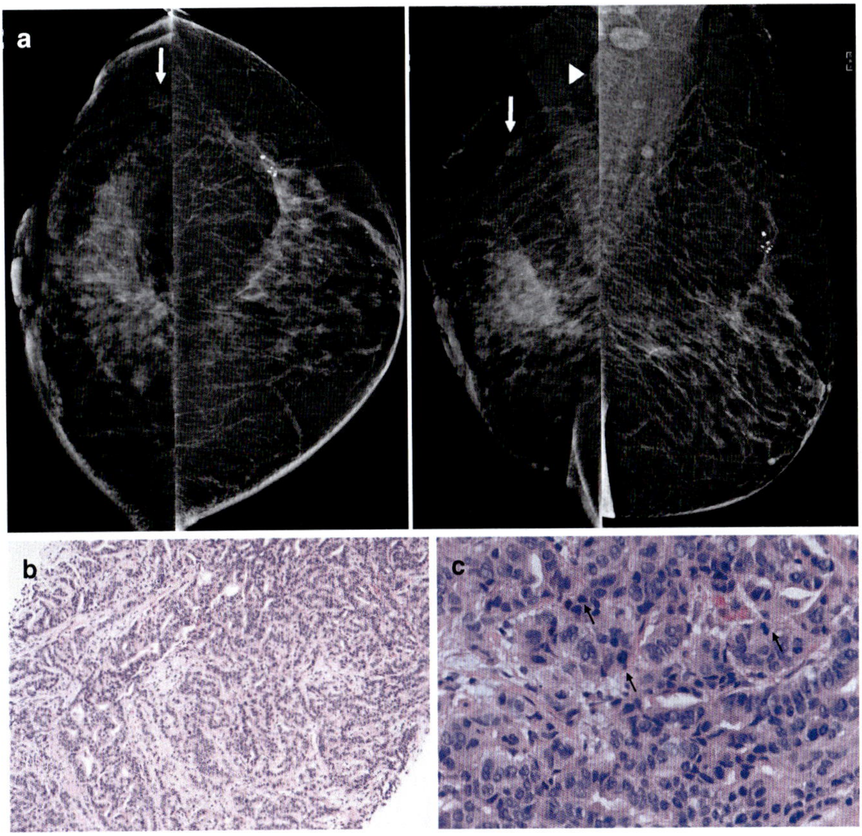

Diffuse, locally advanced invasive ductal carcinoma. (**a**) Diagnostic mammogram in a 64-year-old woman shows the right breast is shrunken, retracted, and edematous with skin and trabecular thickening. There is also global parenchymal asymmetry, on which malignant-type calcifications are superimposed. A second primary is seen as a low-density mass in the upper outer quadrant posteriorly (*arrow*). Axillary adenopathy is partially imaged (*arrowhead*), but evaluated sonographically and subsequently biopsy proven to be metastatic (not shown). (**b** and **c**) Invasive ductal carcinoma with pleomorphic nuclei with coarse chromatin and mitoses (*arrow*)

Case 11

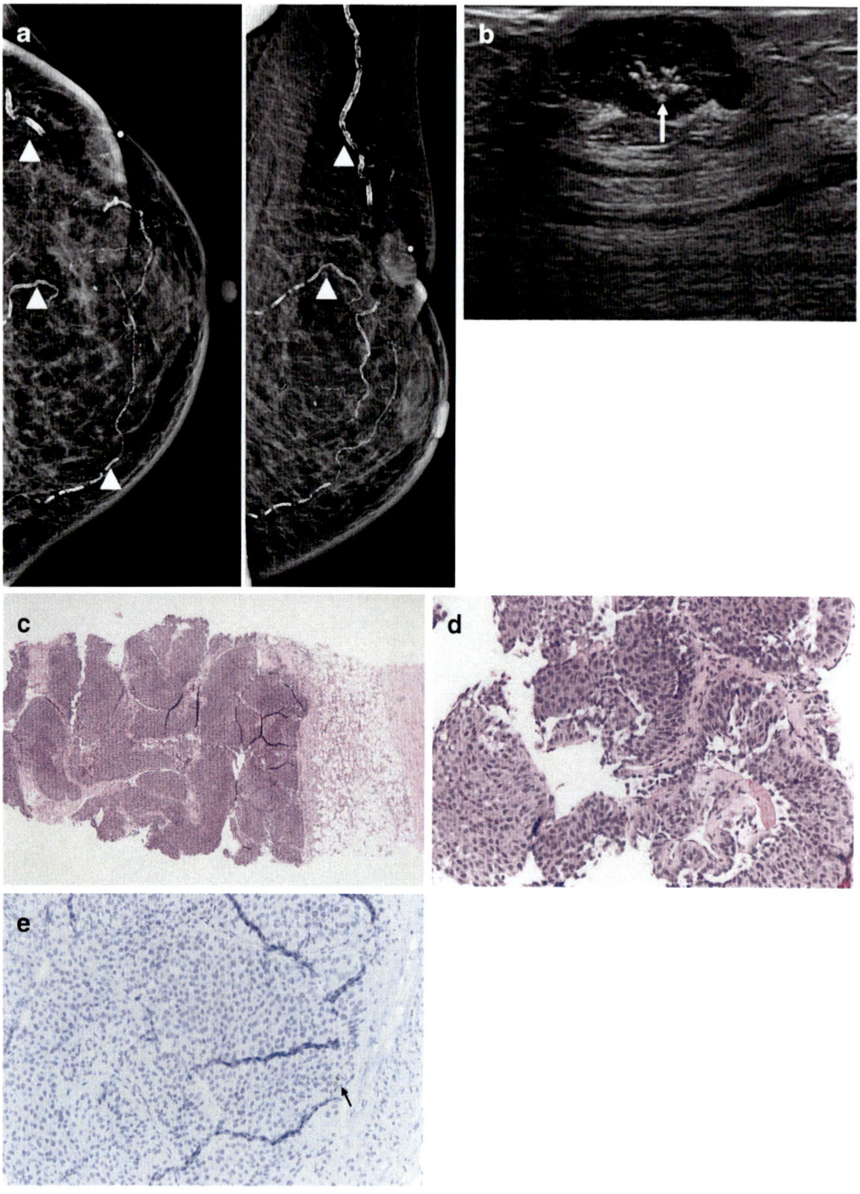

Papillary carcinoma. (**a**) A 77-year-old woman with a palpable mass containing calcifications at prior lumpectomy site, marked on skin with metallic BB. Overlying skin retraction is from surgical scarring. Vascular calcifications incidentally noted (*arrowheads*). (**b**) Lobulated complex solid and cystic mass seen on ultrasound; echogenic foci are calcifications (*arrow*). (**c**–**e**) Needle core biopsies show carcinoma with solid areas arranged around thin fibrovascular cores and collagenized stroma. The circumscribed border is characteristic of solid intraductal papillary carcinoma. Tissue fragmentation is sometimes noted. The p63 stain highlights rare myoepithelial cells at the periphery (*arrow*)

Case 12

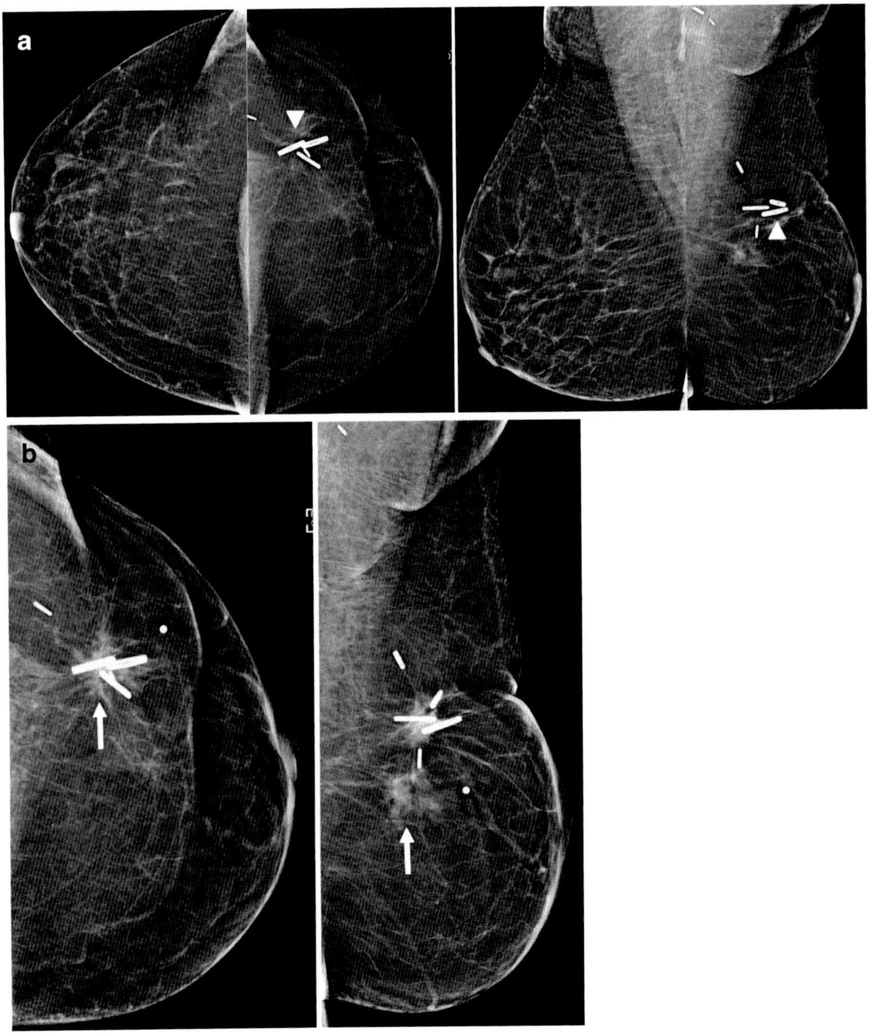

Invasive lobular carcinoma. (**a**) Screening mammogram in a 56-year-old woman. Prior lumpectomy changes in the left breast include smaller size, skin retraction, and architectural distortion amid and inferior to vascular clips (*arrowheads*). (**b**) Palpable developing asymmetry (increasing density amidst the clips) at and inferior to lumpectomy site 1 year later. (**c** and **d**) Core-needle biopsies show solid sheet of discohesive cells, some of which are plasmacytoid (*arrows*). (**e**) Invasive lobular carcinoma may infiltrate as small nests in the breast adipose tissue. (**f**) Tumor cells are usually discohesive and low nuclear grade with single file infiltrative pattern in stromal fibrous tissue (and no desmoplasia), characteristic to lobular carcinoma. The tumor often has a concentric pattern around normal duct (not shown)

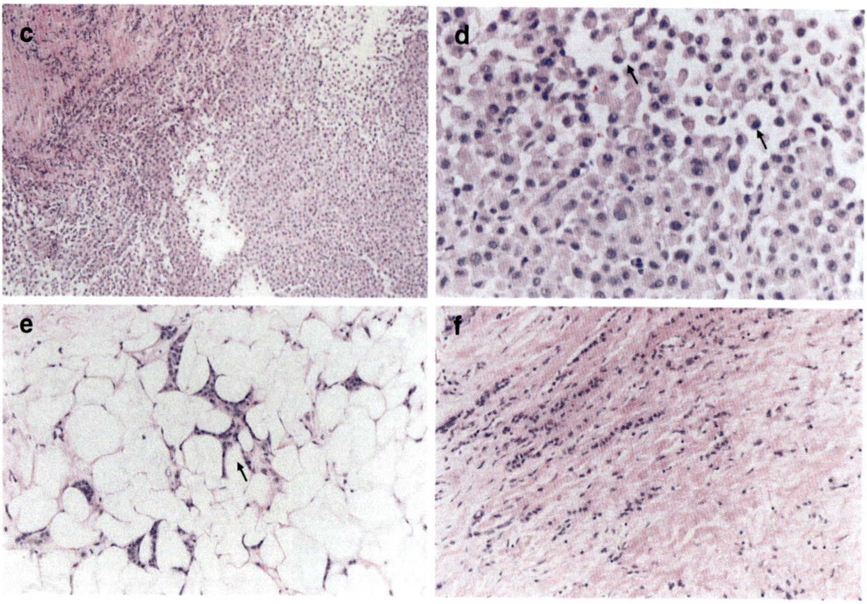
c
d
e
f

Case 13

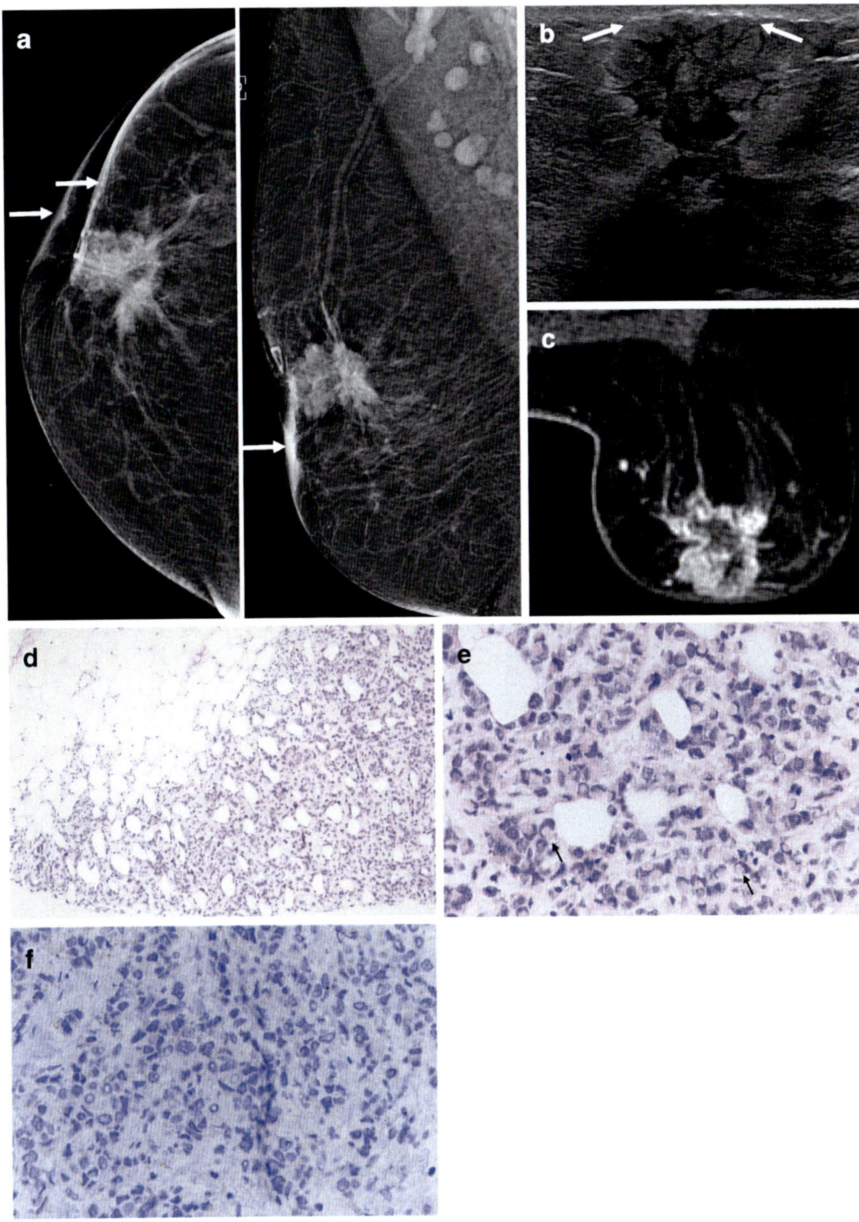

Invasive lobular carcinoma, pleomorphic type. (**a**) Diagnostic mammogram in a 65-year-old woman with a "lump." There is skin thickening and retraction overlying the mass (*arrows*). (**b**) Skin involvement is confirmed on ultrasound, as this heterogeneous mass is inseparable from the deep dermal layer (*arrows*). (**c**) Post-contrast axial MRI image showing an irregular mass with thick rim enhancement extending to the skin. (**d** and **e**) Core-needle biopsies show high nuclear grade invasive carcinoma with eccentrically placed nuclei (*arrow*), infiltrative patterns and apparent discohesion, suggestive of pleomorphic lobular carcinoma and confirmatory negative stain for e-cadherin (**f**)

Case 14

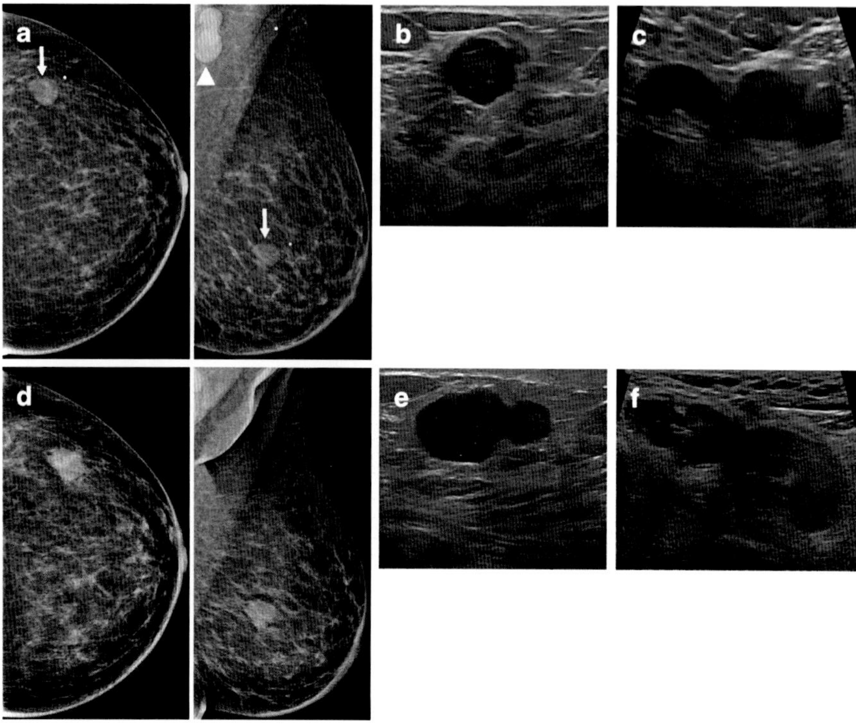

Metaplastic carcinoma with axillary metastases. (**a**) A 50-year-old woman with a palpable mass in the outer central aspect of the left breast (*arrows*) and axillary adenopathy (*arrowhead*). (**b**) Ultrasound shows solid round breast mass and (**c**) axillary adenopathy (enlarged lymph nodes with thickened cortices and no identifiable fatty hila). (**d–f**) Progression of breast mass and axillary metastases after 5 months on chemotherapy. (**g**) PET/CT 7 months into treatment and (**h**) after mastectomy, 11 months into treatment, shows continued progression. (**i**) Core needle biopsies showing atypical spindle cell proliferation. (**j**) The atypical spindle cells are adjacent to or surround non-neoplastic breast epithelium. (**k**) Pleomorphism of the atypical spindle cells is noted in some areas at higher power. (**l** and **m**) The atypical spindle cells are positive for pancytokeratin (**l**) and p63 (**m**)

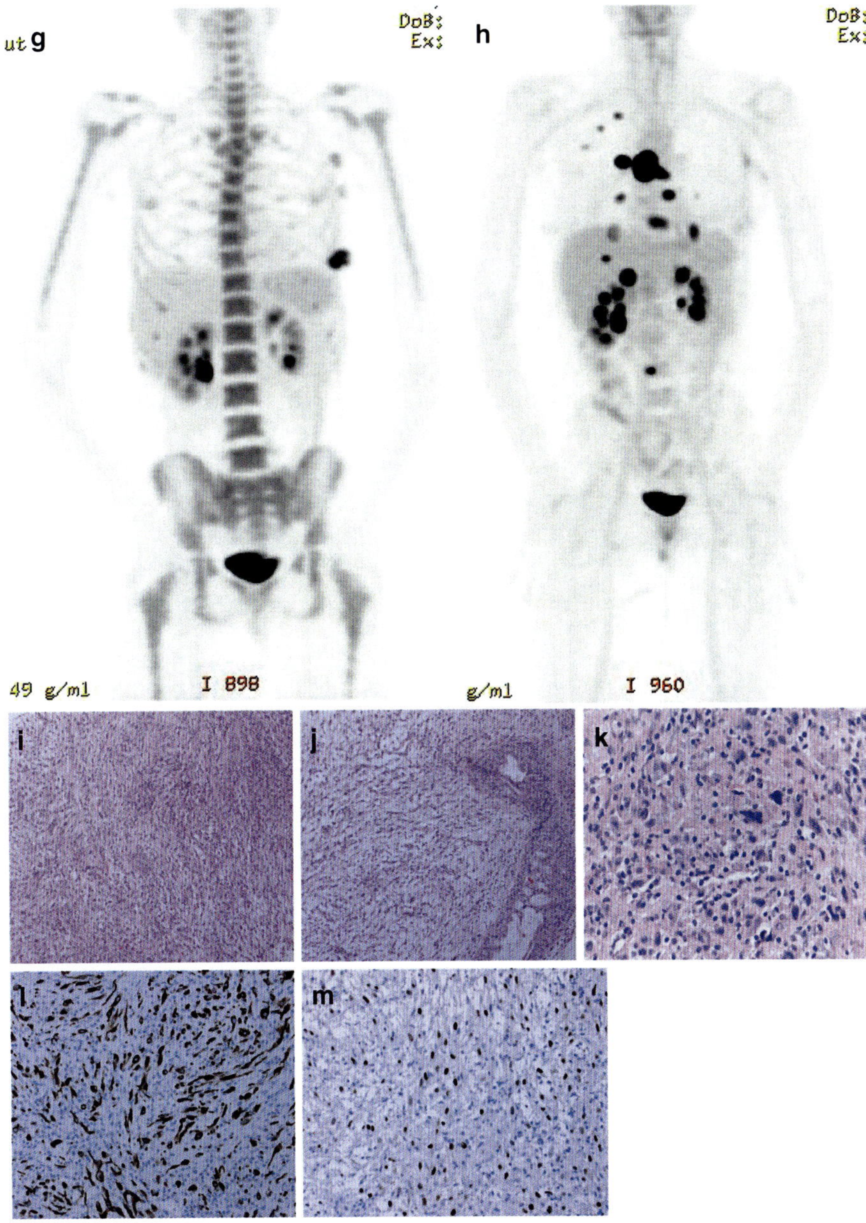
ut g
DoB:
Ex:
h
DoB:
Ex:
49 g/ml
I 898
g/ml
I 960
i
j
k
l
m

Invasive Breast Cancer: Diagnosis and Management Considerations

Breast cancer is the most frequently diagnosed cancer globally and is the leading cause of cancer-related death in women [1]. Although the majority are initially identified by radiologic imaging, however, some suggest that a clinically suspicious mass detected by a patient or physician should also be biopsied, regardless of imaging findings, as about 15 percent of such lesions can be mammographically occult [2]. Breast cancer is a heterogeneous disease which comprises of many biologically different entities with distinct pathological features and clinical implications. These in turn exhibit different behaviors necessitating a tailored approach to their treatment strategies.

Breast Cancer Subtypes and Their Diagnostic Evaluation

All patients diagnosed with breast cancer should be assigned a clinical stage based on its involvement of the breast and/or nodal regions. Staging allows for efficient identification of local and systemic therapy options and provides baseline prognostic information. Pathologists who confirm the diagnosis of invasive cancer should obtain additional biomarkers for estrogen receptors (ER), progesterone receptors (PR), and human epidermal growth factor receptor 2 (HER2) in accordance with protocols laid down by the College of American Pathologists (CAP). An essential component of breast cancer treatment is complete knowledge of extent of disease and its biological features. These factors assist in estimation of risk of cancer recurrence after local therapies and provide information that predicts response to systemic therapy. Multidisciplinary coordination among breast and reconstructive surgeons, radiation and medical oncologists, radiologists, and pathologists facilitates treatment planning and streamlines patient care [3].

An important aspect of initial evaluation of women diagnosed with locally advanced breast cancer or those with persistent symptoms affecting a particular organ system includes assessment of metastatic disease with additional imaging such as CT scan, bone scan, or PET scan. Women with child-bearing potential must be offered fertility counselling. Patients diagnosed with breast cancers that are less than 40 years of age or those who have significant family history suggestive of hereditary syndromes should undergo genetic counselling and testing that may impact their surgical decision.

Classical biomarkers such as ER, PR, and HER2 together with traditional clinicopathological variables including tumor size, tumor grade, and nodal status are conventionally used to determine patient prognosis and management approach. The advent of platforms for gene expression analysis such as microarrays and RT-PCR have shown that response to treatment is not determined merely by anatomical prognostic factors but also by the molecular characteristics of individual tumors [4].

These molecular subtypes of breast cancer are also called intrinsic subtypes. The ER-positive intrinsic subtypes are called luminal tumors since the expression profiles are reminiscent of the luminal epithelial component of the breast. At least two subtypes exist within luminal-like tumors—luminal A and luminal B. Luminal A tumors have higher expression of ER-related genes and lower expression of proliferative genes than luminal B cancers. Luminal B tumors may have HER2 expression. Another intrinsic subtype called HER2-enriched tumors is characterized by overexpression of HER2. A more aggressive subtype called basal-like tumors has expression profiles that mimic that of the basal epithelial cells in normal breast tissue. This subtype is highly proliferative and is characterized by absence of expression of both hormone receptors and HER2 [5]. Despite the growing number of clinically relevant molecular subtypes being identified, current breast cancer management still depends on traditional pathology assessment supplemented with biomarker testing (tumor biology) using validated commercial assays (i.e., Oncotype Dx, MammaPrint, etc.).

Local Therapy for Breast Cancer

Primary therapy for breast cancer should provide optimal local and systemic control of disease and highest cure rate possible as measured by disease-free survival (DFS) and overall survival (OS) rates, while preserving the best possible quality of life. The treatment of breast cancer includes treatment of local disease with surgery, radiation therapy or both, and systemic treatment with chemotherapy, endocrine therapy, biologic agents, or combination of these.

Patients with early-stage breast cancer undergo primary surgery (lumpectomy or mastectomy based on tumor-breast ratio, patient preference, and genetic factors) with or without radiation therapy. Studies have shown that total mastectomy is equivalent to breast-conserving surgery (lumpectomy coupled with whole breast radiation) in terms of survival for the majority of women with stage I and II breast cancers [6]. Women undergoing mastectomy should be offered consultation with plastic surgeons to discuss reconstructive options. Performance of sentinel lymph node mapping and resection in surgical staging of clinically negative axillae is recommended for pathological assessment of axillary nodes in patients with early-stage cancer. Patients with clinically palpable axillary nodes with pathological confirmation of metastases should undergo axillary dissection. Following local therapy, adjuvant systemic therapy may be offered based on patient's tumor characteristics.

Whole breast radiation after breast-conserving surgery helps reduce local recurrence and has been shown to have a beneficial effect on breast cancer-related mortality. CT scan-based treatment planning helps limit radiation exposure to heart and lungs and assures adequate coverage of the lumpectomy site. Chest wall radiation after mastectomy is recommended for patients with tumors larger than 5 cm or pathologically involved margins. Nodal irradiation is considered for patients with macroscopically involved nodes. Addition of radiation to internal mammary nodes and upper axillary nodes including the supraclavicular region has led to reduction in regional and distant recurrence as well as improvement in disease-free survival (radiation therapy to the axilla is avoided in patients who have undergone completion axillary dissection). Accelerated partial breast irradiation (APBI) refers to the use of limited, focused radiation therapy as a more convenient alternative to conventional whole breast radiation for women following breast-conserving surgery. APBI delivers a higher dose of radiation therapy per day to a limited volume of tissue encompassing the lumpectomy bed over a shorter period of time and leading to potentially less late skin toxicity. APBI is used for a highly selected group of patients and is still considered investigational while awaiting results of randomized prospective clinical trials. If adjuvant chemotherapy is indicated, then whole breast radiation is given after chemotherapy is completed; APBI may be delivered before chemotherapy or even intraoperatively.

Neoadjuvant Therapy

In certain clinical scenarios, preoperative (also known as neoadjuvant) systemic therapy is preferred. Randomized trials demonstrate similar long-term outcomes when patients are given the same systemic therapy preoperatively compared to postoperatively [7]. Preoperative systemic therapy can render surgically inoperable tumors operable and improve rates of breast conservation therapy in patients with operable breast cancer. It also allows time to make surgical decisions, particularly when waiting for genetic testing or evaluating options for reconstruction. Preoperative therapy can treat axillary nodal disease and potentially can help avoid axillary dissection in event of a good response resulting in negative sentinel nodes. Neoadjuvant therapy also allows for consideration of additional adjuvant therapy in patients with poor response to initial therapy. Certain subtypes of breast cancer such as HER2-positive and triple-negative disease are considered aggressive and likely to need adjuvant therapy. Preoperative chemotherapy is often elected for these subtypes, as it offers an opportunity to observe clinical and pathological response to systemic therapy which can provide prognostic information. Pathological complete response (pCR) to preoperative therapy is associated with an extremely favorable DFS and OS. The correlation between pCR and long-term outcome is strongest for triple negative breast cancer, followed by HER2-positive cancer and least for ER-positive disease (particularly for luminal A type tumors) [8]. Patients who are ideal candidates for preoperative systemic therapy include those with inoperable cancer, inflammatory breast cancer, bulky or matted lymph nodes, T4 or N3 disease, or patients with high tumor to breast ratio who desire breast conservation.

A number of chemotherapy regimens have activity in the preoperative setting. For most patients with hormone receptor-positive disease, particularly premenopausal patients, we recommend chemotherapy in the neoadjuvant setting rather than endocrine therapy since it is associated with higher response rates in a shorter time period. Preoperative endocrine therapy alone may be considered for selected patients with ER-positive disease based on age, comorbidities, and low-risk luminal biology. In patients with HER2-negative cancers, anthracycline and taxane-based chemotherapy is preferred for hormone receptor positive, node-positive cancers, and triple negative cancers. For those patients in whom the potential cardiotoxic effects of anthracyclines are a primary concern, non-anthracycline regimens are a reasonable alternative. For patients with triple negative cancers, there is some early phase data to incorporate platinum agents, particularly carboplatin, in neoadjuvant therapy since it has improved pathological complete response but comes at the cost of added hematological toxicity and uncertain impact on long-term outcomes [9, 10]. National guidelines do not recommend routine addition of carboplatin to anthracycline and taxane-based chemotherapy, but it may be considered in patients with suboptimal clinical response in triple-negative disease only. Patients with HER2-positive tumors should be treated with preoperative systemic therapy incorporating trastuzumab for at least 9 weeks of preoperative therapy (remainder trastuzumab is completed after surgery for a total of 1 year) [11]. Pertuzumab is added preoperatively for dual HER2 blockade for patients with greater than or equal to T2 lesions and/or N1 disease [12, 13].

Tumor response during neoadjuvant chemotherapy should be assessed routinely with clinical exam to ensure response to therapy. If there is clinical concern for lack of response or progression, then imaging such as breast ultrasound should be considered to confirm clinical exam findings. For patients experiencing progression of disease on neoadjuvant chemotherapy, alternate systemic therapy can be considered or they should be taken for surgery. All patients should undergo surgery following neoadjuvant systemic therapy, even if they have had a complete clinical and/or radiological response. However, trials are in progress to determine whether surgery can be safely omitted in highly selected patients with complete responses and negative biopsies after chemotherapy. The choice between breast conservation and mastectomy after neoadjuvant treatment is dependent on the treatment response (assessed clinically and by posttreatment imaging) and patient's tumor to breast ratio. However, patients who present with a T4 lesions or inflammatory breast cancer should undergo mastectomy following neoadjuvant treatment irrespective of their response due to higher risk for recurrence with breast conservation surgery. Patients with hormone receptor-positive breast cancer should receive adjuvant endocrine therapy to reduce the risk of breast cancer recurrence and breast cancer-related mortality. Additional postoperative chemotherapy following neoadjuvant chemotherapy and surgery is generally not indicated unless the planned course of neoadjuvant therapy could not be completed prior to surgery. There are ongoing trials exploring the role of additional chemotherapy for patients who did not achieve adequate response to neoadjuvant chemotherapy. Some examples of agents that are being studied in this setting include TDM-1 (Ado-trastuzumab emtansine) for HER2-positive patients, capecitabine or carboplatin for triple-negative cancers, and palbociclib for hormone receptor-positive cancers with residual disease after neoadjuvant chemotherapy [14–16].

Adjuvant Chemotherapy

The use of adjuvant systemic therapy is responsible for much of the reduction in cause-specific mortality from breast cancer [17]. Adjuvant chemotherapy refers to the use of cytotoxic chemotherapy after breast cancer surgery, administered with the goal of eradicating microscopic foci of cancer cells that, if left untreated, could grow and recur as metastatic cancer. The data to support adjuvant chemotherapy (versus no treatment) and, specifically, the administration of anthracycline and taxane therapy in the adjuvant setting come from the Early Breast Cancer Trialists' Collaborative Group (EBCTCG). Based on EBCTCG meta-analysis, the use of an anthracycline-containing regimen compared with no treatment resulted in decreased risk of recurrence, breast cancer-specific mortality, and overall mortality [18].

The decision to use adjuvant chemotherapy takes into account tumor histology; expression of ER, PR, and HER2; tumor stage and grade; proliferation index; patient age; as well as high-risk features such as lympho-vascular invasion. Adjuvant chemotherapy is standard for patients with triple-negative breast cancer and either a tumor size greater than 0.5 cm or pathologically involved lymph nodes (regardless of tumor size). Patients with tumors that do not express hormone receptors are not candidates for endocrine therapy, and as the tumor is HER2 negative, they are not candidates for anti-HER2 therapy either. Therefore, our threshold for the use of chemotherapy in these patients is low because this is the only form of adjuvant treatment available to them. The prognosis of small (<0.5 cm), node-negative, triple-negative tumors is generally favorable. For that reason, the benefits of adjuvant chemotherapy are very small and must be weighed against the chances of serious side effects of chemotherapy.

Chemotherapy treatment decision-making for women with ER-/PR-positive, HER2-negative breast cancers is more complex, owing to the variation in prognosis among these tumors, the effectiveness of adjuvant endocrine therapy at reducing recurrence, and the variable sensitivity of ER-positive tumors to chemotherapy treatments. For such patients, the decision to administer chemotherapy is based on an assessment of the composite risk of recurrence and likelihood of benefit (traditional risk factors are taken into account such as patient age and comorbidities, tumor size and grade, lympho-vascular invasion, and lymph node status in addition to the results of gene expression profiles) [19]. Most instances of ER-positive breast cancer less than 1 cm, and all cancers less than 0.5 cm, have a good prognosis with endocrine therapy alone and do not typically require adjuvant chemotherapy. At the other end of the spectrum, most women with stage III breast cancers will warrant adjuvant chemotherapy because of their high risk of recurrence and the likely benefits of chemotherapy.

The use of microarray technology to characterize breast cancer has allowed for development of classifications systems of breast cancer by gene expression profile as mentioned earlier. There are many gene-based assays to predict prognosis such as distant recurrence or survival. The 21-gene assay using reverse transcription polymerase chain reaction (RT-PCR) on RNA isolated from paraffin-embedded breast cancer tissue is amongst the best validated prognostic assays and is most commonly used at our institute. The 21-gene assay recurrence score (RS), also known as Oncotype Dx, has been validated both as a prognostic and a predictive tool. It helps identify those patients with *node-negative*, hormone receptor-positive breast cancer whose prognosis is so favorable that the benefit of chemotherapy is likely to be very low. The optimal RS cutoff for omission of chemotherapy remains unclear since different studies have used different cutoffs [20, 21]. Since the prospective-retrospective studies have validated RS less than 18 as a cutoff to distinguish low from intermediate RS, it is reasonable to avoid adjuvant chemotherapy for patients with node-negative, ER-positive breast cancer and an RS of less than 18. We await outcomes in women with intermediate RS from the TAILORx trial to further clarify the optimal cutoff for adjuvant chemotherapy [22]. An unplanned, retrospective subset analysis from a single, randomized clinical trial in postmenopausal, *node-positive*, ER-positive breast cancer found that RS may provide predictive information for chemotherapy benefit in this population [23]. The SWOG RxPONDER trial, which utilizes RS to assign hormone receptor-positive, HER2-negative, node-positive patients to standard endocrine therapy with or without adjuvant chemotherapy, is ongoing and will clarify the role of RS in node-positive disease.

Another commonly used assay is the 70-gene signature assay which uses microarray technology to analyze gene expression profile from breast tumor tissue to help identify patients with early-stage breast cancer likely to develop distant metastasis [24]. Results from an international randomized trial, the Microarray in Node-Negative Disease May Avoid Chemotherapy (MINDACT) trial, suggest that this profile may identify subsets of patients who have a low likelihood of distant recurrence despite high-risk clinical features. However, it should be noted that the MINDACT study was not powered to exclude a benefit of chemotherapy. This assay has been approved by FDA to assist in assignment of patients with ER-positive or ER-negative breast cancer into a high or low risk for recurrence, but not for predicting benefit from adjuvant systemic therapy [25].

In general, similar chemotherapy regimens are used as adjuvant therapy in patients with ER-/PR-positive, HER2-negative cancer or with triple negative cancers. The regimen of doxorubicin and cyclophosphamide followed by paclitaxel (AC-T) delivered on a dose-dense schedule is the preferred regimen for most patients. For patients with lower-risk disease or a history of cardiac disease, non-anthracycline regimens may be preferable; most commonly employed regimen in this setting is docetaxel and cyclophosphamide (TC). For patients in whom steroid treatment or risk of peripheral neuropathy (both are issues associated with use of taxane therapy) is a particular concern, and where there are concerns about anthracycline exposure due to cardiotoxicity, commonly recommended regimen at our institute is combination of cyclophosphamide, methotrexate, and fluorouracil (CMF). Recently published joint analysis of three adjuvant trials consisting of dose-dense doxorubicin, cyclophosphamide, and paclitaxel compared with docetaxel and cyclophosphamide showed invasive disease-free survival in favor of anthracycline-based therapy [26]. Exploratory analyses for treatment interaction by hormonal status and nodal status suggest that the benefits appear to be clinically meaningful in patients with hormone receptor negative tumors or those with hormone receptor positive tumors and positive axillary nodes.

Treatment directed against the human epidermal growth factor receptor 2 (HER2) is incorporated in the chemotherapy regimen for patients with HER2 overexpression. Initial regimen is then followed by maintenance trastuzumab to complete total therapy for 1 year based on a trial comparing no maintenance versus 1 or 2 years of trastuzumab therapy which favored 1 year of therapy; no additional benefit was derived upon continuation for 2 years [27]. The benefits of adding trastuzumab to adjuvant chemotherapy in patients with HER2-positive tumors were confirmed in a meta-analysis of eight trials of chemotherapy plus trastuzumab versus chemotherapy alone involving nearly 12,000 patients which showed significant improvement in disease-free survival and overall survival [28]. Trastuzumab is associated with cardiotoxicity which necessitates monitoring of cardiac function periodically through treatment. When trastuzumab is combined with an anthracycline-based regimen, there is an expected increase in cardiotoxicity due to overlapping side effects from trastuzumab and anthracyclines. When compared to a non-anthracycline-based chemotherapy regimen, there were more breast cancer recurrences but fewer cardiac events in the non-anthracycline arm [29]. The choice of chemotherapy backbone takes into account patient's age, cardiac risk factors, tumor characteristics, and personal preference. Trastuzumab combined with paclitaxel alone has demonstrated excellent outcomes for patients with node-negative, HER2-positive tumors that are less than 2 cm [30]. HER2-positive tumors that are smaller than 5 mm are less likely to derive benefit from adjuvant therapy including HER2-targeted therapy. There is no data to use pertuzumab in the adjuvant setting at this time, but clinical trial results evaluating this agent along with trastuzumab for 1 year are awaited.

Adjuvant Endocrine Therapy

Patients with ER-/PR-positive invasive cancer should be considered for adjuvant endocrine therapy regardless of their age, tumor type or size, lymph node status, or receipt of adjuvant chemotherapy. In patients receiving both chemotherapy and endocrine therapy, chemotherapy should be given first followed by endocrine therapy. The choice of endocrine therapy is dependent on menopausal status of the patient prior to administration of chemotherapy. Tamoxifen is a commonly used selective estrogen receptor modulator in premenopausal women. In the Suppression of Ovarian Function (SOFT) trial, premenopausal women were randomly assigned to one of three arms: tamoxifen alone, tamoxifen plus ovarian suppression, or exemestane plus ovarian suppression. Ovarian suppression was achieved with the use of the gonadotropin-releasing-hormone agonist triptorelin, oophorectomy, or ovarian irradiation. Compared to tamoxifen alone, tamoxifen plus ovarian suppression did not result in improved outcomes but caused increased toxicity which likely resulted in a higher rate of medication discontinuation. In a subgroup analysis, women at high risk of recurrence, who received prior chemotherapy, had improved outcomes with addition of ovarian suppression [31]. Tamoxifen and Exemestane Trial (TEXT) evaluated comparison between tamoxifen plus ovarian suppression and exemestane plus ovarian suppression. When these two adjuvant endocrine therapy trials (SOFT and TEXT) were combined to compare tamoxifen plus ovarian suppression and exemestane plus ovarian suppression, the latter showed improved rate of freedom from breast cancer at 5 years [32]. Based on the combined results of SOFT and TEXT trials, exemestane plus ovarian suppression is preferred for premenopausal, hormone receptor-positive breast cancer at higher risk of recurrence (patients who are less than 35 years and those that received chemotherapy). Optimal duration of tamoxifen was evaluated by comparing 5 years of tamoxifen to 10 years. Tamoxifen therapy extended to 10 years reduced risk for recurrence and breast cancer-specific mortality at the cost of increased incidence of pulmonary embolism and endometrial cancer [33].

Aromatase inhibitors have consistently been shown to improve outcomes for postmenopausal women with hormone receptor-positive breast cancer compared with tamoxifen. All the available aromatase inhibitor agents (anastrozole, letrozole, and exemestane) have demonstrated similar efficacy and toxicity profiles. Aromatase inhibitors can be utilized as initial adjuvant therapy, or as sequential therapy following 2–3 years of tamoxifen or as extended therapy beyond 5 years of tamoxifen. Sequential therapy of aromatase inhibitor after tamoxifen has been shown to improve overall survival. The extension of treatment with an adjuvant aromatase inhibitor to 10 years resulted in significantly higher rates of disease-free survival and a lower incidence of contralateral breast cancer than those with placebo, but the rate of overall survival was not higher with the aromatase inhibitor than with placebo [34]. Aromatase inhibitors can be associated with hot flashes, musculoskeletal symptoms such as stiffness and joint pain, as well as long-term effects such as osteoporosis and increased cardiovascular risk.

Post-therapy Surveillance

Follow-up care is provided by the members of the treatment team. All women should have a careful history every 3–6 months for the first 3 years after primary therapy, then every 6–12 months for the next 2 years, and then annually. It is recommended that all women should perform monthly breast self-examination. Mammography should be performed annually with first posttreatment mammogram 6 months after completion of radiotherapy [35]. For women who have undergone mastectomy, surveillance is usually performed by physical examination. Because the majority of recurrences occur between scheduled visits, it is prudent to inform women about symptoms of recurrence. Patients on adjuvant tamoxifen with intact uterus should undergo yearly gynecologic assessment and rapid evaluation of abnormal vaginal bleeding due to risk of endometrial cancer associated with tamoxifen use. Patients on aromatase inhibitor (AI) therapy should undergo monitoring of bone health at baseline and periodically thereafter. Bone strengthening agents can be employed for patients on AI therapy who have suboptimal bone health. The data are insufficient to suggest routine laboratory assessments including tumor markers and surveillance imaging in absence of symptoms [35]. Adequate symptom management for women on endocrine therapy improves medication adherence. Reproductive issues may arise during endocrine therapy including sexual dysfunction, fertility, and contraception which need coordination of care with gynecology. Lifestyle modification can be an empowering and effective way to boost physical and mental health in breast cancer survivors and possibly to improve outcomes. Observational data suggest that physical activity to optimize body-mass index and minimization of alcohol intake are associated with a decreased risk of breast cancer recurrence and death in breast cancer survivors [36, 37].

Recurrent or Metastatic Breast Cancer

Recurrent breast cancer can present as local recurrence or distant metastasis. Local recurrence usually presents as a palpable lump in the breast, chest wall, or nodal region, or as new findings on mammography. All patients with local recurrence should undergo biopsy for pathological confirmation and imaging to assess for concurrent distant metastatic disease. In the absence of distant metastases, patients must undergo surgical resection of the recurrence along with nodal sampling followed by involved field radiation therapy if not previously treated or if additional radiation can be administered safely. Based on the CALOR trial, after local treatment, women with local recurrences should be considered for systemic therapy with chemotherapy and/or endocrine therapy if applicable, for a limited duration with similar intent as that of adjuvant therapy. The choice of chemotherapy depends on the biomarkers, previous therapy, and time to recurrent disease [38].

Metastatic breast cancer involving distant sites cannot be cured, but significant improvements in breast cancer-specific survival have been observed with the use of systemic therapies, with some patients achieving long-term remissions [39]. Current practice guidelines recommend that patients with metastatic disease must be biopsied to confirm tumor histology and allow reevaluation of biomarkers. Assessment of ER, PR, and HER2 should be repeated as there may be discordance between the primary and metastatic cancers. This discordance could be related to change in the biology of the tumor, differential effect of prior treatment resulting in clonal selection, or tumor heterogeneity [40, 41]. The treatment strategy is a tailored approach and depends upon tumor biology and biomarkers as well as clinical factors pertaining to the patient such as volume and location of metastatic disease and patient's functional and nutritional status. Although a subset of patients with oligo-metastatic disease may benefit from an intensified locoregional approach, most patients with metastatic breast cancer receive systemic medical therapy consisting of chemotherapy, endocrine therapy, and/or biologic therapies and supportive care measures [42]. The primary goals of systemic treatment for metastatic breast cancer are prolongation of survival, palliation of symptoms, and maintenance or improvement in quality of life.

Women with hormone receptor-positive and HER2-negative metastatic disease should generally be considered for initial endocrine therapy. However, sometimes patients may present with rapidly progressive, symptomatic disease with end-organ dysfunction (visceral crisis which could involve lungs, liver, or compression of important structures), in which case chemotherapy can be chosen over endocrine therapy. Endocrine therapy choices depend on prior exposure to antiestrogen agents. There is some data in postmenopausal women to suggest that aromatase inhibitor therapy appears to have superior outcomes compared to tamoxifen [43, 44]. Fulvestrant (ER down-regulator) when compared to anastrozole as first-line agent in metastatic ER-positive breast cancer who had not received prior hormone therapy showed improved progression-free survival [45]. Compared with anastrozole alone, combination of fulvestrant and anastrozole resulted in an improvement in progression-free and overall survival. On subgroup analysis, the benefit of combination therapy appeared to be limited to endocrine therapy naïve patients [46]. Observation of synergy between CDK 4/6 inhibitors and endocrine therapy has led to emergence of newer combinations for therapy in this population. Palbociclib (CDK 4/6 inhibitor) in combination with letrozole (AI) when compared to letrozole alone showed improved response rates and progression-free survival [47]. Ribociclib, another selective CDK 4/6 inhibitor, in combination with letrozole demonstrated improved efficacy over letrozole alone [48]. CDK 4/6 inhibitors are generally well tolerated, most commonly notable adverse effects include neutropenia, fatigue, derangements of liver function, and nausea. Combination of mTOR inhibitors with endocrine therapy was postulated to overcome resistance to endocrine therapy. An improvement in progression-free survival and response rates was seen with combination of everolimus (mTOR inhibitor) and exemestane (steroidal AI) in patients who had progressed on anastrozole [49]. Everolimus is associated with significant toxicity including stomatitis, pneumonitis, abnormal liver function, hyperglycemia, and fatigue.

Women with hormone receptor-negative metastatic disease or those with hormone receptor-positive disease that have either become refractory to endocrine therapy or have significant tumor burden are considered for chemotherapy. Combination chemotherapy when compared to single agents given sequentially generally provides quicker and higher rates of responses and has longer time to progression but comes at the cost of increased toxicity. There is no compelling evidence that suggests that combination chemotherapy is superior to sequential chemotherapy and the latter is generally preferred for better quality of life. However, combination therapy is preferred in patients with rapidly progressive disease with impending end-organ failure where quicker response is desired. Single-agent chemotherapy is continued until there is evidence for disease progression at which time another agent is chosen based on previous therapy, toxicity profile, logistics of administration, and patient preference. A variety of chemotherapy agents (used as single agents or in combination) are active in breast cancer including anthracyclines (doxorubicin, epirubicin, and pegylated liposomal doxorubicin), taxanes (paclitaxel, docetaxel, and albumin-bound paclitaxel), antimetabolites (capecitabine and gemcitabine), non-taxane microtubule inhibitors (eribulin and vinorelbine), platinum agents (cisplatin and carboplatin), and others such as ixabepilone, cyclophosphamide, and methotrexate. The role of immune therapy in metastatic breast cancer, particularly triple-negative disease, continues to evolve at this time. The duration of chemotherapy should be individualized taking into account the patient's goals of therapy, presence of treatment toxicities, and alternative options that might be available. In general, patients should continue chemotherapy to the best response or disease progression unless toxicity requires discontinuation of treatment sooner. A detailed discussion about the chemotherapy regimens is beyond the scope of this chapter.

For patients with HER2-positive metastatic breast cancer, HER2-directed agents should be a component of treatment. For most patients, HER2-directed agent plus chemotherapy is chosen. However, patients with hormone receptor-positive and

HER2-positive metastatic breast cancer may receive HER2-directed therapy in combination with endocrine therapy, if they have low volume, indolent, and asymptomatic disease, especially in the elderly. The preferred first-line therapy option is combination of trastuzumab, pertuzumab, and docetaxel which has shown improved response rates, progression-free survival, and overall survival when compared to trastuzumab and docetaxel [50, 51]. Common adverse effects from this therapy include febrile neutropenia, diarrhea, rash, mucositis, and edema. There was no increase in the rate of ventricular dysfunction with the combination. After achievement of best response to treatment, cytotoxic chemotherapy is typically discontinued with plan to continue trastuzumab and pertuzumab therapy until disease progression. In patients whose tumors are also hormone receptor positive, endocrine therapy is added to HER2-directed therapy following discontinuation of chemotherapy. Ado-trastuzumab emtansine (T-DM1) is an antibody-drug conjugate composed of trastuzumab, a thioether linker, and a microtubule inhibitor, DM1. This is typically utilized in second-line setting based on improved outcomes in terms of progression-free and overall survival and better toxicity profile when compared to lapatinib plus capecitabine [52]. This could be an alternative first-line treatment for patients unable to receive trastuzumab plus pertuzumab plus taxane, based on non-inferiority and better tolerability of TDM-1 alone or in combination with pertuzumab, when compared to trastuzumab and taxane therapy [53]. The regimen of capecitabine plus lapatinib is an option for patients with HER2-positive disease following progression on trastuzumab containing regimen based on improved time to progression with the combination compared to capecitabine alone [54]. This is reserved as a third-line option after failure of abovementioned regimens.

Distant sites of recurrence may require local therapies to alleviate symptoms and prevent impending complications. Surgery/procedures, radiation, or regional chemotherapy (intrathecal) may be employed as needed for metastatic sites such as brain metastases or leptomeningeal involvement, pleural or pericardial effusion, impending pathological fracture or compression of vital organs, biliary or urinary obstruction, bleeding, cord compression, painful bone metastases, or soft tissue disease.

Monitoring of metastatic disease during therapy is important to make sure that the therapy is providing benefit and the patient does not have toxicity from ineffective therapy. Monitoring of disease entails periodic assessment of symptoms and clinical exam (if disease is easily accessible clinically) to determine response. These are coupled with laboratory tests including serial tumor markers if elevated and periodic imaging (CT scan, bone scan, MRI as indicated) to ensure disease response to therapy. Data on circulating tumor cells suggest their prognostic value, but their use in disease monitoring is controversial and should not be used to influence treatment decisions at this time.

Summary

The therapeutic options for patients with invasive breast cancer are complex. An essential component of patient's management is the multidisciplinary team approach that includes collaboration among breast radiologist, pathologist, breast and reconstructive surgeons, medical and radiation oncologists, palliative care specialist, fertility specialist, genetic counsellors, nurse navigators, and clinical trial coordinators. *The patients and physicians share the responsibility to explore and identify the most appropriate treatment options in order to optimize the chance of cure and minimize toxicity depending on individual patient factors and disease variables.* Participation in clinical trials helps patients access emerging novel therapies and contribute to the improvement in therapeutic outcomes.

References

1. Jemal A, Bray F, Center MM, et al. Global cancer statistics. CA Cancer J Clin. 2011;61:69.
2. Barlow WE, Lehman CD, Zheng Y, et al. Performance of diagnostic mammography for women with signs or symptoms of breast cancer. J Natl Cancer Inst. 2002;94:1151.
3. Chang JH, Vines E, Bertsch H, et al. The impact of a multidisciplinary breast cancer center on recommendations for patient management: the University of Pennsylvania experience. Cancer. 2001;91:1231.
4. Sotiriou C, Pusztai L. Gene-expression signatures in breast cancer. N Engl J Med. 2009;360:790–800.
5. Dai X, Li T, Bai Z, et al. Breast cancer intrinsic subtype classification, clinical use and future trends. Am J Cancer Res. 2015;5(10):2929.
6. Fisher B, Anderson S, Bryant J, et al. Twenty-year follow-up of a randomized trial comparing total mastectomy, lumpectomy and lumpectomy plus irradiation for treatment of invasive breast cancer. N Engl J Med. 2002;347:1233.
7. Rastogi P, Anderson SJ, Bear HD, et al. Preoperative chemotherapy: updates of National Surgical Adjuvant Breast and Bowel Project Protocols B-18 and B-27. J Clin Oncol. 2008;26(5):778.
8. von Minckwitz G, Untch M, Blohmer JU, et al. Definition and impact of pathological complete response on prognosis after neoadjuvant chemotherapy in various intrinsic breast cancer subtypes. J Clin Oncol. 2012;30(15):1796.
9. Sikov WM, Berry DA, Perou CM, et al. Impact of the addition of carboplatin and/or bevacizumab to neoadjuvant once-per-week paclitaxel followed by dose-dense doxorubicin and cyclophosphamide on pathologic complete response rates in stage II to III triple-negative breast cancer: CALGB 40603. J Clin Oncol. 2015;33(1):13.
10. von Minckwitz G, Schneeweiss A, Loibl S, et al. Neoadjuvant carboplatin in patients with triple-negative and HER2-positive early breast cancer (GeparSixto; GBG 66): a randomized phase 2 trial. Lancet Oncol. 2014;15(7):747.
11. Petrelli F, Borgonovo K, Cabiddu M, et al. Neoadjuvant chemotherapy and concomitant trastuzumab in breast cancer: a pooled analysis of two randomized trials. Anti-Cancer Drugs. 2011;22:128.
12. Gianni L, Pienkowski T, Im YH, et al. Efficacy and safety of neoadjuvant pertuzumab and trastuzumab in women with locally advanced, inflammatory, or early HER2-positive breast cancer (Neosphere): a randomised multicenter, open-label, phase2 trial. Lancet Oncol. 2012;13:25.
13. Schneeweiss A, Chia S, Hickish T, et al. Pertuzumab plus trastuzumab in combination with standard neoadjuvant anthracycline-containing and anthracycline-free chemotherapy regimens in patients with HER2-positive early breast cancer: a randomized phase II cardiac safety study (TRYPHAENA). Ann Oncol. 2013;24:2278.
14. A Study of trastuzumab emtansine versus trastuzumab as adjuvant therapy in patients with HER2-positive breast cancer who have residual tumor in the breast or axillary lymph nodes following preoperative therapy (KATHERINE). ClinicalTrials.gov. Identifier: NCT01772472.

15. Platinum based chemotherapy or capecitabine in treating patients with residual triple-negative basal-like breast cancer following neoadjuvant chemotherapy. ClinicalTrials.gov. Identifier: NCT02445391.
16. A study of palbociclib in addition to standard endocrine treatment in hormone receptor positive Her2 normal patients with residual disease after neoadjuvant chemotherapy and surgery (PENELOPE-B). ClinicalTrials.gov. Identifier: NCT01864746.
17. Berry DA, Cronin KA, Plevritis SK, et al. Effect of screening and adjuvant therapy on mortality from breast cancer. N Engl J Med. 2005;353:1784.
18. Early Breast Cancer Trialists' Collaborative Group (EBCTCG), Peto R, Davies C, et al. Comparisons between different polychemotherapy regimens for early breast cancer: meta-analyses of long-term outcome among 100,000 women in 123 randomised trials. Lancet. 2012;379:432.
19. Henry NL, Somerfield MR, Abramson VG, et al. Role of patient and disease factors in adjuvant systemic therapy decision making for early-stage, operable breast cancer: American Society of Clinical Oncology endorsement of Cancer Care Ontario guideline recommendations. J Clin Oncol. 2016;34:2303.
20. Paik S, Shak S, Tang G, et al. A multigene assay to predict recurrence of tamoxifen-treated, node-negative breast cancer. N Engl J Med. 2004;351:2817.
21. Mamounas EP, Tang G, Fisher B, et al. Association between the 21-gene recurrence score assay and risk of locoregional recurrence in node-negative, estrogen receptor-positive breast cancer: results from NSABP B-14 and NSABP B-20. J Clin Oncol. 2010;28:1677.
22. Sparano JA, Gray RJ, Makower DF, et al. Prospective validation of a 21-gene expression assay in breast cancer. N Engl J Med. 2015;373:2005.
23. Albain KS, Barlow WE, Shak S, et al. Prognostic and predictive value of the 21-gene recurrence score assay in postmenopausal women with node-positive, oestrogen-receptor-positive breast cancer on chemotherapy: a retrospective analysis of a randomised trial. Lancet Oncol. 2010;11:55.
24. van de Vijver MJ, He YD, van't Veer LJ, et al. A gene-expression signature as a predictor of survival in breast cancer. N Engl J Med. 2002;347:1999.
25. Cardoso F, van't Veer LJ, Bogaerts J, et al. 70-Gene signature as an aid to treatment decisions in early-stage breast cancer. N Engl J Med. 2016;375:717.
26. Blum JL, Flynn PJ, Yothers G, et al. Anthracyclines in early breast cancer: ABC trials- USOR 06-090, NSABP B-46-I/USOR 07132 and NSABP B-49 (NRG Oncology). J Clin Oncol. 2017; doi:10.1200/JCO.2016.71.4147.
27. Goldhirsch A, Gelber RD, Piccart-Gebhart MJ, et al. 2 years versus 1 year of adjuvant trastuzumab for HER2-positive breast cancer (HERA): an open-label, randomised controlled trial. Lancet. 2013;382:1021.
28. Moja L, Tagliabue L, Balduzzi S, et al. Trastuzumab containing regimens for early breast cancer. Cochrane Database Syst Rev. 2012:CD006243. doi:10.1002/14651858.CD006243.pub2.
29. Slamon D, Eiermann W, Robert N, et al. Adjuvant trastuzumab in HER2-positive breast cancer. N Engl J Med. 2011;365:1273.
30. Tolaney SM, Barry WT, Dang CT, et al. Adjuvant paclitaxel and trastuzumab for node-negative, HER2-positive breast cancer. N Engl J Med. 2015;372:134.
31. Francis PA, Regan MM, Fleming GF, et al. Adjuvant ovarian suppression in premenopausal breast cancer. N Engl J Med. 2015;372:436.
32. Pagani O, Regan MM, Walley BA, et al. Adjuvant exemestane with ovarian suppression in premenopausal breast cancer. N Engl J Med. 2014;371:107.
33. Davies C, Pan H, Godwin J, et al. Long-term effects of continuing adjuvant tamoxifen to 10 years versus stopping at 5 years after diagnosis of oestrogen receptor-positive breast cancer: ATLAS, a randomised trial. Lancet. 2013;381:805.
34. Goss PE, Inge JN, Pritchard KI, et al. Extending adjuvant aromatase-inhibitor therapy to 10 years. N Engl J Med. 2016;375:209.
35. Khatcheressian JL, Hurley P, Bantug E, et al. Breast cancer follow-up and management after primary treatment: American Society of Clinical Oncology clinical practice guideline update. J Clin Oncol. 2013;31:961.

36. Friedenreich CM, Gregory J, Kopciuk KA, et al. Prospective cohort study of lifetime physical activity and breast cancer survival. Int J Cancer. 2009;124:1954.
37. Kwan ML, Kushi LH, Weltzien E, et al. Alcohol consumption and breast cancer recurrence and survival among women with early-stage breast cancer: the life after cancer epidemiology study. J Clin Oncol. 2010;28:4410.
38. Aebi S, Gelber S, Anderson SJ, et al. Chemotherapy for isolated locoregional recurrence of breast cancer (CALOR): a randomised trial. Lancet Oncol. 2014;15:156.
39. Greenberg PA, Hortobagyi GN, Smith TL, et al. Long-term follow-up of patients with complete remission following combination chemotherapy for metastatic breast cancer. J Clin Oncol. 1996;14:2197.
40. Pusztai L, Viale G, Kelly CM, et al. Estrogen and HER2 receptor discordance between primary breast cancer and metastasis. Oncologist. 2010;15:1164.
41. Aurilio G, Disalvatore D, Pruneri G, et al. A meta-analysis of estrogen receptor, progesterone receptor and human epidermal growth factor receptor 2 discordance between primary breast cancer and metastases. Eur J Cancer. 2014;50:277.
42. Pagani O, Senkus E, Wood W, et al. International guidelines for management of metastatic breast cancer: can metastatic breast cancer be cured? J Natl Cancer Inst. 2010;102:456.
43. Nabholtz JM, Buzdar A, Pollak M, et al. Anastrozole is superior to tamoxifen as first-line therapy for advanced breast cancer in postmenopausal women: results of North American multicenter randomized trial. Arimidex Study Group. J Clin Oncol. 2000;18:3758.
44. Gibson L, Lawrence D, Dawson C, et al. Aromatase inhibitors for treatment of advanced breast cancer in postmenopausal women. Cochrane Database Syst Rev. 2009:CD003070. doi:10.1002/14651858.CD003370.pub3.
45. Robertson JF, Bondarenko IM, Trishkina E, et al. Fulvestrant 500 mg versus anastrozole 1 mg for hormone receptor-positive advanced breast cancer (FALCON): an international, randomised, double-blind, phase 3 trial. Lancet. 2016;388:2997.
46. Mehta RS, Barlow WE, Albain KS, et al. Combination anastrozole and fulvestrant in metastatic breast cancer. N Engl J Med. 2012;367:435.
47. Finn RS, Martin M, Rugo HS, et al. Palbociclib and letrozole in advanced breast cancer. N Engl J Med. 2016;375:1925.
48. Hortobagyi GN, Stemmer SM, Burris HA, et al. Ribociclib as first-line therapy for HR-positive, advanced breast cancer. N Engl J Med. 2016;375:1738.
49. Baselga J, Campone M, Piccart M, et al. Everolimus in postmenopausal hormone-receptor-positive advanced breast cancer. N Engl J Med. 2012;366:520.
50. Baselga J, Cortés J, Kim SB, et al. Pertuzumab plus trastuzumab plus docetaxel for metastatic breast cancer. N Engl J Med. 2012;366:109.
51. Swain SM, Baselga J, Kim SB, et al. Pertuzumab, trastuzumab, and docetaxel in HER2-positive metastatic breast cancer. N Engl J Med. 2015;372:724.
52. Verma S, Miles D, Gianni L, et al. Trastuzumab emtansine for HER2-positive advanced breast cancer. N Engl J Med. 2012;367:1783.
53. Perez EA, Barrios C, Eiermann W, et al. Trastuzumab emtansine with or without pertuzumab versus trastuzumab plus taxane for human epidermal growth factor receptor 2-positive, advanced breast cancer: primary results from the phase III MARIANNE study. J Clin Oncol. 2017;35:141.
54. Geyer CE, Forster J, Lindquist D, et al. Lapatinib plus capecitabine for HER2-positive advanced breast cancer. N Engl J Med. 2006;355:2733.

Suggested Readings for the Radiology Section

1. Cardenosa G. Clinical breast imaging: the essentials. Philadelphia, PA: Wolters Kluwer; 2015.
2. Lamb PM, Perry NM, Vinnicombe SJ, Wells CA. Correlation between ultrasound characteristics, mammographic findings and histologic grade in patients with invasive ductal carcinoma

of the breast. Clin Radiol. 2000;55(1):40–4. doi:10.1053/crad.1999.0333. Accessed 26 Feb 2017.

3. Uematsu T, Kasami M, Yuen S. Triple-negative breast cancer: correlation between MR imaging and pathologic findings. Radiology. 2009;250(3):638–47. doi:10.1148/radiol.2503081054. Accessed 23 Feb 2017.
4. Trop I, LeBlanc SM, Davie J, et al. Molecular classification of infiltrating breast cancer: toward personalized therapy. Radiographics. 2014;34:1178–95.
5. Bae MS, Shin S, Ryu HS, et al. Pretreatment MR imaging features of triple-negative breast cancer: association with response to neoadjuvant chemotherapy and recurrence free survival. Radiology. 2016;281(2):392–400. doi:10.1148/radiol.2016152331. Accessed 23 Feb 2017.
6. Cardenosa G, Doudna C, Eklund GW. Mucinous (colloid) breast cancer: clinical and mammographic findings in 10 patients. AJR Am J Roentgenol. 1994;162:1077–9. doi:10.2214/ajr.162.5.8165985. Accessed 23 Feb 2017.
7. Liu H, Tan H, Cheng Y, et al. Imaging findings in mucinous breast carcinoma and correlating factors. Eur J Radiol. 2011;80(3):706–12. doi:10.1016/j.ejrad.2010.06.008. Accessed 23 Feb 2017.
8. Eiada R, Chong J, Kulkarni S, et al. Papillary lesions of the breast: MRI, ultrasound, and mammographic appearances. AJR Am J Roentgen. 2012;198:264–71.
9. Mann RM, Hoogeveen YL, Blickman JG, et al. MRI compared to conventional diagnostic work-up in the detection and evaluation of invasive lobular carcinoma of the breast: a review of existing literature. Breast Cancer Res Treat. 2008;107:1. doi:10.1007/s10549-007-9528-5. Accessed 23 Feb 2017.
10. Leddy R, Irshad A, Rumboldt T, et al. Review of metaplastic carcinoma of the breast: imaging findings and pathologic features. J Clin Imaging Sci. 2012;2:21. www.ncbi.nlm.nih.gov/pmc/articles/PMC3352608/. Accessed 28 Jan 2017
11. Bartella L, Dershaw DD. Magnetic resonance imaging of the invasive breast carcinoma. In: Morris E, Liberman L, editors. Breast MRI: diagnosis and intervention. New York, NY: Springer; 2005.
12. Turnbull L, Brown S, Harvey I, et al. Comparative effectiveness of MRI in breast cancer (COMICE) trial: a randomized controlled trial. Lancet. 2010;375(9714):563–71.
13. Vapiwala N, Hwang WT, Kushner CJ, et al. No impact of breast magnetic resonance imaging on 15-year outcomes in patients with ductal carcinoma in situ or early-stage invasive breast cancer managed with breast conservation therapy. Cancer. 2016. doi:10.1002/cncr.30479. Accessed 25 Feb 2017.
14. Iaconni C, Galman L, Zheng J, et al. Multicentric cancer detected at breast MR imaging and not at mammography: important or not? Radiology. 2016;279(2). doi:10.1148/radiol.2015150796. Accessed 23 Feb 2017.
15. Hollingsworth AB, Stough RG. Multicentric and contralateral invasive tumors identified with pre-op MRI in patients newly diagnosed with ductal carcinoma in situ of the breast. Breast J. 2012;18(5):420–7. doi:10.1111/j.1524-4741.2012.01273.x. Accessed 26 Feb 2017.
16. Fortune-Greeley AK, Wheeler SB, Meyer AM, et al. Preoperative breast MRI and surgical outcomes in elderly women with invasive ductal and lobular carcinoma: a population based study. Breast Cancer Res Treat. 2014;143:203. doi:10.1007/s10549-013-2787-4. Accessed 26 Feb 2017.
17. Alliance for Clinical Trials in Oncology, American College of Radiology Imaging Network Alliance A011104/ACRIN 6694. Effect of preoperative breast MRI on surgical outcomes, costs and quality of life of women with breast cancer NCI Version Date: 04/01/2013.
18. Orel SG, Schnall MD. MR Imaging of the Breast for the Detection, Diagnosis, and Staging of Breast Cancer. Radiology. 2001;220(1):13–30. doi 10.1148/radiology.220.1.r01jl3113. Accessed 6/2/17.
19. Liu PF, Debatin JF, Caduff RF, et al. Improved diagnostic accuracy in dynamic contrast enhanced MRI of the breast by combined quantitative and qualitative analysis. The British Journal of Radiology. 1998;71(845):501–509. doi 10.1259/bjr.71.845.9691895. Accessed 6/2/17.

Miscellaneous Conditions

10

Priti A. Shah and Valentina Robila

Fat Necrosis

There is a saying that fat necrosis can look like anything on imaging. Truly, it may run the gamut of the BI-RADS lexicon and appear as a round, oval, or irregular mass that is fat containing, low, equal, or high density, with circumscribed, indistinct, or spiculated margins mammographically. There may be associated calcifications. The classic appearance, that is unequivocally benign, includes fat containing mass with curvilinear, rim, dystrophic, or lucent centered calcifications, although amorphous, punctate, coarse heterogenous, and fine pleomorphic forms may also be present. Sonographically, the classic appearance is that of a hyperechoic mass with central hypo- to anechoic spaces (Fig. 10.1) [1-4]. Despite its benignity, it may enhance avidly on MRI, mimicking malignancy (as it can on other modalities); although routine fat suppressed images may demonstrate central fat, the morphology and margins may still trigger a biopsy. Unfortunately, even the trauma of a needle biopsy may incite additional changes such that it becomes larger and thus possibly more suspicious in appearance on future studies. Fat necrosis does not usually warrant treatment.

P.A. Shah, MD (✉)
Department of Radiology, Breast Imaging Section, Virginia Commonwealth University Health (VCU HEALTH), Richmond, VA, USA
e-mail: priti.shah@vcuhealth.org

V. Robila, MD, PhD
Department of Pathology, Virginia Commonwealth University Health (VCU HEALTH), Richmond, VA, USA
e-mail: valentina.robila@vcuhealth.org

M.O. Idowu et al. (eds.), *Diagnosis and Management of Breast Tumors*,
DOI 10.1007/978-3-319-57726-5_10

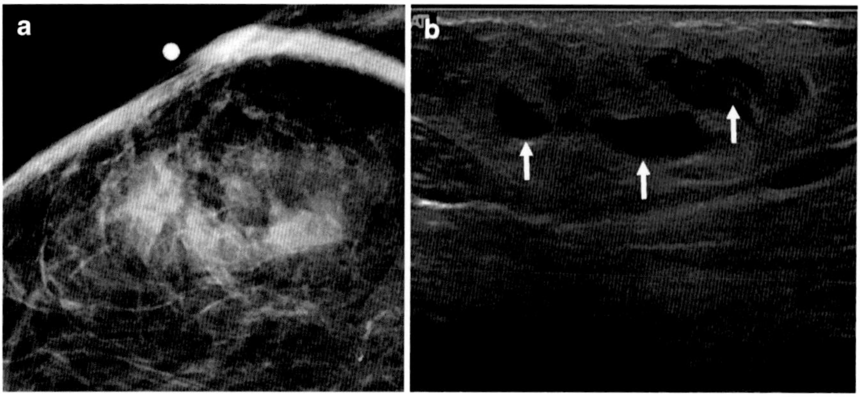

Fig. 10.1 Fat necrosis. (**a**) Spot tangential view at the site of a palpable "lump" (as denoted by metallic BB skin marker) shows an irregular fat containing mass with indistinct margins. (**b**) On targeted ultrasound, an oval, horizontally oriented (*parallel*) mass is imaged in the subcutaneous fat; it is predominantly hyperechoic with central cystic spaces (*arrows*).

Abscess/Mastitis

Subareolar abscesses can be distinguished from peripheral abscesses not only by location but by patient predilection, potential etiologies, imaging appearance, and management.

There are two schools of thought regarding the etiology of subareolar abscesses. One supports the predilection seen in smokers: a metaplastic change in ductal epithelium (supposedly related to cigarettes) resulting in luminal obstruction that makes the patient more susceptible to infection. However, these abscesses are also seen in non-smokers. A second hypothesis is that the process starts as a skin infection, such as a folliculitis, that extends into the breast tissue. This can also be challenged, since some patients may have little skin changes, out of proportion to symptoms and extent of the deeper abscess collection [1].

Clinically, patients with abscesses may feel a painful "lump," overlying which the skin may be erythematous and/or thinned. Depending on the extent of infection, diffuse skin edema, characterized by thickening or peau d'orange change, can be seen, as may purulent drainage.

Subareolar abscesses can be managed with oral antibiotics (more than one course may be required), aspiration, incision and drainage, and/or clinical and ultrasound follow-up. Frustrating to patients and clinicians, even with a good response to initial treatment, they often recur (in 25–40% of patients), requiring (repeat) needle aspiration or incision and drainage acutely, or eventual central duct excision [1, 5]. Recurrent or chronic subareolar abscesses can form fistulous tracts with the skin seen clinically along the areolar margin as draining sinuses. This is known as Zuska disease [6]. Due to repeated bouts of inflammation resulting in fibrosis involving the central ducts, horizontal nipple inversion may eventually occur.

Lactational abscesses can be central or peripheral. These are often managed by the patient's obstetrician/gynecologist, without imaging, and seem to respond better to antibiotics [5, 7].

Peripheral abscesses not related to lactation are more common in diabetics, perhaps related to compromised immune function. These may not involve the skin directly, but be centered in the parenchyma, and therefore be confused with a mass. First-line management is often ultrasound-guided needle aspiration in addition to oral antibiotics. These are less likely to recur.

Imaging Findings

Subareolar abscess: Increased density, focal asymmetry or mass mammographically, possibly with associated skin and/or trabecular thickening (edema). Edema and patient tenderness may limit compression. Sonographically, an irregular fluid collection/complex cystic and solid mass involving the deep dermal layer; tubular extensions can often be seen "funneling" posteriorly, with increased echogenicity and loss of tissue planes that represents parenchymal edema (Fig. 10.2). There is associated skin thickening if not breakdown and drainage. Echogenic foci may represent air if there is an open wound.

Peripheral abscess: A mass or focal asymmetry mammographically, possibly with associated skin (secondarily) and/or trabecular thickening (edema, focal or diffuse). Sonographically, a complex solid and cystic mass, sometimes with mobile internal echoes, and surrounding edema; skin thickening may or may not be apparent. Lactational abscesses also have this appearance; they are more commonly imaged sonographically due to avoidance of radiation while still breastfeeding (Fig. 10.3).

In patients with infectious mastitis, physical exam and imaging findings tend to be diffuse as there may not be a discrete associated fluid collection to suggest an abscess. Focal areas of irregular hypoechoic tissue, or diffusely dilated subdermal lymphatics, may be noted by ultrasound [1]. This clinical picture may overlap that of a locally advanced malignancy more so than with an abscess; therefore, short term follow-up is paramount with biopsy to follow if exam and imaging findings do not resolve with antibiotics. In that vein, direct correlation with clinical signs and symptoms with ultrasound findings are imperative in distinguishing between infectious and malignant processes.

Granulomatous mastitis is a rare noninfectious condition typically seen in women of childbearing age, within several months to years of pregnancy. The etiology is unknown, but some postulate an autoimmune mechanism. It may present

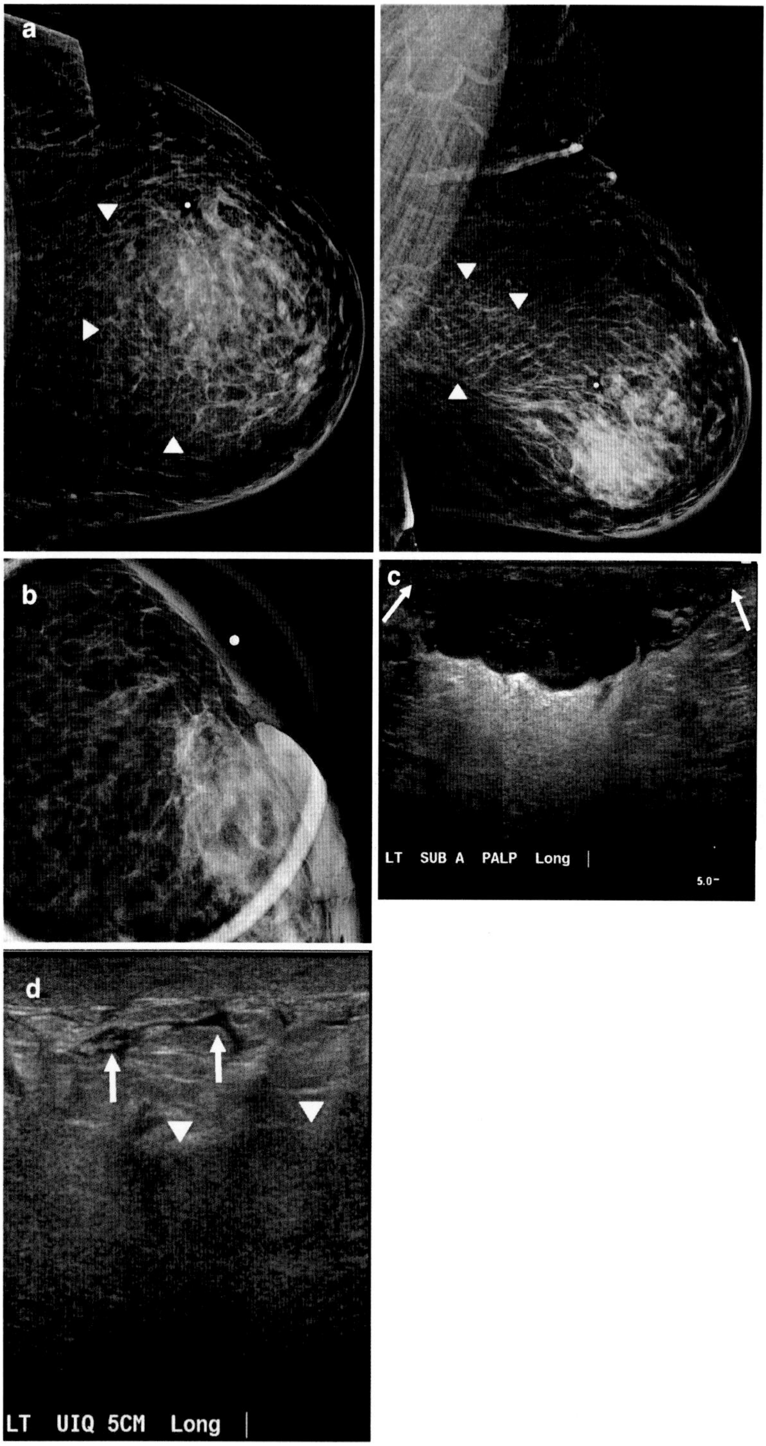
a
b
c
LT SUB A PALP Long
5.0
d
LT UIQ 5CM Long

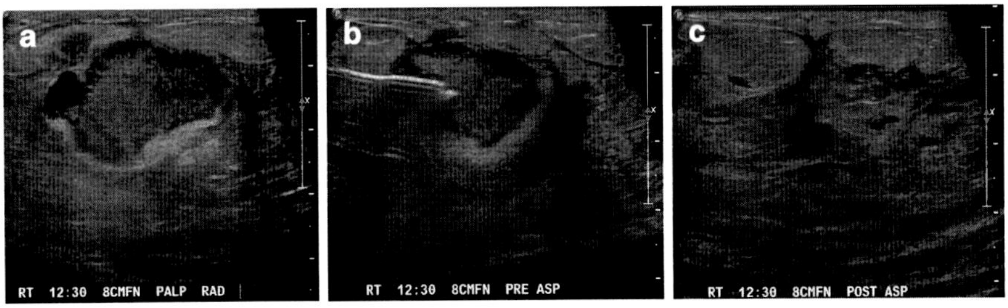

Fig. 10.3 Lactational abscess. (**a**) 41-year-old woman treated empirically with two courses of antibiotics with no decrease in size of a palpable mass and continued decrease in milk production from this side. Targeted ultrasound shows an irregular complex solid (iso-/hyperechoic) and cystic mass and surrounding edema. The internal echoes were mobile in real-time. (**b**) Ultrasound-guided needle aspiration is done, draining the fluid collection to completion. (**c**) Follow-up ultrasound 2 weeks later was normal (not shown).

with a painful, palpable lump, which may overlap the clinical presentation of an abscess. Mammographic findings may include a mass or parenchymal asymmetry; sonographically, masses or hypoechoic tubular densities may be seen (Fig. 10.4), their irregular shape warranting biopsy, on which perilobular noncaseating granulomas would be reported [1, 8]. If the diagnosis is unequivocally confirmed histologically, treatment consists of corticosteroids (if there is any doubt, a course of antibiotics may be tried first to avoid exacerbating a possible infection). Granulomatous mastitis can be recalcitrant even to long-term steroid treatment—and may still require excision [8].

Fig. 10.2 Subareolar abscess and mastitis. (**a**) Standard CC and MLO views of the left breast in a 47-year-old woman show increased mass-like density in the lower central aspect in the area of a painful, erythematous, palpable "lump" denoted by a metallic BB skin marker. There is also increased skin and trabecular (*arrowheads*) thickening reflecting edema more diffusely. (**b**) Spot tangential view better demonstrates the association of the mass with the nipple areolar complex, which is thickened. (**c**) Irregular, complex fluid collection broadly involving the deep dermal layer (*arrows*) with posterior acoustic enhancement. (**d**) Sonography into the upper inner quadrant shows edema: skin thickening, increased interstitial fluid (*arrows*), loss of tissue planes, and ill-defined hypoechoic areas (mastitis, *arrowheads*).

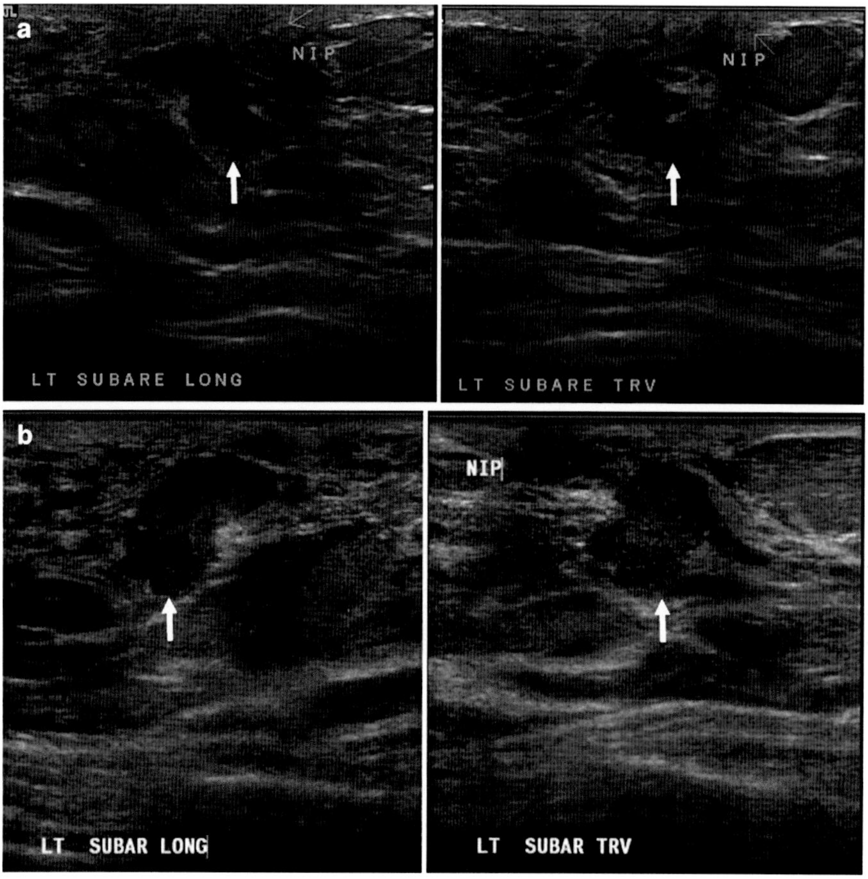

Fig. 10.4 Granulomatous mastitis. (**a**) Orthogonal ultrasound images in a 28-year-old woman with a painful "lump" show an irregular hypoechoic tubular-shaped structure (*arrows*) at the base of the nipple. Histology on core needle biopsy showed a mixed picture of acutely inflamed breast parenchyma with granulomatous features. Even though stains for microorganisms were negative, the patient was started on antibiotics given the acute inflammation reported histologically. (**b**) After 1 month of no clinical improvement and increase in size of the mass, she was started on a course of corticosteroids for presumed granulomatous mastitis given granulomas also seen on pathology. She eventually underwent surgical excision.

Vascular Lesions

These may present clinically as a superficial "lump," or be found incidentally mammographically or sonographically as a round or oval mass, sometimes with calcifications (phleboliths), with vascularity confirmed on color Doppler imaging. They can be hypoechoic to hyperechoic on ultrasound [9]. Common benign lesions include hemangiomas (Fig. 10.5) and angiolipomas. Angiosarcomas in the breast may be primary or secondary—the latter most often related to prior radiation therapy—and present with overlying bluish skin discoloration. These may be more irregular in appearance on imaging and hyperechoic or mixed echogenicity on sonography (Fig. 10.6) [1, 9, 10, 11].

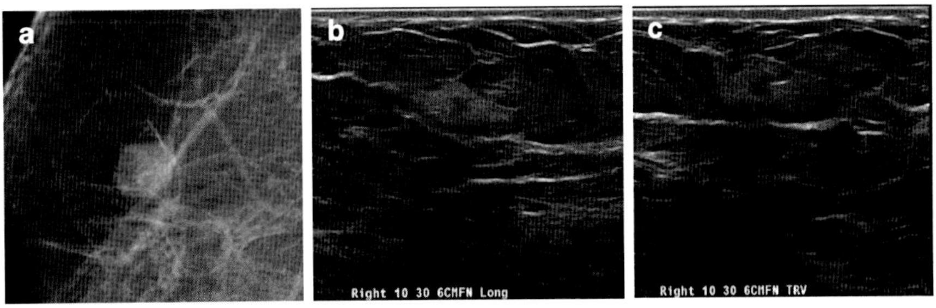

Fig. 10.5 Capillary hemangioma. (**a**) Low-density oval mass with circumscribed margins on spot compression view. (**b** and **c**) Irregular, predominantly hyperechoic mass on ultrasound—this appearance prompted biopsy.

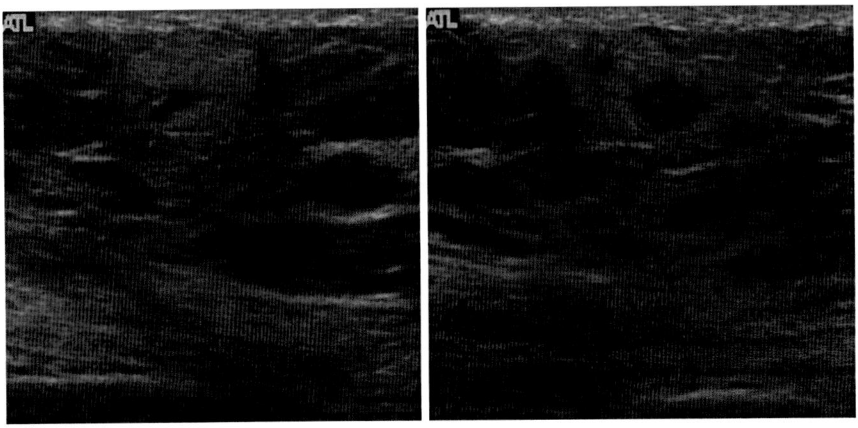

Fig. 10.6 Angiosarcoma. Orthogonal sonographic views show an irregular hyperechoic mass with indistinct margins and central decreased echogenicity in the subcutaneous fat. Given this appearance, and its location deep to a bluish discoloration on the skin in a 52-year-old with a history of radiation following lumpectomy for breast cancer, biopsy was done. An equal density irregular mass was imaged on correlative mammogram (not shown).

Pseudoaneurysm of the breast is rare, and of these, most are post-traumatic, namely, complications from percutaneous biopsies resulting from a disruption in the arterial wall. They may present as a palpable, pulsatile mass and demonstrate swirling internal vascular flow ("yin-yang" sign; Fig. 10.7). Pseudoaneurysms may thrombose spontaneously (self-limited) or be treated under ultrasound with sequential manual compression; thrombin or alcohol injection; embolization with coils, Gelfoam, or glue; or surgically [11, 12].

Lactational adenoma and galactocele

These are two of the more common entities related to the marked physiologic, hormonally mediated, changes of pregnancy and lactation.

Lactational adenoma may be suspected in the third trimester of pregnancy. There is controversy as to whether it arises de novo or transforms from preexisting

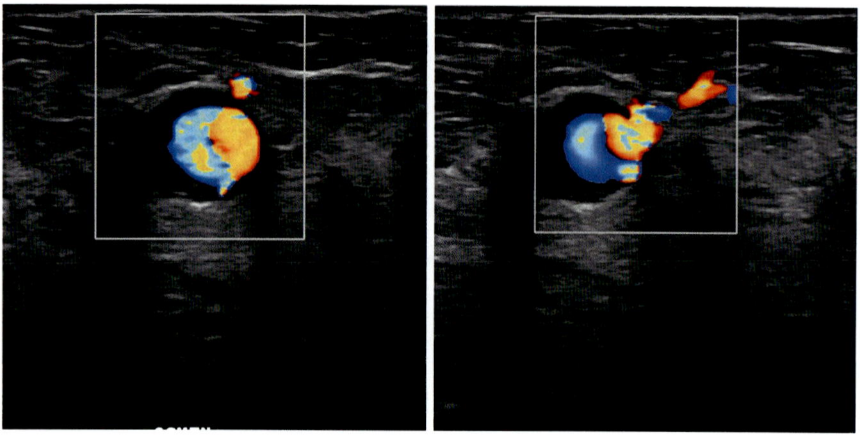

Fig. 10.7 Pseudoaneurysm. Orthogonal sonographic images show a hypoechoic mass with swirling internal vascularity ("yin-yang" sign) and a feeding vessel 2 months after an ultrasound-guided core biopsy with a 14G spring loaded needle; the patient returned because of focal pain. A hematoma (not shown) had been noted at the time of biopsy, and bleeding at that time had stopped with compression. This pseudoaneurysm was treated with percutaneous thrombin injection.

fibroadenoma with the hormonal effects of pregnancy. Sonographically, it may be indistinguishable from a fibroadenoma, having an oval shape, circumscribed margins, parallel (horizontal) orientation, and uniform hypoechogenicity. It may also contain areas of increased echogenicity related to increased lipid (milk) content. With these appearances, one may consider short interval follow up if the patient is otherwise asymptomatic--for example, a repeat ultrasound in 6 months, BI-RADS assessment category 3 (probably benign finding) as with a fibroadenoma. A more heterogeneous appearance may warrant biopsy, however, if pathology is concordant, no further treatment is needed as these regress after delivery and lactation [13].

Galactoceles result from ductal dilation and milk stasis. As this can occur after the cessation of breast feeding, when a mammogram may be a part of the diagnostic work up, one may see an oval mass radiographically, with circumscribed margins and a "fat-fluid" level depending on the lipid and proteinaceous content of the milk [13]. Similarly, sonographically, a fluid-fluid level may be seen as part of a complex solid and cystic mass. Aspiration of milk from the cystic portion is diagnostic, however if the solid portion predominates, or and there are suspicious features, biopsy may be required.

Fibrosis

Fibrosis can run the gamut of benign and malignant features on imaging, from calcifications, to oval or round masses with circumscribed borders, to more irregular shapes with spiculated margins, often with posterior acoustic shadowing sonographically. The latter can mimic the desmoplastic reaction incited by some cancers such that during core needle biopsy, errors in sampling the edge of a malignancy may result in a false negative. In this way, precise targeting of the middle of the lesion is therefore paramount to be confident with regard to radiology-pathology congruence. If there is any doubt with regard to congruence or needle placement, subsequent excisional biopsy may be warranted for a larger sample [14,15].

Pseudoangiomatous Stromal Hyperplasia (PASH) has a wide range of appearances, but more commonly appears as a mass or asymmetry, often in the upper outer quadrant in premenopausal women. When new or developing on imaging, biopsy is indicated, but further treatment is not indicated if concordant and the patient is asymptomatic. PASH can also be diagnosed incidentally at biopsy of another lesion. PASH is a benign mesenchymal proliferation that must be differentiated from angiosarcoma and phyllodes tumors histologically [16].

Selected radiologic-pathologic correlation of miscellaneous lesions is highlighted below.

Case 1

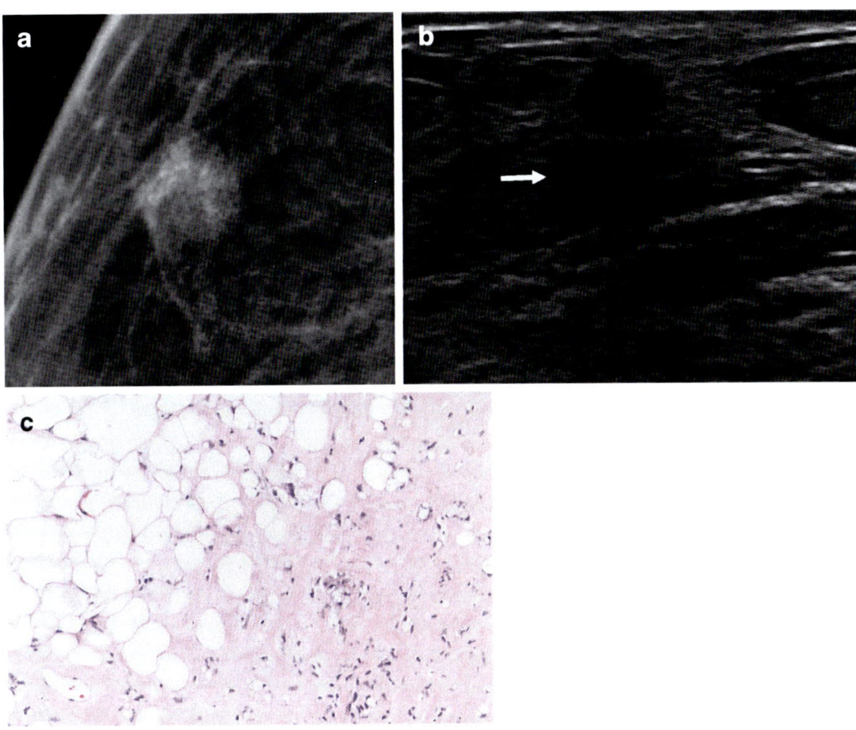

Fat necrosis. (**a**) Palpable low-density round, subcutaneous mass in a 67-year-old woman referred for diagnostic workup. (**b**) Ultrasound shows a hypoechoic mass with circumscribed margins. Despite being nearly anechoic, this is solid, not a cyst, given posterior acoustic shadowing (*arrow*), and biopsy is indicated. (**c**) Fat necrosis. Note the infarcted adipose cells, histiocytes, and associated fibrosis

Case 2

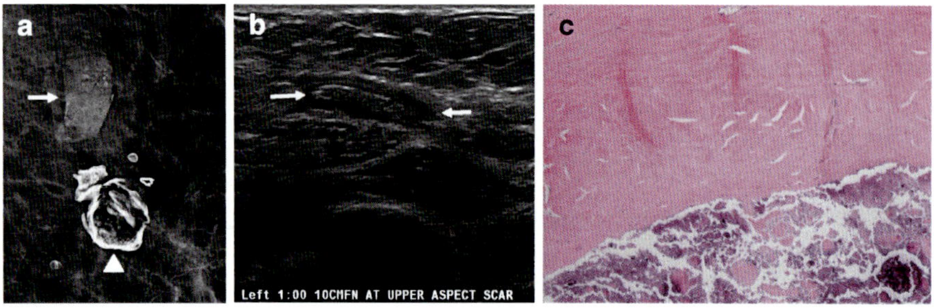

Dense fibrosis presenting as a mass. (**a**) New low-density mass (*arrow*) with amorphous calcifications adjacent to a calcifying oil cyst (*arrowhead*) in a 53-year-old woman undergoing routine mammographic surveillance following lumpectomy for DCIS with calcifications 5 years ago. (**b**) Ultrasound of the new mass shows a horizontally oriented isoechoic to hyperechoic mass (*between arrows*) with circumscribed margins at the upper aspect of the lumpectomy scar; these are benign sonographic features but because the lesion is new, it is assigned a BI-RADS 4 and biopsy is done. (**c**) Dense fibrous tissue with coarse calcifications, possibly calcified fat necrosis. Annual mammography is recommended

Case 3

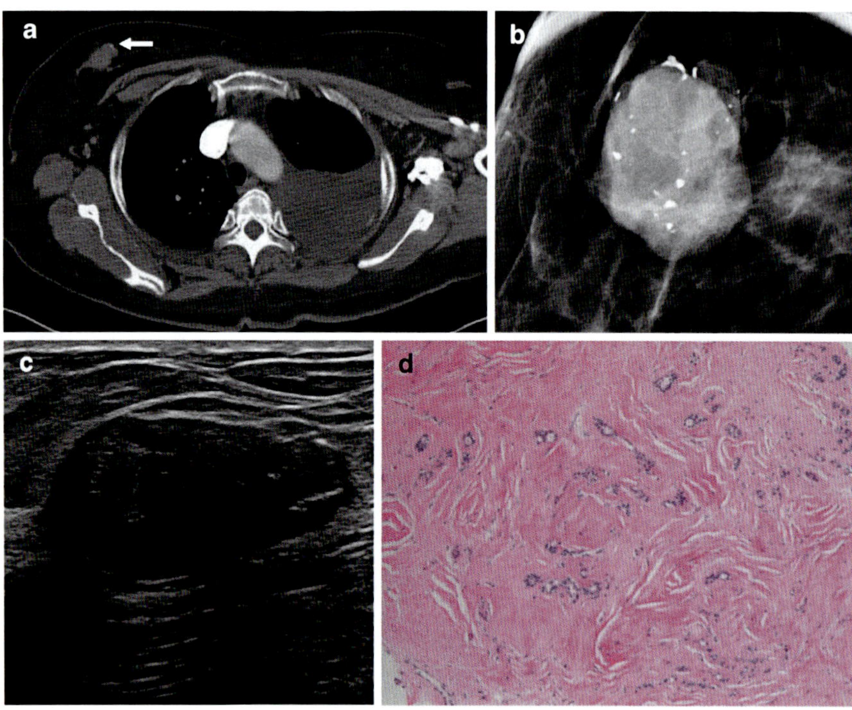

Fibrosis presenting as a mass. (**a**) 56-year-old woman with right breast mass (*arrow*) seen on staging CT for ovarian cancer. Note the focus of increased density in the mass at the tip of the *arrow*, reflecting a large calcification. There is also a large left pleural effusion. (**b**) Associated coarse calcifications and circumscribed margins on mammography support a benign etiology, but there is heterogeneous echogenicity on sonography (**c**). Biopsy is done prior to starting chemotherapy showing (**d**) dense collagenous stromal fibrosis

Case 4

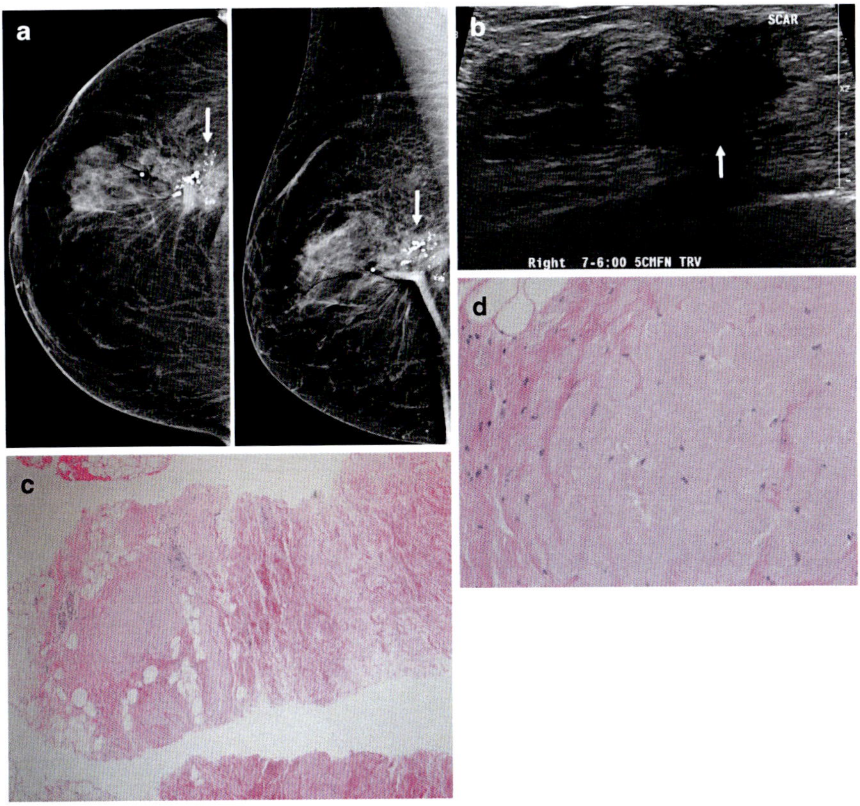

Stromal fibrosis and elastosis presenting as a mass. (**a**) 72-year-old patient with remote history of right lumpectomy. Focal asymmetry, dystrophic calcifications, and overlying skin retraction are postsurgical and radiation changes (*arrows*). A new "lump" anterior to these findings is marked with a metallic BB. (**b**) Ultrasound shows irregular hypoechoic masses corresponding to the mammographic findings, one of which is the surgical scar (*arrow*) and the other is the area of patient concern. Biopsy of the latter was done. (**c**) Needle core biopsies of the mass show stromal fibrosis and elastotic stroma. It may mimic amyloid deposition. (**d**) At higher magnification, note the homogenous areas of amphophilic elastotic stroma

Case 5

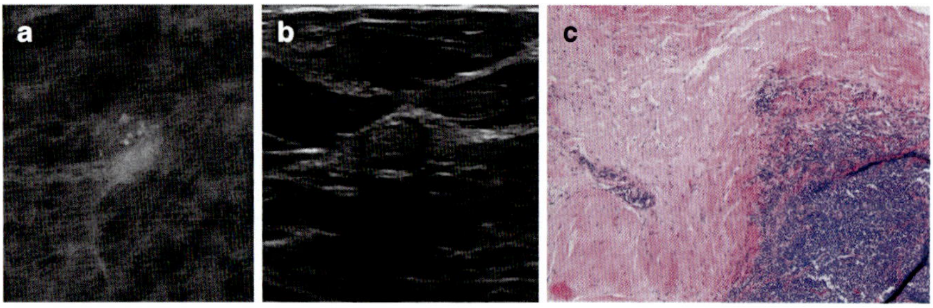

Dense fibrosis and chronic inflammation presenting as a mass. (**a**) Spot compression magnification view in a 40-year-old woman with a known contralateral breast cancer shows an irregular mass with indistinct margins and calcifications. (**b**) On ultrasound this mass has circumscribed margins and is hyperechoic relative to subcutaneous fat. (**c**) Dense fibrous stroma with chronic inflammation

Case 6

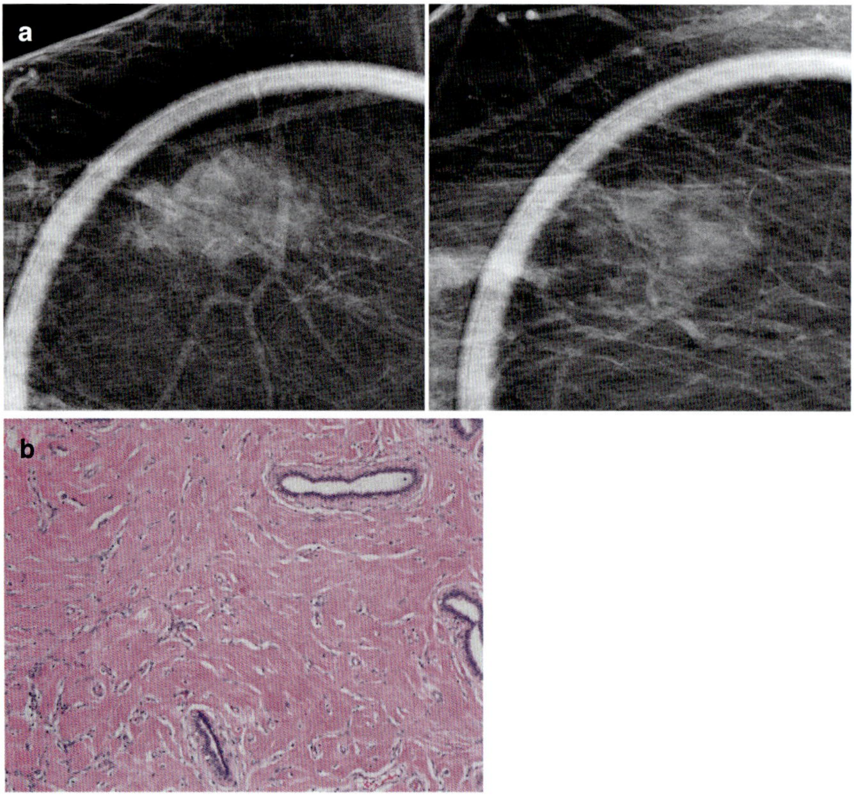

Case 6 Pseudoangiomatous stromal hyperplasia. (a) Orthogonal spot compression mammographic views of a developing nodular focal asymmetry in the upper outer quadrant of the right breast in a 42 year old woman. No corresponding lesion was seen sonographically, so biopsy was done using stereotactic (radiographic) guidance. (b) Pseudoangiomatous stromal hyperplasia showing interconnected slit-like spaces lined by myofibroblasts and are not vascular spaces

Case 7

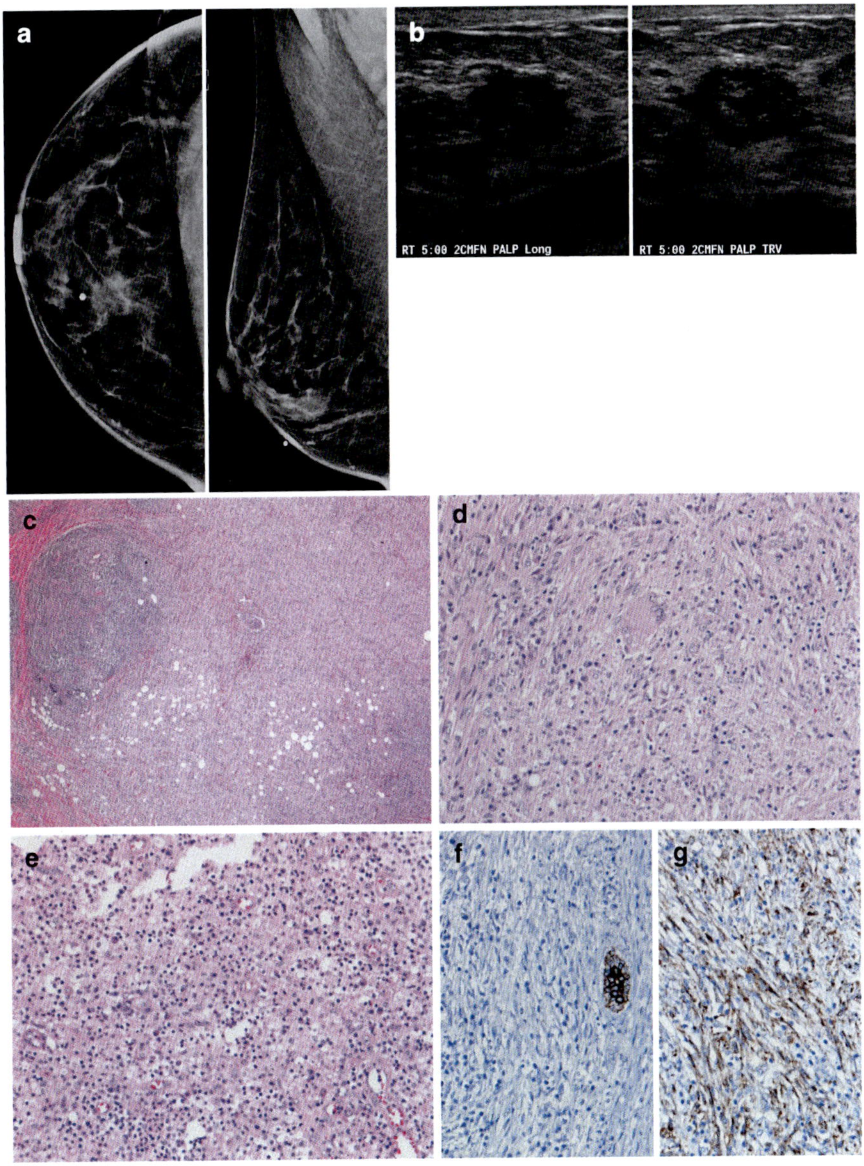

Benign inflammatory condition presenting as a mass: granulomatous mastitis. (**a**) 40-year-old woman presented to the emergency room with a 2-week history of a painful right breast "lump" but no other signs of infection. Mammogram showed an irregular mass in the lower inner aspect deep to the metallic BB skin marker. (**b**) Orthogonal ultrasound images show an irregular mass with heterogeneous echogenicity and angular margins that did not change significantly at 2- and 4-week follow-up ultrasounds (not shown) after a course of antibiotics; therefore, ultrasound core needle biopsy (and subsequent excision) was undertaken. (**c**) Lobulocentric inflammation. (**d**) Histiocytes, lymphocytes, occasional multinucleated giant cells, and eosinophils. (**e**) Microabscesses also seen. Note the negative staining for pancytokeratin (**f**) and positive for CD68 (**g**)

Case 8

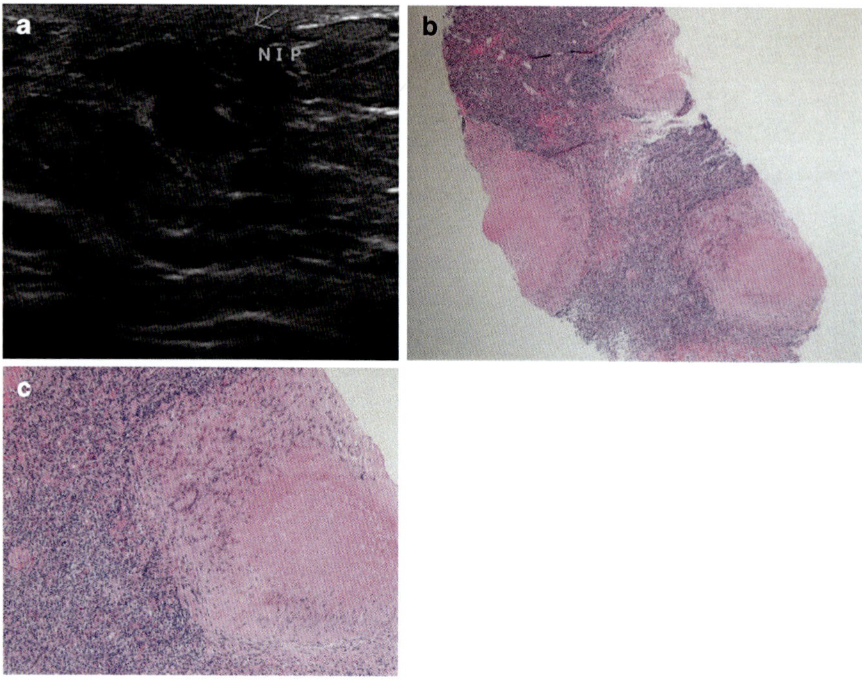

Benign processes presenting as a mass: Granulomatous mastitis. (**a**) Ultrasound of a different patient with granulomatous mastitis shows another sonographic appearance, that of an irregular hypoechoic tubular shaped structure at the base of the nipple. (**b**) Breast tissue with granulomatous inflammation. (**c**) Note the central necrosis surrounded by epithelioid histiocytes and lymphocytes. The stains for fungal organisms and acid-fast bacilli were negative

Case 9

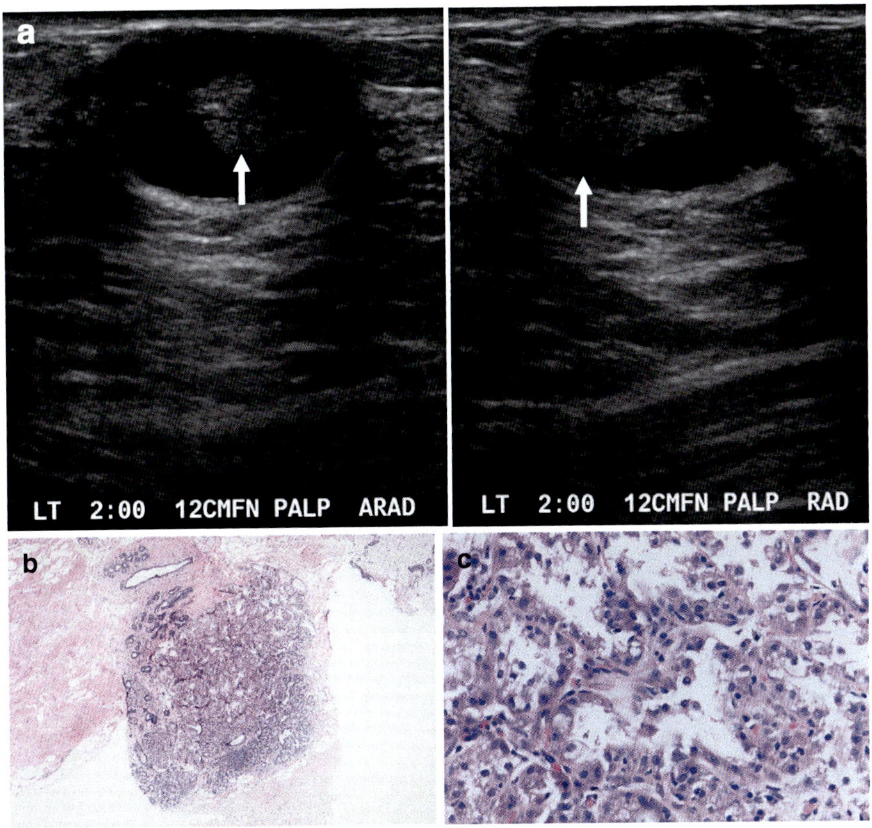

Lactating Adenoma. (**a**) Orthogonal sonographic images of a palpable "lump" in 28-year-old woman who is breastfeeding show a complex cystic and solid mass with circumscribed margins. Biopsy of the solid portion (arrows) is done after aspiration of the fluid in the cystic portion. (**b** and **c**) Enlarged epithelial cells with cytoplasmic vacuolization protrude in lumen; the myoepithelial cells are inconspicuous

Case 10

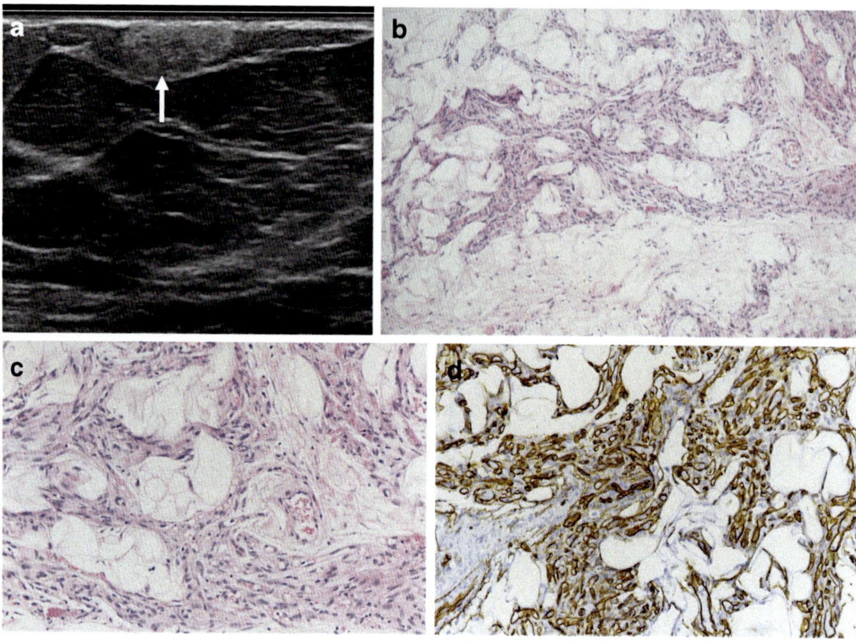

Capillary hemangioma. (**a**) Ultrasound of a palpable finding in this 81 year old woman shows a horizontally oriented, predominantly hyperechoic, mixed echogenicity mass (*arrow*) with circumscribed margins in the subcutaneous fat. Despite benign imaging features, it was increasing in size, and so biopsy was undertaken. (**b** and **c**) Needle-core biopsy shows a capillary proliferation. (**d**) Confirmed by CD34- positive staining of endothelial cells

Case 11

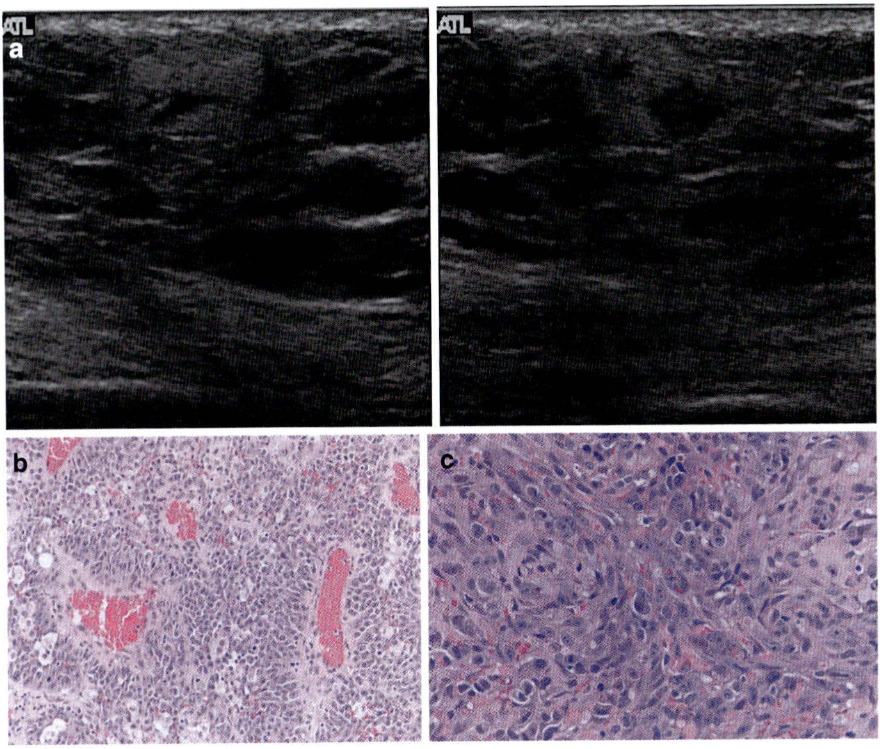

Angiosarcoma. (**a**) Orthogonal sonographic views show an irregular hyperechoic mass with indistinct margins and central decreased echogenicity in the subcutaneous fat. Given this appearance, and its location deep to a bluish discoloration on the skin in a 52 year old with a history of radiation following lumpectomy for breast cancer, biopsy was done. An equal density irregular mass was imaged on correlative mammogram (not shown). (**b**, **c**) Histology shows a solid proliferation of spindle cells, with pleomorphism, vesicular nuclei and prominent nucleoli. CD34 (not pictured) confirms vascular neoplasm consistent with high grade angiosarcoma

References

1. Cardenosa G. Clinical breast imaging: the essentials. Philadelphia: Wolters Kluwer; 2015.
2. Hogge JP, Robinson RE, Magnant CM, Zuurbier RA. The mammographic spectrum of fat necrosis in the breast. Radiographics. 1995;15(6):1347–56. doi:10.1148/radiographics.15.6.8577961. Accessed 25 Feb 2017.
3. Soo MS, Kornguth PJ, Hertzberg BS. Fat necrosis in the breast: sonographic features. Radiology. 1998;206(1):261–9. doi:10.1148/radiology.206.1.9423681. Accessed 25 Feb 2017.
4. Upadhyaya VS, Uppoor R, Shetty L. Mammographic and sonographic features of fat necrosis of the breast. Indian J Radiol Imaging. 2013;23(4):366–72. doi:10.4103/0971-3026.125619. Accessed 25 Feb 2017.
5. Trop I, Dugas A, David J, et al. Breast abscesses: evidence-based algorithms for diagnosis, management, and follow up. Radiographics. 2011;31(6):1683–99. doi:10.1148/rg.316115521. Accessed 23 Feb 2017.
6. Zuska JJ, Crile G, Ayres WW. Fistulas of lactiferous ducts. Am J Surg. 1951;81(3):312–7. doi:10.1016/0002-9610(51)90233-4. Accessed 26 Feb 2017.
7. Sabate JM, Clotet M, Torrubia S, et al. Radiologic evaluation of breast disorders related to pregnancy and lactation. Radiographics. 2007;27:S101–24. doi:10.1148/rg.27si075505. Accessed 23 Feb 2017.
8. Sabate JM, Clotet M, Gomez A, et al. Radiologic evaluation of uncommon inflammatory and reactive breast disorders. Radiographics. 2005;25(2):411–24. doi:10.1148/rg.252045077. Accessed 23 Feb 2017.
9. Jesinger RA, Lattin GE, Ballard EA, et al. Vascular abnormalities of the breast: arterial and venous disorders, vascular masses, and mimic lesions with radiologic-pathologic correlation. Radiographics. 2011;31(7):E117–37. doi:10.1148/rg.317115503. Accessed 25 Feb 2017.
10. Yang WT, Hennessy BT, Dryden MJ, et al. Mammary angiosarcomas: imaging findings in 24 patients. Radiology. 2007;242(3):725–34. doi:10.1148/radiol.2423060163. Accessed 23 Feb 2017.
11. Ingram AD, Mahoney MC. An overview of breast emergencies and guide to management by interventional radiologists. Tech Vasc Interv Radiol. 2014;17(1):55–63. doi:10.1053/j.tvir.2013.12.009. Accessed 23 Feb 2017.
12. Bazzocchi M, Francescutti GE, Zuiani C, et al. Breast pseudoaneurysm in a woman after core biopsy: percutaneous treatment with alcohol. AJR Am J Roengenol. 2002;179(3):696–8. doi:10.2214/ajr.179.3.1790696. Accessed 25 Feb 2017.
13. Sabate JM, Clotet M, Torrubia S, et al. Radiologic evaluation of breast disorders related to pregnancy and lactation. Radiographics. 2007;27(Suppl 1):S101–24. doi: 10.1148/rg.27si075505 Accessed 5 June 2017
14. Geraldine Revelon, Mark E. Sherman, Olga M. B. Gatewood, Rachel F. Brem, (2000) Focal Fibrosis of the Breast: Imaging Characteristics and Histopathologic Correlation. Radiology 216 (1):255-259 doi: 10.1148/radiology.216.1.r00jl16255 Accessed 5 June 2017
15. Kopans DB. Breast Imaging, 3rd ed. Philadelphia: Williams and Wilkins. 2007
16. Erin Bowman, Gabriela Oprea, Joel Okoli, Kathleen Gundry, Monica Rizzo, Sheryl Gabram-Mendola, Upender Manne, Geoffrey Smith, Stefan Pambuccian, Harvey L. Bumpers, (2012) Pseudoangiomatous Stromal Hyperplasia (PASH) of the Breast: A Series of 24 Patients. The Breast Journal 18 (3):242-247 doi: 10.1111/j.1524-4741.2012.01230.x Accessed 5 June 2017

Index

M.O. Idowu et al. (eds.), *Diagnosis and Management of Breast Tumors*,
DOI 10.1007/978-3-319-57726-5